Informed Consent in Predictive Genetic Testing

Jessica Minor

Informed Consent in Predictive Genetic Testing

A Revised Model

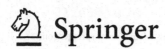 Springer

Jessica Minor
Greenville
South Carolina
USA

ISBN 978-3-319-38558-7   ISBN 978-3-319-17416-7 (eBook)
DOI 10.1007/978-3-319-17416-7

Springer Cham Heidelberg New York Dordrecht London
© Springer International Publishing Switzerland 2015
Softcover reprint of the hardcover 1st edition 2015

Printed on acid-free paper

Springer International Publishing is part of Springer Science+Business Media (www.springer.com)

Preface

This book grew from my PhD dissertation. I wanted to write about a topic that was cutting edge and would be applicable for several years. I had been thinking about the ethics of predictive genetic testing (PGT), particularly direct-to-consumer testing, for a while. Eventually I decided that even though I had heard some stories about predictive testing ending badly, I could not clearly say that the testing was unethical. Then I started to evaluate what was troubling in regards to PGT. Especially in the cases that did not turn out well, it seemed that one of the main issues was a lack of understanding. I believe PGT can be a great tool for medicine, but if there is a lack of understanding about the test, potential treatments, or long-term outcomes, then there is the potential for significant harm. While considering these issues, I remembered a plenary speaker in one of the American Society for Bioethics & Humanities conferences addressing future issues and concerns for bioethicists. One of the issues discussed was informed consent. After considering PGT some more, I decided that a more robust discussion on informed consent and PGT could prove valuable to the areas of bioethics, genetic testing, and genetic counseling research.

After doing some more research I decided that a revised model of informed consent would be more appropriate for PGT, since there are some characteristics that differentiate PGT from other types of testing. These characteristics are: the difficulty in understanding genetic risks and probabilities; the problem of treatment options for diagnosed genetic traits; and the concern with family-related genetic information. All three of these characteristics are incorporated into a revised model of informed consent for PGT.

This book focuses on four components: comprehension, disclosure, voluntariness, and patient safety. First, PGT involves a risk analysis of the related probabilities that can be complicated for patients to comprehend. This point develops the importance of understanding in the current model. Second, there are complex treatment options, including no treatment for some diseases, that require genetic counseling to select an appropriate option. This point develops the importance of disclosure in the current model. Third, PGT involves family-related information with accompanying implications that can compromise voluntariness. This third point develops the importance of avoiding coercion of both the patient and the patient's family when information is presented. Fourth, the revised model of consent requires an additional component to the traditionally recognized three components (comprehension, disclosure, voluntariness): the culture of patient safety. That is, the revised model of consent enhances the traditional components of consent within a medical culture that emphasizes patient safety.

While the first chapter goes into more depth about the purpose and distinctiveness of the book, I did not find many books that addressed specific issues of informed consent that arise from PGT. None of the literature has merged the current components of consent (understanding, disclosure, and voluntariness) with the distinguishing characteristics of PGT. I believe this book's thesis is distinctive, because it establishes a revised model by aligning the three distinguishing characteristics of PGT with the three widely recognized components in the current model.

In the book, I explain what PGT is, address several misconceptions of genetic risks and probabilities, evaluate the idea of treatment options or the lack of treatment options, and call attention to some family-related issues due to genetics. There is also a very in-depth history of informed consent from both a clinical and research standpoint. I discuss how the current components of consent arose, and then compare and contrast the current model with the revised model of consent for PGT. At the end, I apply the revised model of informed consent to direct-to-consumer genetic testing and pleiotropic genetic testing.

While this book focuses on proposing a revised model of informed consent, I believe it can also be useful for those interested in genetic testing both personally and professionally. This book addresses some important questions people need to consider before participating in PGT. I also feel that the points raised in this book can promote increased dialogue among health professionals about how the requirement of informed consent for PGT can be met both legally and ethically.

I would like to acknowledge Dr. Gerard Magill, my advisor during the dissertation process. Dr. Magill always offered extremely helpful comments and was a wise and generous mentor.

Contents

Contents

Chapter 1
Introduction

Genetic testing has been used for many years, but recently genetic testing has been used not as a diagnostic tool but as predictive measures. Francis Collins, Director of the National Human Genome Research Institute at the National Institutes of Health, says "virtually every human illness has a hereditary component."[1] Because of this and the technology that has been developed, now everyone is a patient. Neil Sharpe and Ronald Carter in their book, *Genetic Testing: Care, Consent, and Liability,* say that the result of this genetic technology is "more information (accurate or not) from more sources (biased or not) available to more patients (receptive or not) every day."[2] Because of this sometimes the actual value and utility of genetic information can be questioned.[3] The article "Evaluating the Utility of Personal Genomic Information" by Morris Foster, John Mulvihill, and Richard Sharp states that the evaluation of such testing "shifts from examining the value of asking a specific question about a particular gene for which variants are known to examining the value of a vast amount of information that includes multiple known variants and variants that are unknown, ambiguous, or have no significance."[4]

Predictive genetic testing (PGT) can have implications on many different aspects of a person's life whether it's medical, social, emotional, or psychological. Many times people do not comprehend completely the results and impact the testing will have on themselves and their family. One woman illustrates this point further after she received the results of a test for the breast cancer mutation, the BRCA gene. She said the following:

> I am a carrier of a BRCA2 gene mutation. My genetic status is now as much a part of my personal identity as are my age (47 years old), my religion (Jewish), and my educational training (a master's in community health). I have one sister who won the coin toss and did

---

[1] Abigail L Rose, Nikki Peters, Judy A. Shea, et al., "Attitudes and Misconceptions about Predictive Genetic Testing for Cancer Risk," 148.

[2] Neil Sharpe and Ronald Carter, *Genetic Testing: Care, Consent, and Liability,* 2.

[3] Wylie Burke, Ronald Zimmern, and Mark Kroese, "Defining Purpose: A Key Step in Genetic Test Evaluations," 675.

[4] Morris Foster, John Mulvihill, and Richard Sharp, "Evaluating the Utility of Personal Genomic Information," 570.

© Springer International Publishing Switzerland 2015
J. Minor, *Informed Consent in Predictive Genetic Testing*,
DOI 10.1007/978-3-319-17416-7_1

not inherit the mutation. My husband and I have two adult children, a son and a daughter, both of whom intend to learn their genetic status some day. Without a doubt, this genetic journey has been not only one of the greatest challenges of my life but also one of the loneliest.[5]

While some of the information can be helpful, sometimes the information that is returned has no direct value or medical benefit for the patient.[6] The technology and information can be premature, running ahead of treatment options and ethical implications. Neil Sharpe and Ronald Carter say that there is an "unfortunate technological lag between our theoretical knowledge of a given genetic disease and our systemic ability to provide effective therapy."[7]

Because the individual has not yet manifested symptoms of a specific disease or illness, informed consent should have different regulations and goals for PGT. In reference to informed consent, Lewis Vaughn in his book, *Bioethics: Principles, Issues, and Cases*, says "At the simplest level, the term refers to the action of an autonomous, informed person agreeing to submit to medical treatment or experimentation."[8] Informed consent can be viewed as a "cornerstone for the development of the discipline of bioethics," and it is one of the most essential and debated aspects of medicine today.[9]

The next section will give a description of the thesis statement. While the ideals and goals for informed consent can be complicated to discuss, implement, and establish ethical procedures, this book seeks to address some of those issues by developing a revised model of informed consent for PGT.[10] The need for this model arises from distinguishing characteristics of PGT, which make it distinctive from other forms of health-related testing. These characteristics are: the difficulty in understanding genetic risks and probabilities; the problem of treatment options for diagnosed genetic traits; and the concern with family-related genetic information. The second chapter explains PGT to identify these characteristics that shape the revised model of consent. The third chapter explores the history of consent to identify the widely recognized components of consent (understanding, disclosure, and voluntariness) that represent the current model. The fourth chapter explains the revised model by aligning the three distinguishing characteristics of PGT with the three widely recognized components in the current model. The fifth chapter applies the revised model to direct-to-consumer and pleiotropic genetic testing. The sixth chapter gives a conclusion about the revised model of informed consent for PGT.

To explain the significance of the revised model of consent, the following main categories are discussed. First, PGT involves a risk analysis of the related probabilities that can be complicated for patients to comprehend. This point develops the

---

[5] Neil Sharpe and Ronald Carter, *Genetic Testing: Care, Consent, and Liability*, 291.

[6] Morris Foster, John Mulvihill, and Richard Sharp, "Evaluating the Utility of Personal Genomic Information," 570.

[7] Neil Sharpe and Ronald Carter, *Genetic Testing: Care, Consent, and Liability*, 2.

[8] Lewis Vaughn, *Bioethics: Principles, Issues, and Cases*, 144.

[9] Neil C. Manson and Onora O'Neill, *Rethinking Informed Consent in Bioethics*, 1–2; Robert M. Arnold and Charles W. Lidz, "Informed Consent: Clinical Aspects of Consent in Health Care," 4.

[10] Lewis Vaughn, *Bioethics: Principles, Issues, and Cases*, 144.

importance of understanding in the current model. Risk assessment involves calculating probabilities to determine the likelihood of developing a disease. To accomplish this, the relation between autonomy and comprehension is crucial. The current model uses an approach to autonomy that is standardized and generic, focusing on consent by providing a signature to accept or reject a test. The revised model enhances patient involvement by adopting a more extensive approach, described as a process rather than as an event. Typically the current model does not offer a large amount of time to comprehending risk assessments. The additional time and complexity involved in comprehending the connection between risk and probability has significant implications for patient education by the doctor, thereby developing the meaning of the doctor-patient relationship. For example, the emergence of the so-called Nocebo Effect needs to be considered here.

Second, there are complex treatment options, including no treatment for some diseases, that require genetic counseling to select an appropriate option. This point develops the importance of disclosure in the current model. Typically the current model emphasizes appropriate disclosure of information. The revised model takes this further and recognizes that this disclosure needs to be accompanied with genetic counseling both before and after testing to enhance decision making about a suitable option. Appropriate genetic counseling must include patient assessment and feedback mechanisms.

Third, PGT involves family-related information with accompanying implications that can compromise voluntariness. This third point develops the importance of avoiding coercion of both the patient and the patient's family when information is presented. The third distinctive characteristic of PGT is the relevance of genetic information for the patient's family. In the current model, family-related coercion is often difficult to identify. The revised model ensures voluntary consent by establishing procedures to avoid two forms of coercion: pressure by the family for the patient to be tested (eg, if there is a family genetic trait already known, there can be pressure upon a child to be tested to ascertain if s/he is a carrier etc); and pressure upon the family regarding the testing outcome (eg, if a trait emerges that affects other siblings, a process needs to be undertaken to ascertain whether the sibling wants to know).

The revised model of consent requires an additional component to the traditionally recognized three components (comprehension, disclosure, voluntariness): the culture of patient safety. That is, the revised model of consent enhances the traditional components of consent within a medical culture that emphasizes patient safety. This safety culture requires nationally established systems of accountability for PGT that implement the revised components of consent in a transparent manner to foster trust in the emerging system of genetic-related services.

This next section will situate the thesis of the book within the current state of the question in the literature. The state of the question exists to explain the distinctiveness of this work within the context of the current literature on informed consent and predictive genetic testing (PGT). The debate on PGT usually covers the science, ethics, and the public's understanding of PGT. Ruth Hubbard and R.C. Lewontin's article, "Genetic Testing for Disease Predisposition, Pitfalls of Genetic Testing," talks about many issues of PGT including genetic determinism, possible misunderstandings, and social influences and factors like discrimination. Neil Sharpe and Ronald Carter in their book *Genetic Testing: Care, Consent, and Liability* discuss genetic testing in relation to communication, duty of care, family influences, informed consent, and confidentiality and discrimination.

The history of informed consent focuses on a discussion of the background and emerging components of informed consent. Both Albert Jonsen's book *The Birth of Bioethics* and Tom Beauchamp and James Childress' book *Principles of Biomedical Ethics* discuss the history and background of informed consent and address the cases that shaped the discussion for medicine and research.

The debate on the current model of informed consent focuses on three common components, understanding, disclosure, and voluntariness. Authors Neil Manson and Onora O'Neill in their book, *Rethinking Informed Consent in Bioethics,* address the issue of inadequate understanding of risk predictions, because of misconceptions or not enough patient education.[11] Stephen Wear's book *Informed Consent* and Thomas Goetz's book *The Decision Tree* analyze disclosure and communication. The current model emphasizes disclosure for decision making. Elizabeth Chapman's article "Ethical Dilemmas in Testing for Late Onset Conditions: Reactions to Testing and Perceived Impact on Other Family Members" demonstrates genetic testing can have an influence on an entire family. Neil Sharpe and Ronald Carter in their book *Genetic Testing: Care, Consent, and Liability* discuss family-related implications of genetic testing.

The application of direct-to-consumer (DTC) genetic testing is analyzed in Daniel Farkas and Carol Holland's article "Direct-to-Consumer Genetic Testing: Two Sides of the Coin." Peter Kraft and David Hunter's article "Genetic Risk Prediction—Are We There Yet?" looks at the science and background of DTC genetic testing. Cynthia Marietta and Amy McGuire's article "Direct-to-Consumer Genetic Testing: Is It the Practice of Medicine?" looks at DTC testing in relation to medical practice and the emphasis on medical treatment and the doctor-patient relationship.

The following articles focus on the current problems of informed consent for pleiotropic genetic testing. Ellen Wright Clayton's article "Incidental Findings in Genetics Research Using Archived DNA" and Elizabeth Chapman's article "Ethical Dilemmas in Testing for Late Onset Conditions: Reactions to Testing and Perceived Impact on Other Family Members" focus on the ethics, background information, and disclosure of pleiotropic genetic testing. Zachary Cooper, Robert Nelson, and Lainie Ross's article "Informed Consent for Genetic Research Involving Pleiotropic Genes: An Empirical Study of ApoE Research" focuses on the challenges of pleiotropic testing, mainly communication, understanding, and patient safety.

While all of these books promote foundational aspects of informed consent, there are few books that address specific issues of informed consent that arise from PGT. Some books like *Rethinking Informed Consent in Bioethics, Genetic Testing: Care, Consent, and Liability,* and *The Decision Tree* linked informed consent and genetic testing briefly, but did not address PGT. Even though Neil Sharpe and Ronald Carter's book *Genetic Testing: Care, Consent, and Liability* develops a ge-

---

[11] Neil C. Manson and Onora O'Neill, *Rethinking Informed Consent in Bioethics,* 144.

netics model of consent, that model does not take into consideration all of the other important factors that can arise from PGT. The current model focuses on more of a transactional, event model of consent, and does not adequately address the characteristics of PGT which make it distinctive from other forms of medical testing. None of the literature has merged the current components of consent (understanding, disclosure, and voluntariness) and the distinguishing characteristics of PGT together in order to form a revised model. Given the setting of the literature, the book's thesis is distinctive, because it establishes a revised model by aligning the three distinguishing characteristics of PGT with the three widely recognized components in the current model.

The last section will provide a summary of the chapters. Each of the next sections will give a description and synopsis of what the chapters will discuss and analyze within the debate on PGT and informed consent.

A. Chapter 2: Predictive Genetic Testing

The second chapter explains PGT to identify the distinguishing characteristics of PGT that shape the revised model of consent. This chapter will look at the science behind PGT, genetic risks and probabilities, treatment options, and family-related genetic information.

1. Science Behind PGT

The first part of this chapter looks at the science of PGT. PGT analyzes DNA and genetics to identify whether a person will develop or already has an at-risk gene that causes them to have a higher or lower than an average risk of developing a specific disease. This chapter will look at PGT and the science behind it including issues of new genetic technologies and understanding genetic information associated with specific diseases. In identifying the distinguishing characteristics of genetics, the chapter will highlight the power and limitations of genetic information.

2. Understanding Genetic Risks and Probabilities

The second part of the chapter looks at genetic risks and probabilities. Since risk predictions are very complex with difficult ideas to convey, genetic tests can result in misunderstandings and ambiguous results.[12] Authors Neil Manson and Onora O'Neill ask, "How can people give adequate consent to acts that use genetic information if (as is acknowledged) they have false beliefs about genetic information

---

[12] Chris Berdik, "Genetic Tests Give Consumers Hints About Disease Risk; Critics Have Misgivings," 1–2.

or understand it poorly?"[13] The authors clearly illustrate the problem of adequate understanding and the ethics of consent. In order to have solid informed consent, it is important to increase public education on potential choices. One of the questions to address is whether or not patients and the public understand genetic risks and probabilities. By combing the science and ethics of PGT, this chapter will seek to address possible misunderstands of genetic information and PGT risk assessments.

3. Treatment Options

The next section will discuss and analyze possible treatment options for genetic tests. PGT often has complicated treatment options for diagnosed genetic traits, because sometimes there are no treatments available for certain diseases. As a result, the disclosure of possible options is crucial in order to make appropriate decisions for PGT. This section will look at the standards of establishing adequate disclosure of treatment options for diagnosed genetic traits.[14] There are three general standards: a reasonable physician standard, reasonable patient standard, and a subjective standard. Overall there is not a specific formula for knowing how much information a patient needs to be informed, but this section addresses disclosure of treatment options for PGT.[15]

4. Family-Related Genetic Information

The last section will look at the concern of family-related genetic information. Because genetic information can relate to the entire family, often there are problems that can arise as a consequence. Possessing genetic information can result in discrimination, privacy concerns, a burden of knowledge, and coercion.[16] Confidentiality and discrimination can be a concern with genetics, but since the passing of the Genetic Information Non-discriminatory Act (GINA), genetic discrimination has not been as problematic. However discrimination can still be an unintended consequence for the patient and the patient's family and can play a role in informed consent and PGT.

---

[13] Neil C. Manson and Onora O'Neill, *Rethinking Informed Consent in Bioethics*, 144.

[14] Neil F. Sharpe and Ronald Carter, *Genetic Testing: Care, Consent, and Liability*, 131.

[15] Robert M. Arnold and Charles W. Lidz, "Informed Consent: Clinical Aspects of Consent in Health Care," 11.

[16] Regina Ensenauer, M.D., Virginia Michels M.D., and Shanda Reinke M.S, "Genetic Testing: Practical, Ethical, and Counseling Considerations," 63; Bert Heinrichs, "What Should We Want to Know About Our Future? A Kantian View on Predictive Genetic Testing. Medicine," 29; Michael Burgess PhD, Claude Lanberg, MD, PhD, Bartha Maria Knoppers, LLD, "Bioethics for Clinicians: 14. Ethics and Genetics in Medicine," 1309; Brita Arver, Aina Haegermark, Ulla Platten, et. al., "Evaluation of Psychosocial Effects of Pre-Symptomatic Testing for Breast/Ovarian and Colon Cancer Pre-Disposing Genes: a 12-Month Follow-Up," 109.

Often in the case of genetic testing, people cite the problem of the right to know versus the right not to know one's genetic makeup. Because of the complexity of genetic information, there are also family concerns that are raised by the right to know or not to know. The foundation of this argument can stem from the debate on genetic exceptionalism versus normal medical information. Genetic exceptionalism is the idea that genetic information is special, distinctive, and different than other types of medical information. Reasons for and against genetic exceptionalism will be presented and discussed further in this section. This area demonstrates the importance genetic information has on consent for the patient and the patient's family. As a result appropriate measures are needed to ensure the responsibility of genetic information especially in areas that can have potential side effects on others.[17]

B. Chapter 3: History and Components of Informed Consent

The third chapter explores the history of consent to identify the widely recognized components of consent (understanding, disclosure, and voluntariness) that represent the current model. Informed consent is needed when an "activity is already subject to ethical, legal, and other requirements," because consent is not needed for something you are allowed to do already.[18] This chapter will look at the cases that have shaped informed consent in both the medical and research fields and the components of the current model of informed consent.

1. Background of Informed Consent

The first part of chapter three will look at the background cases of informed consent. The beginning of informed consent started with principles that originated around 1914 with the case of Schloendorff v. society of New York hospital which emphasized the idea of autonomy. This case resulted in the idea that people have a right to determine what treatment they want. Salgo v. Leland Stanford Junior University Board of Trustees discussed physician disclosure of information in 1957. Several cases in the 1960s developed the ideas and addressed the basic features of informed consent, which include the nature and risks of the procedure, alternatives, expected benefits, and conditions of consent.[19] These initial ideas started the consent procedures of today. There were also several research cases that resulted in stronger regulations for informed consent such as the Tuskegee syphilis study, Willowbrook, and Guatemala. These cases all included a level of manipulation and/or coercion of vulnerable individuals, inadequate disclosure, and a lack of clinical equipoise. In

---

[17] Neil C. Manson and Onora O'Neill, *Rethinking Informed Consent in Bioethics*, 144.
[18] Neil C. Manson and Onora O'Neill, *Rethinking Informed Consent in Bioethics*, 72.
[19] Lewis Vaughn, *Bioethics: Principles, Issues, and Cases*, 144–146.

the Tuskegee study, people were treated solely as research subjects for information purposes, and the best interests of the individuals were not emphasized. The pediatricians in the Willowbrook case conducted research on mentally retarded children instead of treating the sick children. With research studies the focus changes to information and scientific research instead of clinical treatment; research studies also have a different goal and differing standards of consent. The Helsinki Declaration differentiates clinical research and nonclinical research, and this chapter will analyze the change of focus from research consent to clinical patient consent. This book will adopt both a research subject and patient treatment model of consent for PGT. Since PGT can return useful information on diseases and has the opportunity to help other researchers, the model of research subject is applicable. While both approaches will be used in certain situations, the main focus of PGT will be on the patient treatment model. The rest of this section will further develop the approach for the patient treatment and research subject model.[20]

2. Emergence of Components of Informed Consent

The last section will look at the emergence of informed consent components including the areas of comprehension, disclosure, and voluntariness. This section will analyze and discuss the history and major ideas included within each of the components of informed consent.

a. Comprehension

The first major component of informed consent is comprehension. The relationship between comprehension and autonomy has continued to emerge through the history of informed consent. Tom Beauchamp and James Childress address the connection between autonomy and comprehension in *Principles of Biomedical Ethics*.[21] Autonomy is often cited as a major principle of informed consent, because it has had a role in the development of many informed consent procedures. Autonomy was seen in the Schloendorff case, and this idea was developed into the self-determination of competent patients. Informed consent has the potential to help respect individual autonomy, because obtaining consent exhibits at least a minimal form of autonomy. In order to have comprehension and understanding of information, the patient needs to be presented with information about risk information and the physician should encourage patient education. Comprehension and autonomy is encouraged by increased patient participation in the process. Consent should have an adequate

---

[20] Tom Beauchamp and James Childress, *Principles of Biomedical Ethics*, 96, 322–323, 326–327, 428–430; Albert Jonsen, *The Birth of Bioethics*, 136, 138, 147, 150, 152, 180–181.
[21] Tom Beauchamp and James Childress, *Principles of Biomedical Ethics*, 127.

understanding of the information. This section will further analyze the development of comprehension within the history of informed consent.[22]

b. Disclosure

The second main component is disclosure. Disclosure often addresses possible treatment and testing options of the current medical diagnosis and medical outlook. Salgo v. Leland Stanford Junior University Board of Trustees in 1957 and several cases in the 1960s discuss the emergence of physician disclosure of alternatives, risks, and benefits.[23] While disclosing all the applicable information is helpful and necessary, disclosure by itself does not always encourage appropriate decision-making.[24] More information does not always lead to a better informed consent. Manson and O'Neill state, "Signatures, let alone ticks in boxes, may have legal weight, but they lack ethical weight, and often do not provide evidentiary weight that genuinely informed consent has been given."[25] Informed consent is an ethical ideal where doctors are required to "tell patients about possible medical interventions and to respect their choices regarding them. It is also a legal requirement, compelling health care providers to disclose information about interventions to patients and obtain their permission before proceeding."[26] The link between disclosure and decision-making is addressed in the *Principles of Biomedical Ethics*.[27] The specific history of disclosure and genetic counseling will be discussed further in relation to informed consent.

c. Voluntariness

The last component is voluntariness. Voluntariness of consent is often a major principle for genetic testing. The Tuskegee syphilis study, Willowbrook, and Guatemala experiments and research all have principles of voluntariness and coercion within them. These studies all involve a type of manipulation, coercion, and/or discrimination of vulnerable populations. The Willowbrook study raised the issue of voluntariness of parents consenting for their children to enter research studies. Often medical testing has the ability to coerce and discriminate in order to get people involved in research studies or testing trials. When voluntariness of individuals is not emphasized, often the best interests of patients are ignored.[28] The connection between

---

[22] Neil C. Manson and Onora O'Neill, *Rethinking Informed Consent in Bioethics*, 70, 185; Lewis Vaughn, *Bioethics: Principles, Issues, and Cases*, 144–147; Robert M. Arnold and Charles W. Lidz, "Informed Consent: Clinical Aspects of Consent in Health Care," 9.

[23] Lewis Vaughn, *Bioethics: Principles, Issues, and Cases*, 144–47.

[24] Neil C. Manson and Onora O'Neill, *Rethinking Informed Consent in Bioethics*, 69–70.

[25] Neil C. Manson and Onora O'Neill, *Rethinking Informed Consent in Bioethics*, 192.

[26] Lewis Vaughn, *Bioethics: Principles, Issues, and Cases*, 144.

[27] Tom Beauchamp and James Childress, *Principles of Biomedical Ethics*, 121.

[28] Albert Jonsen, *The Birth of Bioethics*, 147, 150; Tom Beauchamp and James Childress, *Principles of Biomedical Ethics*, 96, 322–323, 326–327, 428–430.

voluntariness is analyzed further in the book by Tom Beauchamp and James Childress, *Principles of Biomedical Ethics*.[29] Also since genetic information can have an impact on the patient and the patient's family, informed consent needs to take into account the patient and patient's family concerns, values, and beliefs about genetic testing. Some of the important aspects of informed consent can be family factors and the voluntariness of patients.[30] People should have the ability to consent voluntarily about treatment.[31] The rest of this section will look at cases and illustrations of the voluntariness of informed consent for medical and genetic testing.

C. Chapter 4: Revised Model of Informed Consent

The fourth chapter explains the revised model by aligning the three distinguishing characteristics of PGT with the three widely recognized components in the current model. This chapter aligns understanding risk probabilities with comprehension, treatment options with disclosure, and family-related information with voluntariness. Then the revised model adds another component to informed consent, which is patient safety.

The practice of the current model of informed consent in matters related to genetics tends to be more of an event, disclosure model.[32] The revised model is an "ongoing process where patient insight is developed and re-assessed."[33] To explain the significance of the revised model of consent, the following main categories of comprehension, disclosure, voluntariness, and patient safety are discussed.

1. Comprehension

First, PGT involves a risk analysis of the related probabilities that can be complicated for patients to comprehend. This point develops the importance of understanding in the current model. Risk assessment involves calculating probabilities to determine the likelihood of developing a disease. To accomplish this, the relation between autonomy and comprehension is crucial. Autonomy is emphasized in the current model by letting the patient decide whether or not to get tested. The current model uses an approach to autonomy that is standardized and generic, focusing on consent by providing a signature to accept or reject a test. The revised model

---

[29] Tom Beauchamp and James Childress, *Principles of Biomedical Ethics*, 132.

[30] Neil Sharpe and Ronald Carter, *Genetic Testing: Care, Consent, and Liability*, 131.

[31] Lewis Vaughn, *Bioethics: Principles, Issues, and Cases*, 145.

[32] Stephen Wear, *Informed Consent: Patient Autonomy and Clinician Beneficence within Health Care*, 100; Neil C. Manson and Onora O'Neill, *Rethinking Informed Consent in Bioethics*, 69–71; Robert M. Arnold and Charles W. Lidz, "Informed Consent: Clinical Aspects of Consent in Health Care," 8.

[33] Stephen Wear, *Informed Consent*, 95.

enhances the link between risk and understanding. This model enhances patient involvement by adopting a more extensive approach, described as a process rather than as an event. This model takes into consideration the fact that PGT has risks and values at stake that can only be evaluated by the specific patient.[34] Typically the current model does not offer a large amount of time to comprehending risk assessments. The additional time and complexity involved in comprehending the connection between risk and probability has significant implications for patient education by the doctor, thereby developing the meaning of the doctor-patient relationship. For example, the emergence of the so-called Nocebo Effect will be considered here. This Effect says that providing patients too much information can result in harm when the patients are not able to handle the amount of information properly.[35]

2. Disclosure

Second, there are complex treatment options, including no treatment for some diseases, that require genetic counseling to select an appropriate option. This point develops the importance of disclosure in the current model. Typically the current model emphasizes appropriate disclosure of information. While patients can be educated about the procedure, selecting an appropriate treatment option can be more difficult. Genetic counseling can supplement disclosure and help to enhance selection of an appropriate option, but it is not required in the current model.[36] In this model, genetic counseling and disclosure for decision-making purposes can be more difficult, since there are limited mechanisms in place to assess the patient. The current model also has challenging reimbursement policies which make it difficult for genetic counseling to take place. The revised model takes this further and recognizes that this disclosure needs to be accompanied with genetic counseling both before and after testing to enhance decision making about a suitable option. Appropriate genetic counseling must include patient assessment and feedback mechanisms. A couple of feedback mechanisms and patient assessments will be discussed and analyzed, including feedback loops, a decision tree, linear steps, and nomagrams. Through the use of a decision tree, patients can better internalize the risks, benefits, and future impact of their decision in order to facilitate appropriate decision making. Also the revised model has more of an emphasis on prevention, which can help to facilitate appropriate institutional and reimbursement policies for counseling and education.[37]

---

[34] Stephen Wear, *Informed Consent,* 37–38.

[35] Rebecca Erwin Wells and Ted J. Kaptchuk, "To Tell the Truth, the Whole Truth, May Do Patients Harm: The Problem of the Nocebo Effect for Informed Consent," 22–29.

[36] Stephen Wear, *Informed Consent,* 62, 66, 95–96; Neil C. Manson and Onora O'Neill, *Rethinking Informed Consent in Bioethics,* 70, 80.

[37] Thomas Goetz, *The Decision Tree,* xiv–xvii, 141–142, 197, 215; Stephen Wear, *Informed Consent,* 62, 122.

3. Voluntariness

Third, PGT involves family-related information with accompanying implications that can compromise voluntariness. Since the results can impact the entire family, there is an opportunity for external pressures. This third point develops the importance of avoiding coercion of both the patient and the patient's family when information is presented. The third distinctive characteristic of PGT is the relevance of genetic information for the patient's family. In the current model, family-related coercion is often difficult to identify. *Patient Autonomy and the Ethics of Responsibility* by Alfred Tauber briefly discusses coercion in the doctor-patient relationship.[38] The revised model shifts the focus from coercion of the patient alone to family-related coercion regarding PGT. Often coercion and a lack of voluntary consent can come in many forms, "some subtle, some not so subtle."[39] Even the subtle forms of negative influences like ostracism and peer pressure can arise among anyone applying "compelling pressure" such as the patient's family.[40] The revised model ensures voluntary consent by establishing procedures to avoid two forms of coercion: pressure by the family for the patient to be tested (eg, if there is a family genetic trait already known, there can be pressure upon a child to be tested to ascertain if s/he is a carrier etc); and pressure upon the family regarding the testing outcome (eg, if a trait emerges that affects other siblings, a process needs to be undertaken to ascertain whether the sibling wants to know).

4. Patient Safety

Lastly, the revised model of consent requires an additional component to the traditionally recognized three components (comprehension, disclosure, voluntariness): the culture of patient safety. That is, the revised model of consent enhances the traditional components of consent within a medical culture that emphasizes patient safety. This safety culture requires nationally established systems of accountability for PGT that implement the revised components of consent in a transparent manner to foster trust in the emerging system of genetic-related services. In order for this model to implement appropriate systems of accountability and transparency, a shift from treatment and diagnosis to prevention and early detection needs to occur. This shift will in turn emphasize a culture of patient safety in the area of PGT. Programs to ensure accountability will look at measures within laboratories and testing clinics to confront regulatory challenges that can increase false accountability.[41] The revised model will promote consistent, appropriate institutional policies that ensure enhanced accountability measures. The revised model adheres to transparency

---

[38] Alfred Tauber, *Patient Autonomy and the Ethics of Responsibility*, 63.

[39] John Kilner, Rebecca Pentz, Frank Young, eds., *Genetic Ethics,* 240.

[40] Linda Farber Post, Jeffrey Blustein, and Nancy Neveloff Dubler, *Handbook for Health Care Ethics Committees*, 42–43.

[41] Thomas Goetz, *The Decision Tree,* xiv, xvi–xvii, 117.

measures that focus specifically on PGT. Trust is developed in the revised model by measures ensuring accountability of PGT and transparency in implementation.[42]

D. Chapter 5: Application

The end of the book applies the revised model of informed consent to both direct-to-consumer (DTC) and pleiotropic genetic testing. Each area will give a background of the genetic test, and then it will apply the revised model of consent to the test.

1. DTC Genetic Testing

The first section looks at DTC genetic testing and applies the revised model to this field. The beginning of the chapter will look at the background of testing, and then the end of the chapter will apply the revised model to DTC genetic testing.

a. Background of DTC Genetic Testing

DTC genetic testing is a little different than the typical genetic testing, because a physician is not required to be involved, and it has both a research subject and patient treatment model of consent. Peter Kraft, Ph.D. and David Hunter's article, "Genetic Risk Prediction—Are We There Yet?" looks at the implications of this testing on patients and analyzes whether or not the science behind the testing is adequate. This article argues that DTC genetic testing could be a little premature, because the results can easily be misunderstood and the research is still in the beginning stages. Cynthia Marietta and Amy McGuire's article "Direct-to-Consumer Genetic Testing: Is It the Practice of Medicine?" discusses the question of physician or counselor involvement. The authors suggest that if the DTC genetic testing companies are involved in practicing medicine, then physicians should be involved. Some of the risks with this type of testing include misinterpretation of results and a lack of necessary follow-up.[43] But advocates say it can help consumers feel empowered by knowing their genetic makeup and helping with future treatment plans. Advocates say that once a person knows that he or she is at an increased risk for a particular disease, then the person will take precautionary measures such as having more screening tests or changing lifestyle habits.[44]

---

[42] Neil C. Manson and Onora O'Neill, *Rethinking Informed Consent in Bioethics*, 157–158; Robert M. Arnold and Charles W. Lidz, "Informed Consent: Clinical Aspects of Consent in Health Care," 10; Stephen Wear, *Informed Consent,* 72, 81.

[43] Cynthia Marietta, Amy McGuire, "Direct-to-Consumer Genetic Testing: Is It the Practice of Medicine?" 370–371; Emily Singer, "Off-the-Shelf Genetic Testing on Display," 1.

[44] Chris Berdik, "Genetic Tests Give Consumers Hints About Disease Risk; Critics Have Misgivings," 1–2; Leslie Pray, "DTC Genetic Testing: 23andMe, DNA Direct and Genelex," 4; Cynthia Marietta, Amy McGuire, "Direct-to-Consumer Genetic Testing," 370.

b. Application of the Revised Model

The second part of this section will apply the revised model to DTC genetic testing. This section will apply the areas of comprehension, disclosure, voluntariness, and patient safety to DTC genetic testing. Then it will conclude with a case study of DTC genetic testing.

1). Comprehension

The fist area of application is comprehension. DTC genetic testing recognizes the importance of autonomy and self- determination. Since DTC genetic testing is different than some of the other types of testing in that it focuses on a patient and research subject model of consent, the application of autonomy can be a little different in this approach. This model emphasizes more patient involvement through a process of increased education in order to fully understand the risk assessments for DTC genetic testing. The doctor-patient relationship is a little different with DTC genetic testing, because often there is no direct contact with a physician. Companies encourage discussing the results with a physician, but risk assessment discussions are limited with DTC genetic testing. The revised model encourages more patient and physician education concerning DTC genetic testing risks assessments.

2). Disclosure

The next area for DTC genetic testing is disclosure. The revised model includes both medical and non-medical information within the disclosure processes. One additional area of disclosure with DTC genetic testing should be disclosing the level of research the results are based on. In order to establish better predictions, DTC genetic testing companies need to have a broad range of samples.[45] In order to protect against unsubstantiated claims, the revised model encourages adopting a research confidence rating system to illustrate the difference between preliminary and confirmed research.[46] Genetic counseling is needed in the consideration of whether to initiate testing and after the testing in order to evaluate the results.[47] Post-test counseling ensures the patient meets to assess the results with either the DTC testing company or the patient's personal physician. Also genetic counseling should include patient assessment and feedback mechanisms.

---

[45] Peter Kraft, Ph.D. and David Hunter, "Genetic Risk Prediction—Are We There Yet?" 1701.

[46] Kristine Goodwin, "Information Overload? National Conference of State Legislatures."

[47] Kathy Beal, "Statement on Direct-to-Consumer Genetic Testing: Genetics Professionals Should Be Part of Genetic Testing Process Says American College of Medical Genetics," 1–2; Dr. Hsien-Hsien Lei, "Dr. Robert Marion on Direct-to-Consumer Genetic Testing," August 26, 2009; Jane Kaye, "The Regulation of Direct-to-Consumer Genetic Tests," R180.

3). Voluntariness

The third area of application is voluntariness. The voluntary nature of consent is crucial in order to ensure a meaningful consent for DTC genetic testing.[48] Sometimes external influences can actually support and benefit a person's decision-making by giving additional information, but other times external influences exhibit deception, weakened choices, and faulty reasoning.[49] The revised model of informed consent for DTC genetic testing seeks to avoid these types of detrimental influences. Tom Beauchamp and James Childress in the book *Principles of Biomedical Ethics* says that professionals in the healthcare and medical research areas should "probe for and ensure understanding and voluntariness" of consent.[50] The revised model seeks to avoid coercion of both the patient and the family. This model ensures voluntary consent by adhering to procedures that decrease pressure by the family for the patient to be tested. The revised model also ensures voluntary consent by adhering to procedures that decrease pressure upon the family regarding the testing outcome.

4). Patient Safety

Finally, the area of patient safety is applied to DTC genetic testing. Risks from false assurances and unreliable results can be minimized by adhering to the patient safety component within the revised model for PGT. One article in the *Journal of Molecular Diagnostics* said "It is the consumer's responsibility to exercise caution to avoid becoming a victim of marketing ploys that prey on humanity's innate curiosity and fears."[51] While ultimately DTC genetic testing is up to the consumer, there should also be mechanisms in place to ensure accountability, transparency, and trust in order to promote patient safety. DTC genetic testing labs will be required to participate in some type of genetics quality assurance program. This can help to ensure accountability, accuracy, and validity of materials and results.[52] The revised model of consent also recognizes and emphasizes the significance of transparency in implementation. One company, 23andMe, started a star system for "research confidence rating—with one star for preliminary research and four stars for established research."[53] When consumers see the accountability and transparency measures that 23andMe is starting to take right now, there can be a certain level of trust with that company. This section will end with a case study on DTC genetic testing and informed consent.

---

[48] Tom Beauchamp and James Childress, *Principles of Biomedical Ethics,* 79.

[49] Linda Farber Post, Jeffrey Blustein, and Nancy Neveloff Dubler, *Handbook for Health Care Ethics Committees*, 42–43.

[50] Tom Beauchamp and James Childress, *Principles of Biomedical Ethics*, 64.

[51] Daniel Farkas and Carol Holland, "Direct-to-Consumer Genetic Testing: Two Sides of the Coin," 3.

[52] Thomas Goetz, *The Decision Tree,* xvi-xvii, 117; Bernard Lo, *Resolving Ethical Dilemmas*, 273.

[53] Kristine Goodwin, "Information Overload? National Conference of State Legislatures."

2. Pleiotropic Genetic Testing

The second section of this chapter is pleiotropic genetic testing. This section will
look at the background of pleiotropic genetic testing, and then apply the revised
model of informed consent to pleiotropic genetic testing.

a. Background of Pleiotropic Genetic Testing

Pleiotropy is where multiple diseases can be expressed from one gene; one
example is a test for Apolipoprotein E (ApoE), which can give a risk assessment for both coronary artery disease (CAD) and Alzheimer's disease. Doctors generally run the test to find out about the risk of coronary artery disease
(CAD), but the results can also show the risk of developing Alzheimer's disease. Normally the patient has only given consent to find out about CAD, but
now the doctor has to determine whether or not the patient should know the
rest of the results. Zachary Cooper, Robert Nelson, and Lainie Ross's article
"Informed Consent for Genetic Research Involving Pleiotropic Genes: An Empirical Study of ApoE Research," concludes that most of the time, informed
consent for pleiotropic testing is not adequate, because many times the physicians and/or investigators have not disclosed what pleiotropy means and the
possible consequences of the testing. Since there is no significant treatment
for Alzheimer's disease, knowing a person is at risk might make pleiotropic
genetic testing more of a problem.[54]

b. Application of the Revised Model

The second part of pleiotropic genetic testing is the application of the revised model
of informed consent. This part will apply the areas of comprehension, disclosure,
voluntariness, and patient safety. The end of the chapter will conclude with a case
study on the revised model of informed consent for pleiotropic genetic testing.

1). Comprehension

The first aspect of the revised model is comprehension of risk and probabilities.
Informed consent for pleiotropic genetic testing cites autonomy as one of the foundational principles of testing. The ideas behind autonomy and pleiotropic testing are

---

[54] Robert Wachbroit, "The Question Not Asked: The Challenge of Pleiotropic Genetic Tests," 131,
133; Zachary Cooper, Robert Nelson, and Lainie Ross, "Informed Consent for Genetic Research
Involving Pleiotropic Genes: An Empirical Study of ApoE Research," 1; Ruth Hubbard and R.C.
Lewontin, "Genetic Testing for Disease Predisposition, Pitfalls of Genetic Testing," 360–362;
Lewis Vaughn, *Bioethics: Principles, Issues, and Cases*, 465–66.

that patients have the right to decide for themselves whether or not to be tested for the pleiotropic gene.[55] The revised model of consent encourages patient involvement through a more extensive process of consent. This model promotes additional conversations and education of the patient in order to cultivate comprehension and understanding of the patient when thinking about risk assessments. The revised model of consent looks at education and communication in order to ensure additional understanding and comprehension.

2). Disclosure

The second area of application is disclosure. Because PGT has many complex treatment options, the revised model requires disclosure and genetic counseling in order to select an appropriate option. If the nature of pleiotropic genes were not clearly communicated antecedently, disclosure of this type of information can be difficult to communicate; patients might not be expecting to hear about additional risks of Alzheimer's disease.[56] Disclosure should focus on what testing means and discuss the nature of Alzheimer's disease and pleiotropic genes. The pre-test counseling should focus on what the information will mean to the patient, since the test returns results for two diseases.[57] The counselor can also ask about disclosure of results; does the patient want to know his Alzheimer's risk.[58] By focusing on genetic counseling and patient feedback mechanisms, the revised model should ensure appropriate decision making.

3). Voluntariness

The third area of the revised model is voluntariness of family-related information. In pleiotropic genetic testing, coercion can arise from family members with strong opinions on either wanting or not wanting to know additional at-risk information for possible Alzheimer's disease. Also voluntariness can be impacted by the way a doctor or relative explains the information or views of pleiotropic genetic testing.[59] The revised model ensures voluntary consent by establishing procedures to avoid two forms of coercion: pressure by the family for the patient to be tested (eg, if heart

---

[55] Lewis Vaughn, *Bioethics: Principles, Issues, and Cases*, 465–66.

[56] KG Fulda and Lykens K, "Ethical Issues in Predictive Genetic Testing: A Public Health Perspective," 143–7.

[57] Robert Wachbroit, "The Question Not Asked: The Challenge of Pleiotropic Genetic Tests," 131–133; Lewis Vaughn, *Bioethics: Principles, Issues, and Cases*, 465–66; Annelien L. Bredenoord, Hester Y. Kroes, Edwin Cuppen, et al., "Disclosure of Individual Genetic Data to Research Participants: The Debate Reconsidered," 41–42.

[58] Ruth Hubbard and R.C. Lewontin, "Genetic Testing for Disease Predisposition, Pitfalls of Genetic Testing," 360–362; Lewis Vaughn, *Bioethics: Principles, Issues, and Cases*, 465–66; Robert Wachbroit, "The Question Not Asked: The Challenge of Pleiotropic Genetic Tests," 133–136.

[59] Tom Beauchamp and James Childress, *Principles of Biomedical Ethics*, 95.

disease runs in the family, there can be pressure upon a younger individual to be tested in to see if s/he is at-risk etc); and pressure upon the family regarding the testing outcome (eg, if the patient finds out s/he is at an increased risk for Alzheimer's disease, there can be pressure on other individuals in the family to get tested for the disease as well).

4). Patient Safety

The last part of this chapter is the application of patient safety in the revised model of informed consent for pleiotropic genetic testing. The revised model applies systems changes in order to increase patient safety and decrease risk for informed consent of pleiotropic genetic testing. The revised model seeks to establish accountability measures for pleiotropic genetic testing procedures and results.[60] This model promotes accountability by encouraging additional communication between the doctors and laboratories performing the tests. Often specific accountability and transparency measures are hard to identify in informed consent, but the revised model seeks to enhance and clarify those measure for pleiotropic genetic testing.[61] Transparency can be maintained by the doctors and counselors when educating and communicating with the patient about pleiotropic testing. When discussing risks and options with patients, doctors and counselors should be especially attentive to bringing out the differences of pleiotropic genetic testing in order to promote transparency of information and procedures. After establishing additional measures, trust is easier to build and maintain in the revised model of informed consent. The end of the section will have a case study on informed consent and pleiotropic genetic testing.

E. Chapter 6: Conclusion

The last chapter of the book is the conclusion. This book demonstrates the need for a revised approach to consent for PGT. The revised process model should be a continual "process where patient insight is developed and re-assessed" instead of the bureaucratic interferences.[62] The revised model of informed consent for PGT tries to emphasize and clarify the expectations, goals, and challenges of implementation to encourage better medical treatment for individuals. An article in the American Psychological Association Ethics Rounds suggests there is a relationship between

---

[60] Thomas Goetz, *The Decision Tree*, xvi–xvii, 117; Bernard Lo, *Resolving Ethical Dilemmas*, 273.

[61] KG Fulda and Lykens K., "Ethical Issues in Predictive Genetic Testing: A Public Health Perspective," 143–7.

[62] Robert M. Arnold and Charles W. Lidz, "Informed Consent: Clinical Aspects of Consent in Health Care," 4–5; Stephen Wear, *Informed Consent*, 95.

ethics and clinical care. Dr. Stephen Behnke of the American Psychological Association says "good ethics can promote good clinical care."[63] While the informed consent process can help improve patient decisions and communication, the consent process will not lead to perfect decisions. It can only improve ethical decision-making about proposed treatments and testing.[64] The last chapter will summarize and will provide practical ways for implementation of the revised model.

References

Arnold, Robert M. and Charles W. Lidz. "Informed Consent: Clinical Aspects of Consent in Health Care." In *Taking Sides: Clashing Views on Bioethical Issues*, edited by Carol Levine, 4–14. Boston: McGraw Hill Higher Education, 2010.

Arver, Brita, Aina Haegermark, Ulla Platten, et al. "Evaluation of Psychosocial Effects of Pre-Symptomatic Testing for Breast/Ovarian and Colon Cancer Pre-Disposing Genes: a 12-Month Follow-Up." *Familial Cancers* 3:2 (2004): 109–116.

Beal, Kathy. "Statement on Direct-to-Consumer Genetic Testing: Genetics Professionals Should Be Part of Genetic Testing Process Says American College of Medical Genetics." *American College of Medical Genetics* (September 24, 2007): 1–2.

Beauchamp, Tom and James Childress. *Principles of Biomedical Ethics*. New York: Oxford University Press, 2001.

Behnke, Stephen, Dr. "Informed Consent and APA's New Ethics Code: Enhancing Client Autonomy, Improving Client Care." *Ethics Rounds. American Psychological Association* 35: 6(June 2004): 80–81.

Berdik, Chris. "Genetic Tests Give Consumers Hints About Disease Risk; Critics Have Misgivings." *Washington Post.* (January 26, 2010): Special, 1–2.

Bredenoord, Annelien L., Hester Y. Kroes, Edwin Cuppen, et al. "Disclosure of Individual Genetic Data to Research Participants: The Debate Reconsidered." *Trends in Genetics* 27: 2(February 2011): 41–47.

Burgess, Michael, PhD, Claude Lanberg, MD, PhD, Bartha Maria Knoppers, LLD. "Bioethics for Clinicians: 14. Ethics and Genetics in Medicine." *Canadian Medical Association Journal* 158:10 (1998): 1309–1313.

Burke, Wylie, Ronald Zimmern, and Mark Kroese. "Defining Purpose: A Key Step in Genetic Test Evaluations." *Genetics in Medicine* 9: 10(October 2007): 675–681.

Cooper, Zachary, Robert Nelson, and Lainie Ross. "Informed Consent for Genetic Research Involving Pleiotropic Genes: An Empirical Study of ApoE Research." *IRB: Ethics and Human Research* 28:5 (September/October 2006): 1–11.

Ensenauer, Regina E., Virginia V. Michels, and Shanda S. Reinke. "Genetic Testing: Practical, Ethical, and Counseling Considerations." *Mayo Clinic Proceedings* 80: 1(January 2005): 63–73.

Farkas, Daniel, and Carol Holland. "Direct-to-Consumer Genetic Testing: Two Sides of the Coin." *Journal of Molecular Diagnostics* 11:4 (2009): 263–265.

Foster, Morris, John Mulvihill, and Richard Sharp. "Evaluating the Utility of Personal Genomic Information." *Genetics in Medicine* 11:8 (2009): 570–574.

Fulda, KG and Lykens K. "Ethical Issues in Predictive Genetic Testing: A Public Health Perspective." *Journal of Medical Ethics* 32: 3(March 2003): 143–147.

---

[63] Dr. Stephen Behnke, "Informed Consent and APA's New Ethics Code: Enhancing Client Autonomy, Improving Client Care," 80–81.

[64] Robert M. Arnold and Charles W. Lidz, "Informed Consent: Clinical Aspects of Consent in Health Care," 5.

Goetz, Thomas. *The Decision Tree*. New York: Rodale Inc., 2010.

Goodwin, Kristine. "Information Overload? National Conference of State Legislatures." *State Legislatures Magazine*, September 2008. Accessed December 10, 2011. http://www.ncsl.org/issues-research/health/state-legislatures-magazine-information-overload.aspx.

Heinrichs, Bert. "What Should We Want to Know About Our Future? A Kantian View on Predictive Genetic Testing. Medicine." *Health Care and Philosophy* 8:1 (2005): 29–37.

Hubbard, Ruth and R.C. Lewontin. "Genetic Testing for Disease Predisposition, Pitfalls of Genetic Testing," In *Intervention and Reflection*, edited by Ronald Munson, 352–354. Belmont, CA: Wadsworth Publishing, 2007.

Jonsen, Albert. *The Birth of Bioethics*. New York: Oxford University Press, 1998.

Kaye, Jane. "The Regulation of Direct-to-Consumer Genetic Tests." *Human Molecular Genetics* 17:2 (2008): R180–183.

Kilner, John, Rebecca Pentz, Frank Young, eds. *Genetic Ethics*. Grand Rapids, MI: William B Eerdmans Publishing Company, 1997.

Kraft, Peter, Ph.D., David Hunter. "Genetic Risk Prediction—Are We There Yet?" *The New England Journal of Medicine*. 360: 17 (April 23, 2009): 1701–1703.

Lei, Hsien-Hsien, Dr. "Dr. Robert Marion on Direct-to-Consumer Genetic Testing." *Books About DNA, DNA Testing, Personalities with DNA*, August 26, 2009. Accessed September 2, 2011. www.eyeondna.com/2009/08/26/dr-robert-marion-on-direct-to-consumer-genetic-testing/.

Lo, Bernard. *Resolving Ethical Dilemmas*. Philadelphia, PA: Lippincott Williams and Wilkins, 2005.

Manson, Neil C. and Onora O'Neill. *Rethinking Informed Consent in Bioethics*. New York: Cambridge University Press, 2007.

Marietta, Cynthia and Amy McGuire. "Direct-to-Consumer Genetic Testing: Is It the Practice of Medicine?" *Journal of Law, Medicine & Ethics* 37: 2(Summer 2009): 369–374.

Post, Linda Farber, Jeffrey Blustein, and Nancy Neveloff Dubler. *Handbook for Health Care Ethics Committees*. Baltimore: The John Hopkins University Press, 2007.

Pray, Leslie. "DTC Genetic Testing: 23andMe, DNA Direct and Genelex." *Nature Education* 1:1 (2008): 1–4.

Rose, Abigail L., Nikki Peters, Judy A. Shea, et al. "Attitudes and Misconceptions about Predictive Genetic Testing for Cancer Risk." *Community Genetics* 8 (2005): 145–151.

Sharpe, Neil F. and Ronald Carter. *Genetic Testing: Care, Consent, and Liability*. Hoboken, New Jersey: John Wiley & Sons, Inc., 2006.

Singer, Emily. "Off-the-Shelf Genetic Testing on Display." *Technology Review*, June 9, 2009. Accessed October 2, 2011. http://www.technologyreview.com/news/413745/off-the-shelf-genetic-testing-on-display/2/.

Tauber, Alfred. *Patient Autonomy and the Ethics of Responsibility*. Cambridge, MA: The MIT Press, 2005.

Vaughn, Lewis. *Bioethics: Principles, Issues, and Cases*. New York: Oxford University Press, 2009.

Wachbroit, Robert. "The Question Not Asked: The Challenge of Pleiotropic Genetic Tests." *Kennedy Institute of Ethics Journal* 8: 2(June 1998): 131–144.

Wear, Stephen. *Informed Consent: Patient Autonomy and Clinician Beneficence within Health Care*. Washington, DC: Georgetown University Press, 1998.

Wells, Rebecca Erwin and Ted J. Kaptchuk. "To Tell the Truth, the Whole Truth, May Do Patients Harm: The Problem of the Nocebo Effect for Informed Consent." *American Journal of Bioethics* 12: 3(March 2012): 22–29.

Chapter 2
Predictive Genetic Testing

The second chapter gives an introduction to and analysis of predictive genetic testing (PGT). This chapter explains PGT to identify the distinguishing characteristics of PGT that shape the revised model of consent in future chapters.

In order to fully understand the distinguishing characteristics, the beginning of the chapter will focus on the science of PGT. Having an understanding of the science behind this testing will help to elicit and further develop the three distinctive characteristics for this and future chapters. This chapter will introduce each of the three characteristics that arise from the science of PGT. As a result, this chapter establishes the foundation of the analysis for all the subsequent chapters.

The first part of Chap. 2 focuses on the background and science of PGT in order to get a better idea of the technical aspects behind genetic testing. The second part deals with the first distinguishing characteristic of PGT, understanding genetic risks and probabilities. Because genetic risks and probabilities are typically unique to PGT, this section will look at possible misunderstandings that can arise from not fully understanding genetic information. The third part looks at treatment options for diagnosed genetic traits. PGT can be different from other medical tests in that this testing can return results for diseases that have no treatment or preventative measures. This section will analyze that fact and identify some possible treatments that might help with PGT. The fourth area analyzes family-related genetic information. While some medical tests can involve family information, PGT has significant implications for family members of the individuals being tested. This section will discuss different styles of communication and disclosure of test results, and it will also look at the different concerns of family-related information for genetics. Then this fourth area will analyze the ideas of genetic exceptionalism versus normal medical information in regards to family-related genetic information. The fifth section will conclude with a summary of the implications and the distinguishing characteristics of PGT. By identifying the distinguishing characteristics of genetics, the chapter will highlight the power and limitations of genetic information and testing. The conclusion will bring together all the aspects of PGT that can influence the revised model of informed consent.

© Springer International Publishing Switzerland 2015
J. Minor, *Informed Consent in Predictive Genetic Testing*,
DOI 10.1007/978-3-319-17416-7_2

A. The Science Behind PGT

This section will look at PGT and the science behind it including issues of new genetic technologies and genetic information associated with specific diseases. Predictive genetic testing (PGT) looks at those at risk, the asymptomatic people.[1] One of the differences between PGT and a typical medical diagnostic test is the fact that PGT looks at the future while a diagnostic test gives information concerning the present.[2]

An article by Philip Mitchell, Bettina Meiser, Alex Wilde, et al. defines genetic testing as a test "used to identify a particular genotype (or set of genotypes) for a particular disease in a particular population for a particular purpose."[3] Philip Mitchell, Bettina Meiser, Alex Wilde, et al. go on to say that population is important because of the positive predictive value (PPV). The predictive value of a test is influenced by how often that disease occurs in a specific population. Generally there are three concepts used to evaluate a test: analytical validity, clinical validity, and clinical utility. The article by Philip Mitchell, Bettina Meiser, Alex Wilde, et al. says that analytical validity is related to the reliability and accuracy of a specific test. In genetic testing this is the ability of the test to identify the specific genotype. Analytical validity answers the question of does the genetic test actually identify what it is supposed to identify such as a Huntington's mutation or the BRCA mutation. Clinical validity is "determined by: (1) the strength of evidence for the link between genotype and disease; and (2) test performance characteristics such as sensitivity, specificity, positive and negative predictive values, and likelihood ratios."[4] Clinical validity looks at the accuracy and consistency of test performance. Clinical utility looks at the actual value of the test. This area answers the question of whether or not the test provides information that could be useful to the patient. There are 8 areas that should be analyzed in clinical utility. The testing purpose should look at areas of legitimacy, efficacy, effectiveness, and appropriateness. The possibility of testing should analyze areas of acceptability, efficiency of economic evaluation, optimality of economic evaluation, and equity of resources.[5]

This science behind PGT will look at four different areas including the science, utility, benefits, and risks of testing. The science will look at the technical aspects of testing, the utility will provide the basic value and purpose of testing, and then the benefits and risks of testing will be analyzed.

---

[1] Anita Silvers and Michael Ashley Stein, "An Equality Paradigm for Preventing Genetic Discrimination," 1342; Michael J. Green and Jeffrey R. Botkin, "'Genetic Exceptionalism' in Medicine: Clarifying the Differences between Genetic and Nongenetic Tests," 571.

[2] James Evans, Cecile Skrzynia, and Wylie Burke, "The Complexities of Predictive Genetic Testing," 1053.

[3] Philip Mitchell, Bettina Meiser, Alex Wilde, et al., "Predictive and Diagnostic Genetic Testing in Psychiatry," 227–228.

[4] Philip Mitchell, Bettina Meiser, Alex Wilde, et al., "Predictive and Diagnostic Genetic Testing in Psychiatry," 227–228.

[5] Philip Mitchell, Bettina Meiser, Alex Wilde, et al., "Predictive and Diagnostic Genetic Testing in Psychiatry," 227–228.

1. Science

The purpose of PGT is to assess an individual's risk of developing a specific disease. PGT analyzes DNA and genetics to identify whether a person will develop or already has an at-risk gene that causes them to have a higher or lower than an average risk of developing a specific disease. In order to make predictions about a person's risk for developing a specific disease, scientists analyze areas in a person's genes and chromosomes for genetic variants and mutations.[6] PGT looks at "polymorphisms that increase the probability of disease development."[7] Mutations can be identified by looking at segments of genes and chromosomes in order to identify genes that are different from the normal size and shape of a specific gene.[8] Currently, studies have identified the genetic variants that might be linked to a higher risk of at least 40 diseases.[9] Also studies have identified over 1000 genetic variants associated with a risk of disease.[10] The genetic variants make up what is called a single nucleotide polymorphism (SNP).Generally companies predict genetic risks by "calculating how often that condition occurs among people of the customer's general age, sex and ethnicity, then factor in the presence or absence of the relevant SNP."[11] It is important to note that the results depend on what genetic variants the laboratory decides to use when analyzing the predicted risk of disease.[12] One company could be analyzing 9 variants, while the other company is analyzing 13 variants. The number of variants analyzed can make a difference in the results as well. Once a genetic variant is associated with a risk of a particular disease, tests can be run to look at the SNPs in a specific sample in order to determine risk. If the individual does have the mutation, then it means that that individual has a higher chance of developing that specific disease or cancer than a person without that mutation.[13]

Diseases can be caused by a number of genetic and environmental factors. An important aspect to predicting disease is the fact that there can be several variants in a gene and those variants can be linked to several different diseases.[14] SNPs can be associated with many different areas. One SNP could be more common in a person

---

[6] Anita Silvers and Michael Ashley Stein, "An Equality Paradigm for Preventing Genetic Discrimination," 1346–1347.

[7] Michael J. Green and Jeffrey R. Botkin, "'Genetic Exceptionalism' in Medicine: Clarifying the Differences between Genetic and Nongenetic Tests," 571.

[8] Abigail L. Rose, Nikki Peters, Judy A. Shea, et al., "Attitudes and Misconceptions about Predictive Genetic Testing for Cancer Risk," 146.

[9] Peter Kraft, Ph.D. and David Hunter, "Genetic Risk Prediction—Are We There Yet?" 1701.

[10] Pauline C. Ng, Sarah S. Murray, Samuel Levy, et al., "An Agenda for Personalized Medicine," 724–725.

[11] Chris Berdik, "Genetic Tests Give Consumers Hints About Disease Risk; Critics Have Misgivings," 2.

[12] Francis Collins, *The Language of Life,* xxi–xxii.

[13] Abigail L. Rose, Nikki Peters, Judy A. Shea, et al., "Attitudes and Misconceptions about Predictive Genetic Testing for Cancer Risk," 146.

[14] Anita Silvers and Michael Ashley Stein, "An Equality Paradigm for Preventing Genetic Discrimination," 1346, 1385.

with breast cancer, Parkinson's disease, or another type of cancer.[15] The BRCA 1/2 gene mutations were identified in 1994 and 1995.[16] These mutations increase the likelihood of developing breast and/or ovarian cancer. Generally many different genes are involved in the development of a disease. For example, Anita Silvers and Michael Ashley Stein in the *Vanderbilt Law Review* say that researchers have found over eight hundred gene mutations that are linked to cystic fibrosis. Since there are so many different variations and mutations for this disease, the predictability of developing cystic fibrosis can vary greatly from variation to variation. One genetic mutation can impact the severity of the disease while another mutation might not impact the disease at all. Anita Silvers and Michael Ashley Stein in the *Vanderbilt Law Review* state that "identical mutations in such genes will affect individuals from different populations to different degrees because of variations in environmental factors."[17] Each mutation does not carry the same weight.

Huntington's disease is more of a unique disease for PGT in that the test has a higher degree of certainty for predicting. In 1993, the genetic variation for Huntington's disease was identified, and as a result PGT was offered for at-risk individuals. Huntington's disease is an incurable neurodegenerative disease with no medical treatments available to slow the progression.[18] There are approximately 30,000 individuals with Huntington's disease, but it is suggested that there are another 200,000 that have not been tested yet and are at risk in the United States. This disease is generally categorized as a late-onset condition, because typically the disease manifests itself around 40 years old. The test for Huntington's disease has 100 % penetrance, which means if the gene is present, then the individual will develop Huntington's disease at some point in his or her life. On the other side, if the gene is not present, then the individual is not at risk for Huntington's disease. With this disease, either the Huntington's gene is present or it is absent. Because of the certainty and the predictive value of testing for Huntington's disease, the results for PGT are more clear cut. The science behind PGT for Huntington's disease is not as complicated as other diseases. However, there are other issues to consider with this testing such as the non-existent treatment options and the difficult family implications of this predictive testing, and both of these issues will be discussed in later sections.[19]

The confidence in predictive genetic testing can be both over- and underestimated at times. Most genetic tests will not predict with certainty the likelihood of develop-

---

[15] Chris Berdik, "Genetic Tests Give Consumers Hints About Disease Risk; Critics Have Misgivings," 2; Marion Harris, Ingrid Winship, and Merle Spriggs, "Controversies and Ethical Issues in Cancer-Genetics Clinics," 301.

[16] Abigail L. Rose, Nikki Peters, and Judy A. Shea, et al., "Attitudes and Misconceptions about Predictive Genetic Testing for Cancer Risk," 145.

[17] Anita Silvers and Michael Ashley Stein, "An Equality Paradigm for Preventing Genetic Discrimination," 1385.

[18] Susan M. Cox, "Stories in Decisions: How At-Risk Individuals Decide to Request Predictive Testing for Huntington Disease," 258.

[19] Kathryn Holt, "What Do We Tell the Children? Contrasting the Disclosure Choices of Two HD Families Regarding Risk Status and Predictive Genetic Testing," 254–255.

ing a specific disease, because most diseases have a number of genetic and environmental aspects to them. Huntington's disease, however, has a genetic test that will predict with a high degree of certainty that a person will develop the disease in the future. But even with a disease like Huntington's, there is no way to predict how the disease will affect an individual person. Many of the tests are subject to uncertainty, false positives or negatives, and possible misinterpretation. Anita Silvers and Michael Ashley Stein in the *Vanderbilt Law Review* say "neither now nor in the future will someone's genetic makeup forecast that person's future health condition with certainty."[20] There are many factors that can influence the development and severity of the disease or illness. Some of the factors that influence the predictive value of the test include the differences of gene expression, accuracy of the specific test, and reliability of the research. But on the other side, Anita Silvers and Michael Ashley Stein in the *Vanderbilt Law Review* say "it is equally misleading to say that basing health predictions on genetic testing is 'little more than medical speculation.'"[21] So while PGT cannot attest to the severity and/or certainty of a specific disease, this testing does have a certain value and legitimacy for medical care.[22]

Also included within the science of PGT are the inheritance patterns for disease. If one parent is homozygous for a specific disease, then he or she has two copies of the mutation. If a parent is heterozygous for a disease, then he or she has one copy of the mutation and one copy of the normal gene. Because there are different patterns of inheritance, not all disease inheritance is the same. For example, Huntington's disease is an autosomal dominant disease. The inheritance pattern for Huntington's disease is easy, because it is only concerned with one gene. Because it is dominant, the disease will be passed down to the children if any of the children inherit one mutated gene. The Punnett square below further illustrates this concept. The capital "H" is the mutation causing Huntington's disease, while the lower case "h" represents the normal gene (Table 2.1).

The box represents one parent with Huntington's disease (Hh in bold) and one parent without Huntington's disease (hh in italic). When children are born, each child will have a 50% chance of inheriting Huntington's disease (Hh) and a 50% chance of not having Huntington's disease (hh). This is a basic representation of genetic inheritance patterns. While this seems fairly easy, the inheritance pattern for

Table 2.1 Punnett square for Huntington's disease		**H**	**h**
	h	Hh	hh
	h	Hh	hh

---

[20] Anita Silvers and Michael Ashley Stein, "An Equality Paradigm for Preventing Genetic Discrimination," 1347–1348.

[21] Anita Silvers and Michael Ashley Stein, "An Equality Paradigm for Preventing Genetic Discrimination," 1347–1348.

[22] Susan Wolf and Jeffrey Kahn, "Genetic Testing and the Future of Disability Insurance: Ethics, Law & Policy," 8; Anita Silvers and Michael Ashley Stein, "An Equality Paradigm for Preventing Genetic Discrimination," 1347–1348.

Huntington's disease is probably one of the easiest. Most other diseases that can be predicted with PGT are multifactorial diseases. There are several factors that influence the inheritance of the BRCA mutation. Even if a person has the mutation, it is not necessarily a positive diagnosis since there are other influencing factors such as the environment and the individual's lifestyle.[23]

2. Utility

Sometimes PGT is recommended based on the utility of the testing, and other times it is not recommended because of a lack of insufficient evidence of testing benefit. Some instances of increased utility include the following: "high morbidity and mortality of disease, effective but imperfect treatment, high predictive power of the genetic test (high penetrance), high cost or onerous nature of screening and surveillance methods, and preventive measures that are expensive or associated with adverse effects."[24] On the other hand, decreased utility for predictive genetic testing include: "low morbidity and mortality of disease, highly effective and acceptable treatment, poor predictive power of the genetic test (low penetrance), availability of inexpensive, acceptable, and effective screening and surveillance methods, and preventive measures that are inexpensive, efficacious, and high acceptable—for example, vaccination."[25] James Evans, Cecile Skrzynia, and Wylie Burke in "The Complexities of Predictive Genetic Testing," from the British Medical Journal say that the usefulness of the test can decrease if the disease is curable. For example, James Evans, Cecile Skrzynia, and Wylie Burke suggest that when breast and colon cancer are able to be cured or treated by effective and safe measures, then the benefit of testing is reduced. However, if the disease is curable and is identified earlier, then the disease might be able to be cured earlier rather than later. Evans, Skrzynia, and Burke also suggest that if there are successful and economical screening tools in place for certain diseases, then the utility of PGT will decrease. One example given is of hypertension. Since there are acceptable screening methods that are not expensive, there is not a need to participate in PGT for hypertension. James Evans, Cecile Skrzynia, and Wylie Burke suggest that if the cost of screening is much higher, then PGT will be more economical and attractive to individuals. Evans, Skrzynia, and Burke also suggest that in order for PGT to have higher utility, the preventive measures would generally have some problems and/or be fairly costly. For example, the utility of PGT typically can increase when a person is at risk for breast cancer and is considering a prophylactic mastectomy. James Evans, Cecile

---

[23] Heidi Chial, "Mendelian Genetics: Patterns of Inheritance and Single-Gene Disorders;" Susan Wolf and Jeffrey Kahn, "Genetic Testing and the Future of Disability Insurance: Ethics, Law & Policy," 8.
[24] James Evans, Cecile Skrzynia, and Wylie Burke, "The Complexities of Predictive Genetic Testing," 1054.
[25] James Evans, Cecile Skrzynia, and Wylie Burke, "The Complexities of Predictive Genetic Testing," 1054–1055.

Skrzynia, and Wylie Burke say "when prevention is simple, however, the value of testing decreases," and the example of a vaccination is given.[26] Since vaccinations are so easy to prevent diseases, there is no need for PGT of diseases like measles, mumps, and rubella. The utility of PGT can play an important role in the utilization of testing and the risks and benefits of testing.

3. Benefits

Reasons to undergo testing include motivational and emotional. Motivational reasons include "early detection, prevention, and control."[27] The goal of PGT is to identify which people have the mutation so that additional monitoring can take place for those at risk. Identification and monitoring of at-risk individuals will hopefully "lead to reduced morbidity and mortality through targeted screening, surveillance, and prevention."[28] If there is additional monitoring, then the hope is that there can be early diagnosis of the disease. PGT can help to monitor those at increased risk and decrease the amount of screening for those that are not at risk or are low risk. Possible prevention and treatment plans are another benefit of testing. Sometimes there can be surgeries or chemotherapy that can help to decrease a person's risk for a specific disease.[29] Also PGT could help with future plans and "may lead individuals to alter their diet or avoid exposure to certain chemicals in an attempt to avoid future disease."[30] The hope is that people will avoid "risk-inducing behaviors."[31] Shoshana Shiloh and Shiri Ilan, the authors of "To Test or Not To Test? Moderators of the Relationship Between Risk Perceptions and Interest in Predictive Genetic Testing," described a study about risk perceptions and testing utilization. The study concluded that the high interest in the test was associated with "both motivations and especially with emotional-reassurance motivation, but not with risk perceptions, health/illness orientations, and cancer anxiety."[32] The study demonstrated that risk perceptions did not necessarily lead to increased test utilization or interest in PGT. Shoshana Shiloh and Shiri Ilan say that understanding the perceived risk is crucial but that is not enough to alter behaviors including fitness modifications. In order to change behaviors and goals, there needs to be psychological changes as well. The

---

[26] James Evans, Cecile Skrzynia, and Wylie Burke, "The Complexities of Predictive Genetic Testing," 1054–1055.

[27] Clara L. Gaff, Veronica Collins, Tiffany Symes, et al., "Facilitating Family Communication about Predictive Genetic Testing: Probands' Perceptions," 133.

[28] James Evans, Cecile Skrzynia, and Wylie Burke, "The Complexities of Predictive Genetic Testing," 1052.

[29] Neil Sharpe and Ronald Carter, Genetic Testing: Care, Consent, and Liability, 269–70.

[30] Susan Wolf and Jeffrey Kahn, "Genetic Testing and the Future of Disability Insurance: Ethics, Law & Policy," 8.

[31] Neil Sharpe and Ronald Carter, Genetic Testing: Care, Consent, and Liability, 269–70.

[32] Shoshana Shiloh and Shiri Ilan, "To Test or Not To Test? Moderators of the Relationship Between Risk Perceptions and Interest in Predictive Genetic Testing," 471.

article by Shoshana Shiloh and Shiri Ilan concludes that in order to have informed consent and decision making, there needs to be objective and reasonable information about the possible risks and benefits. Also there can be psychological and emotional benefits of testing. Emotional motivations include eliminating uncertainty, gaining support or hope, and preparing emotionally.[33] Finding out that a person is not at risk or is at a very low risk of developing a certain disease can often decrease his or her anxiety levels. This can also lead to a greater "self-perception." Knowing a person's risk status can help to alter or reinforce their view of themselves. Sometimes PGT can result in a greater "sense of control," because the person at risk can follow certain procedures and/or treatments that could potentially decrease their risk.[34] In some people's minds, PGT can help to gain control by knowing their risk status and/or organizing events in their life and future.[35] Motivational and emotional reasons for testing can be benefits of PGT.

There can also be future benefits. Anita Silvers and Michael Ashley Stein in the *Vanderbilt Law Review* suggest that some genetic variants and mutations could have different functions and outcomes than originally thought. "In the future, scientists could discover that having a particular breast cancer gene mutation correlates with immunity from AIDS (as sickle-cell trait correlates with heightened immunity to malaria)."[36] Even with emotional, motivational, and future benefits, sometimes there can also be anxiety, worry, and discrimination that can impact themselves and their family.[37]

4. Risks

Shoshana Shiloh and Shiri Ilan in their article, "To Test or Not To Test? Moderators of the Relationship Between Risk Perceptions and Interest in Predictive Genetic Testing," say that while PGT can promote encouragement and hope, it can also "cause considerable distress to others from premature knowledge of likely illness."[38] Discrimination and psychological harms are often cited as the main harms, but there can be others associated with PGT. Sometimes there can be false assurances which can cause problems for future treatment. False assurances come from getting a lower risk than what is actually true. On the other hand, there can be problems from getting a higher risk than what is actually true. If a woman is told she

---

[33] Shoshana Shiloh and Shiri Ilan, "To Test or Not To Test? Moderators of the Relationship Between Risk Perceptions and Interest in Predictive Genetic Testing," 471–472, 476–477.

[34] Neil Sharpe and Ronald Carter, *Genetic Testing: Care, Consent, and Liability,* 269–70.

[35] Abigail L. Rose, Nikki Peters, Judy A. Shea, et al., "Attitudes and Misconceptions about Predictive Genetic Testing for Cancer Risk," 148.

[36] Anita Silvers and Michael Ashley Stein, "An Equality Paradigm for Preventing Genetic Discrimination," 1385.

[37] Abigail L. Rose, Nikki Peters, Judy A. Shea, et al., "Attitudes and Misconceptions about Predictive Genetic Testing for Cancer Risk," 148.

[38] Shoshana Shiloh and Shiri Ilan, "To Test or Not To Test? Moderators of the Relationship Between Risk Perceptions and Interest in Predictive Genetic Testing," 469.

has a high risk for developing breast cancer, then she will make decisions based on that information such as having a prophylactic double mastectomy. Problems arise when people adopt "irreversible, risk-inducing or expensive risk prevention strategies based upon incorrectly high estimations of risk."[39] Also sometimes people can have feelings of powerlessness. People often have no control over whether or not they develop a certain disease, and this can cause additional problems emotionally and even physically by not following recommended protocols. The possibility of discrimination and stigmatization can also be a risk of this information.[40]

Discrimination can occur in many areas including employment, insurance, and social situations. Genetic discrimination "arises when individuals with no symptoms or signs receive less favorable or adverse treatment because of their genotype."[41] If the concern about discrimination is high, then sometimes people might not participate in PGT, because he or she is concerned about his family's insurance premiums. If the tests are not conducted, then the individual could be missing out on possible treatment options. In a study with 163 cancer geneticists, about 68% of the geneticists said that if a person underwent testing for BRCA1 or 2 or hereditary non-polyposis colorectal cancer (HNPCC) they would not bill insurance so that there would be no discrimination. Also with this study, 26% of the geneticists said that they were in favor of using an alias for testing so as not to cause potential discrimination.[42] Another study conducted by phone found that people were also discriminated against because a family member had a hereditary genetic disease. Anita Silvers and Michael Ashley Stein in the *Vanderbilt Law Review* say that having a negative test result could result in other prospects. Anita Silvers and Michael Ashley Stein continue to say that "Proof that they are not at risk will reassure them of their ability to succeed in endeavors aversive for people who develop the disease."[43] Sometimes people who are at-risk will not participate in certain events or careers in life, because the individuals assume there is nothing he or she can do. Other times, people do not allow individuals to participate, because people consider those individuals to be at risk.[44] Discrimination can occur in many different areas and activities. At the beginning, individual and family discrimination played a significant part in PGT, but in 2003, the Genetic Information Non Discrimination Act (GINA) was established. This act tries to eliminate employment and insurance discrimination.[45] How

---

[39] Neil Sharpe and Ronald Carter, *Genetic Testing: Care, Consent, and Liability,* 270.

[40] Douglas Martin and Heather Greenwood, "Public Perceptions of Ethical Issues Regarding Adult Predictive Genetic Testing," 107.

[41] Marion Harris, Ingrid Winship, Merle Spriggs, "Controversies and Ethical Issues in Cancer-Genetics Clinics," 304–305.

[42] Marion Harris, Ingrid Winship, Merle Spriggs, "Controversies and Ethical Issues in Cancer-Genetics Clinics," 304–305.

[43] Anita Silvers and Michael Ashley Stein, "An Equality Paradigm for Preventing Genetic Discrimination," 1349.

[44] Anita Silvers and Michael Ashley Stein, "An Equality Paradigm for Preventing Genetic Discrimination," 1349.

[45] Marion Harris, Ingrid Winship, Merle Spriggs, "Controversies and Ethical Issues in Cancer-Genetics Clinics," 305; Cynthia Marietta and Amy McGuire, "Direct-to-Consumer Genetic Testing: Is It the Practice of Medicine?" 370.

ever, Susan Wolf and Jeffrey Kahn in "Genetic Testing and the Future of Disability Insurance: Ethics, Law & Policy," say that the "fear of discrimination is important, as individuals may decide to forego genetic testing (even when it might prove medically useful) in order to protect themselves against insurance discrimination."[46]

Another possible concern about knowing a person is at risk is psychological harms.[47] Marita Broadstock, Susan Michie, and Theresa Marteau in "Psychological Consequences of PGT: A Systematic Review" from the *European Journal of Human Genetics*, suggest that there were no significant changes in the emotional suffering for the carriers and non-carriers in a period of 3 years after PGT. The authors suggest a couple of reasons for this finding. In this study, there could be general psychological defense methods that had already been started. Broadstock, Michie, and Marteau say that research suggests that the people participating in testing are often stronger emotionally and are more capable of handling information. By already deciding to take a PGT and coming forward for testing, people tend to have thought about the testing in advance. Another study found that people getting tested for Huntington's disease (HD) generally "had higher ego strength, were more socially extroverted, and had more positive coping strategies than the general population."[48] Often the people considering getting tested for HD have increased experiential knowledge about this disease. Another study with HD looked at those who decided not to undergo testing and then compared them to those who came forward for testing. The study suggested that those who did not undergo HD testing were more pessimistic about the future. The most common attitudes presented in those who participated in the study were denial of the results or test, elimination of uncertainty, or both. Also sometimes people from at-risk families already had strong coping methods. Broadstock, Michie, and Marteau concluded that as genetic testing is increasingly brought into routine medical care, "some of the protective factors associated with the research environment are likely to be reduced," and likely there will be more psychological harms.[49]

However on the other hand, in "Predictive Genetic Testing in Children and Adults: A Study of Emotional Impact" from the *Journal of Medical Genetics,* S. Michie, M. Bobrow, and T. M. Marteau suggest that there is a significant level of anxiety after getting a positive test result. S. Michie, M. Bobrow, and T. M. Marteau say that this conclusion is especially important in adults with not as many psychological resources.[50] One article by Regina E. Ensenauer, Virginia V. Michels, and Shanda S. Reinke, "Genetic Testing: Practical, Ethical, and Counseling Consider-

---

[46] Susan Wolf and Jeffrey Kahn, "Genetic Testing and the Future of Disability Insurance: Ethics, Law & Policy," 11.

[47] Neil Sharpe and Ronald Carter, *Genetic Testing: Care, Consent, and Liability,* 270.

[48] Marita Broadstock, Susan Michie, Theresa Marteau, "Psychological Consequences of Predictive Genetic Testing: A Systematic Review," 735–736.

[49] Marita Broadstock, Susan Michie, Theresa Marteau, "Psychological Consequences of Predictive Genetic Testing: A Systematic Review," 735–736.

[50] S. Michie, M. Bobrow, and T. M. Marteau, on behalf of the FAP Collaborative Research Group, "Predictive Genetic Testing in Children and Adults: A Study of Emotional Impact," 520, 526.

ations," illustrates the importance of genetic information and possible psychosocial implications when it says "Once genetic testing results are learned, it is something that will stay with that patient throughout her/his lifetime."[51] As a result, additional counseling and assessments could be helpful to decrease any potential anxiety.[52]

B. Understanding Genetic Risks and Probabilities

Since risk predictions are very complex with difficult ideas to convey, genetic tests can result in misunderstandings and ambiguous results.[53] PGT and risk assessments are often "complicated and confusing."[54] Authors Neil Manson and Onora O'Neill ask, "How can people give adequate consent to acts that use genetic information if (as is acknowledged) they have false beliefs about genetic information or understand it poorly?"[55] The authors clearly illustrate the problem of adequate understanding and the ethics of consent. In order to have solid informed consent, it is important to increase public education on potential choices. One of the questions to address is whether or not patients and the public understand genetic risks and probabilities.

This section on understanding will look at three ideas. The first discussion is on interpreting test results, and this area will look at both positive and negative results of testing. The second area will look at misunderstandings of genetic information and PGT risk assessments, and this section will seek to identify and address those misunderstands. The third area of discussion is education, and this analyzes both patient and public education of genetic risks and probabilities.

1. Interpreting Test Results

Having a positive result on the prostate cancer test does not mean that a person has prostate cancer right now nor is it certain that he will ever get prostate cancer in the future. A positive test is not a clinical diagnosis at the time. A positive test means that a person has an increased risk for developing a certain disease or illness.[56] A positive test means that there was some kind of variance in a chromosome or gene, and depending on how that gene functions determines what type of increased risk

---

[51] Regina E. Ensenauer, Virginia V. Michels, and Shanda S. Reinke, "Genetic Testing: Practical, Ethical, and Counseling Considerations," 70.

[52] S. Michie, M. Bobrow, and T. M. Marteau, on behalf of the FAP Collaborative Research Group, "Predictive Genetic Testing in Children and Adults: A Study of Emotional Impact," 526.

[53] Chris Berdik, "Genetic Tests Give Consumers Hints About Disease Risk; Critics Have Misgivings," Special, 1.

[54] Maxwell Mehlman, "Predictive Genetic Testing in Urology: Ethical and Social Issues," 433.

[55] Neil C. Manson and Onora O'Neill, *Rethinking Informed Consent in Bioethics*, 144.

[56] AMA, "Direct-to-Consumer Genetic Testing;" Regina E. Ensenauer, Virginia V. Michels, and Shanda S. Reinke, "Genetic Testing: Practical, Ethical, and Counseling Considerations," 66.

a consumer will have.[57] Also it is important to remember that mutations in genes or chromosomes can manifest themselves differently to different people. In genetics, having a certain gene or genotype does not always translate into specific symptoms or traits for each person.[58] Another important factor to remember is that most diseases are multifactorial, in that the disease takes into account several areas including family history and environmental responses.[59]

Negative results carry the same weight. Just because a person received a negative result, does not mean the person will be absent of that disease.[60] It simply means that the test did not find a genetic variance in the gene or chromosome.[61] Negative test results do not mean that the person will never develop the disease, but that there is still a normal "population risk" for that disease.[62] For those undergoing BRCA testing, if the results are negative, then that means the individual has the same level of risk for breast and/or ovarian cancer as the general public. Those individuals have an average risk. However, while the person is at an average risk, there are no testing procedures that will "remove this background risk."[63] The only thing that can help a person with an average risk like the general public are the screening recommendations which include clinical breast exams and mammograms at the scheduled time. While most negative results mean the person did not have the mutation, a negative result could also be evidence of a false assurance. False assurances generally mean that either the genetic variance has not been identified yet or the test failed to detect the genetic variance.[64] With BRCA 1/2, "contrary to possible patient and physician expectations, no current single technology can identify all mutations."[65]

An article by Jon Emery, Kristine Barlow-Stewart, and Sylvia A. Metcalfe entitled, "There's Cancer in the Family," says that genetics most likely influences all cancers to an extent, but "certain cancers, such as breast, colorectal and ovarian are more likely to demonstrate familial clustering."[66] The BRCA1 gene, affecting 1 out

---

[57] Cynthia Marietta, Amy McGuire, "Direct-to-Consumer Genetic Testing: Is It the Practice of Medicine?" 370; Neil Sharpe and Ronald Carter, *Genetic Testing: Care, Consent, and Liability*, 269.

[58] AMA, "Direct-to-Consumer Genetic Testing;" Regina E. Ensenauer, Virginia V. Michels, and Shanda S. Reinke, "Genetic Testing: Practical, Ethical, and Counseling Considerations," 66–67.

[59] Cynthia Marietta and Amy McGuire, "Direct-to-Consumer Genetic Testing: Is It the Practice of Medicine?" 370.

[60] AMA, "Direct-to-Consumer Genetic Testing;" Neil Sharpe and Ronald Carter, *Genetic Testing: Care, Consent, and Liability*, 268.

[61] Cynthia Marietta and Amy McGuire, "Direct-to-Consumer Genetic Testing: Is It the Practice of Medicine?" 370.

[62] Marion Harris, Ingrid Winship, and Merle Spriggs, "Controversies and Ethical Issues in Cancer-Genetics Clinics," 302.

[63] Janice Berliner and Angela Fay, "Risk Assessment and Genetic Counseling for Hereditary Breast and Ovarian Cancer: Recommendations of the National Society of Genetic Counselors," 256.

[64] AMA, "Direct-to-Consumer Genetic Testing;" Cynthia Marietta and Amy McGuire, "Direct-to-Consumer Genetic Testing: Is It the Practice of Medicine?" 370.

[65] Neil Sharpe and Ronald Carter, *Genetic Testing: Care, Consent, and Liability*, 268.

[66] Jon Emery, Kristine Barlow-Stewart, and Sylvia A. Metcalfe, "There's Cancer in the Family," 194.

of 1000 people, has increased risks for developing breast and ovarian cancer. Those with this gene have a 40–80% chance of developing breast cancer and a 10–60% chance of developing ovarian cancer. This gene, BRCA1, is also associated with a higher risk of developing prostate cancer. However, it is important to note though that even with the increased risk from the BRCA 1/2 mutations, only 5–10% of all breast cancer is linked to these genetic mutations.[67] Also another example, those with a mutation in the mismatch repair (MMR) gene have a chance of developing hereditary non-polyposis colorectal cancer (HNPCC). Typically there is a 1 in 1000 chance of having this mutation in the general public. But if a person has this hereditary mutation, then there is a 70–90% chance that he or she will develop colorectal cancer by the age of 75. Also if a person has this mutation, then there is a chance he or she could develop other cancers as well such as endometrial, ovarian, stomach, urinary tract, small intestine, pancreatic, and/or biliary tree cancer. These other cancers have a lower risk of developing, but there is still a risk.[68]

2. Misunderstandings

Sometimes there is confusion about what the results of PGT, risk assessments, and genetic tests in general mean. At times the media can contribute to some of the misleading information about genetics and genetic testing.[69] One example of the media contributing to misunderstanding is illustrated in a story in the *New York Times*. With PGT there will always be a level of uncertainty. Uncertainty is included in whether or not an individual will get the disease, when the disease will occur, and/or the severity of the disease; however, the idea of uncertainty is generally not presented. The *New York Times* discussed a "genetic report card," and said that this "would predict a baby's health history at birth."[70]

There can also be faulty views of genetics by the general public or even medical professionals. Possible misunderstandings about genetics include confusion about facts like genes are in human cells, there are 46 chromosomes, and the genes are in chromosomes. There are also misunderstandings with the idea of risk probabilities like problems in measuring risk and/or overestimating risk. Robert Klitzman in "Misunderstandings Concerning Genetics Among Patients Confronting Genetic Disease" analyzes some common misconceptions of genetics and genetic testing. He identifies three categories of misconceptions: genetic tests, genetic mechanisms, and statistics. Misconceptions about genetic tests include ideas that genetics can

---

[67] Abigail L. Rose, Nikki Peters, Judy A. Shea, et al., "Attitudes and Misconceptions about Predictive Genetic Testing for Cancer Risk," 145–146.

[68] Jon Emery, Kristine Barlow-Stewart, and Sylvia A. Metcalfe, "There's Cancer in the Family," 194, 196–197.

[69] Abigail L. Rose, Nikki Peters, Judy A. Shea, et al., "Attitudes and Misconceptions about Predictive Genetic Testing for Cancer Risk," 149.

[70] James Evans, Cecile Skrzynia, and Wylie Burke, "The Complexities of Predictive Genetic Testing," 1053.

predict behavior and genetic tests have more predictive power than they really do. One misconception of genetic testing is that genetics can predict behavior. One person says "You hear a lot about predispositions for drug addiction and alcoholism, and "the gay gene"—folk information. My wife works with scientists. They know what's going on, but are the minority."[71] This idea can be linked to genetic exceptionalism which can be seen in media stories and the news. Also, people often think that genetic tests can predict with certainty the odds of developing a particular disease.[72] The complexity of this idea is illustrated in the following statement:

> People think the test will tell you whether you will get the disease or not, rather than it being a piece of information that says, "You're probably at higher risk for getting this disease, but it doesn't mean you're going to get it." Intellectually, I understand that. But emotionally, even that is hard to wrap my head around.[73]

While many times the predictive value is overestimated, Susan Michie, John Weinman, Julie Miller, et al. suggests the opposite. Michie, Weinman, Miller, et al. in "Predictive Genetic Testing: High Risk Expectations in the Face of Low Risk Information," analyze uncertainty and categorize this area as test representation. While the article by Michie, Weinman, Miller, et al. was written towards the beginning of PGT, there is still some relevance to "seeing is believing" as stated by those in the study comparing bowel screening to genetic test. Screening for a disease can tell if there is an actual tumor, but PGT on the other hand looks to genetics to predict when or if the disease will develop in the future. Sometimes physical evidence proves more valuable to people. Michie, Weinman, Miller, et al. suggest that the confidence level for this type of testing can be lower than other types, which can lead to a higher perception of risk. Those with more uncertainty about the confidence of results thought they had a higher level of risk than what was actually true, which suggests that there is a greater perception of risk when there is lower confidence in testing results.[74] Both Klitzman and Michie, Weinman, Miller, et al. illustrate that PGT results can be overestimated and underestimated.

Misconceptions also exist for genetic mechanisms. There are five popular areas including: homozygous and heterozygous, inheriting physical characteristics and diseases together, families passing on more genes to certain children, metaphysics of genetics, and implications for beliefs about scientific and non-scientific mechanisms. The first, homozygotic and heterozygotic, relates to the dominant and recessive inheritance patterns previously discussed. One woman illustrates the confusion that exists when she said "I don't know: Is there such a thing as genes being just

---

[71] Robert Klitzman, "Misunderstandings Concerning Genetics Among Patients Confronting Genetic Disease,"434.

[72] Robert Klitzman, "Misunderstandings Concerning Genetics Among Patients Confronting Genetic Disease," 430–433.

[73] Robert Klitzman, "Misunderstandings Concerning Genetics Among Patients Confronting Genetic Disease," 433.

[74] Susan Michie, John Weinman, Julie Miller, et al., "Predictive Genetic Testing: High Risk Expectations in the Face of Low Risk Information," 36, 46; Maxwell Mehlman, "Predictive Genetic Testing in Urology: Ethical and Social Issues," 433.

slightly there—you have this gene in a minute way, not a more dominant way? I don't know how that works."[75] If inheritance of disease is not adequately addressed, there can be confusion and anxiety. The second issue is common views about inheritance of genetic mutations and physical traits. This is demonstrated by the following quote: "I always thought that because I looked more like my mother, I was at risk of getting the disease."[76] People can think that because they look more like the person with a disease, they have similar risks for that disease. Following this logic, people who did not look or act like the affected person, thought the gene skipped them. Similarly, the third misconception is the idea that a person can have more "biological material" from a parent than another individual. It is assumed that since a child looks more like one parent that child has more of the parent's genes, and as a result will develop similar diseases. When growing up children hear things like:

> "You're just like me when I was a kid." So you assume: if I look more like him or her, then I'm probably going to get what he or she has. In high school, hereditary means: two parents come together and pass on what they have. Whatever they have, you have. So, if you look like your dad, then most likely, if he has green eyes, I have green eyes. My dad's got big teeth, I got big teeth.... Now, you hear my dad has that disease and it's hereditary, so "I got the disease." You explain it in your head by saying, "I probably have more of his cells than her cells."[77]

The fourth misunderstanding, metaphysics and the power of positive thinking, emphasizes the power of the mind. In this area, the mind can control the body. People might think that if the mind is powerful enough, the disease will not manifest. If a person hopes really hard, then maybe certain people might not get sick. A woman said the following about Huntington's disease (HD):

> I had this real strong feeling that my dad had come to clean it up, to finish off this nasty, ugly business, and that my sister and I were going to be fine. He took this thing on, and was gonna wrestle it down for us. I also thought that if anybody has it, it would probably be her. Three days after my dad's funeral, she was going to get her results. She sat in front of me in the car. I put my hands on her, and thought, "Take it away. Make me have it, so you don't have to." My dad was the best support I ever had. I just really thought that he wouldn't have given me such a thing.[78]

She thought her dad had a decision about whether or not to give HD to the family. The fifth misconception is fitting the scientific and nonscientific views together. When a person has a misconception, it can be difficult to understand something that seems contradictory. One woman tried to rationalize this by saying "I suppose I look more like my father's family on the inside, and my mother's side on the

---

[75] Robert Klitzman, "Misunderstandings Concerning Genetics Among Patients Confronting Genetic Disease," 435.

[76] Robert Klitzman, "Misunderstandings Concerning Genetics Among Patients Confronting Genetic Disease," 435.

[77] Robert Klitzman, "Misunderstandings Concerning Genetics Among Patients Confronting Genetic Disease," 436.

[78] Robert Klitzman, "Misunderstandings Concerning Genetics Among Patients Confronting Genetic Disease," 437.

outside."[79] When beliefs seem to conflict with tests, the individual can either realize their perception was wrong or come up with a new beliefs that fit both the test
results and their prior misconceptions. Sometimes misconceptions have a stronger
impact than people realize.

The next common area of misunderstandings is statistics. The study found four
main categories including: "percentages vs. proportions, absolute vs. relative risks,
each "toss of the coin" being independent, and the existence of two options meaning that the odd must be 50/50."[80] The first is about percentages and proportions.
Many people do not necessarily understand the implications of percentages, and
so it is important to make the numbers "real." There is a one in 4 chance that you
could develop this disease. The second area is absolute and relative risks. This issue can be complicated for both patients to comprehend and health care workers
to communicate. One person with degrees in Mathematics and Business gave the
following example. A health care worker "said that if I took Tamoxifen, I was going
to double my chances of uterine cancer."[81] After talking with the medical staff, the
patient realized that doubling his chances meant that his chances would be two in
10,000 instead of 1 in 10,000. The patient continued to say that "People sometimes
throw numbers out, and if you don't understand or question it, it could be pretty
scary."[82] Absolute risks are the typical general population risks associated with getting a disease like the one in 10,000 above. Relative risk is a ratio of the person's
risk, which takes into account other factors like taking tamoxifen above. Also, risk
is not static; risks can fluctuate according to new research or models. Sometimes
doctors assume patients understand, but often they do not.[83] The third area in statistics is the idea of statistics in relation to a coin toss. Since there is a 50% chance
of getting the gene, some people think that if there are two siblings, one will get the
disease, and one will not. However, this is not true, because each flip of the coin is
independent of each other. Therefore each sibling has a 50% chance of developing
the disease. One man said that he was scared when his brother did not have the gene,
because he thought "for sure we couldn't both get away unscathed. I know they're
independent events, so the fact that he tested negative does not influence my testing
at all. But emotionally, it didn't feel that way at all."[84] People need to be reminded
that there is the same level of risk with each flip of the coin. The fourth area is the
idea that the presence of two options has to indicate that there is a 50/50% chance.
Since a person can have or not have the gene, people think there is a 50% chance of

---

[79] Robert Klitzman, "Misunderstandings Concerning Genetics Among Patients Confronting Genetic Disease," 437.

[80] Robert Klitzman, "Misunderstandings Concerning Genetics Among Patients Confronting Genetic Disease," 437.

[81] Robert Klitzman, "Misunderstandings Concerning Genetics Among Patients Confronting Genetic Disease," 438.

[82] Robert Klitzman, "Misunderstandings Concerning Genetics Among Patients Confronting Genetic Disease," 438.

[83] Neil Sharpe and Ronald Carter, *Genetic Testing: Care, Consent, and Liability,* 361–362.

[84] Robert Klitzman, "Misunderstandings Concerning Genetics Among Patients Confronting Genetic Disease," 438.

getting a disease. While there is a 50% chance of Huntington's if it runs in the family, the general risk for breast cancer is 12%. The risk for the BRCA 1/2 mutations is 0.24% in Caucasians and 1.2% in the Ashkenazi population. The rate of BRCA 1/2 in those already diagnosed with breast cancer is about 8.3% in the Ashkenazi Jewish, 2.2% in the non-Hispanic Caucasian, and 1.3% in the African-American population. Having the BRCA mutation is significantly lower than a 50% chance.[85]

Also Klitzman suggests that education, emotions, concepts of responsibility, penalties, and social aspects will play a role. First, the level of education can have a positive or negative effect. Some common misconceptions can be eliminated if a person has had some education in science and/or statistics. Second, sometimes even after presenting a patient with a negative or lower than average risk, he or she might still perceive that risk to be more intimidating due to emotional issues.[86] The third factor is beliefs about punishment. Sometimes people think the inheritance of a disease was a result of something he or she did, fate, or karma. The fourth factor is the role of social contexts. People can feel embarrassed, because their views are thought to be unreasonable. One person felt embarrassed by being a part of a group that believed "some people came into the world to extinguish a genetic disease from the family."[87] Social beliefs can play a large part in forming people's perception. All of the previous misunderstandings can have some serious implications. First, misunderstandings can impact the decision to get tested and treated. One person said: "I thought: if I didn't have a mammogram, I wouldn't have breast cancer... So I've never had a mammogram."[88] If people are confused about testing, then their choices could result in inappropriate treatment decisions. Second, misunderstandings can have a big impact on a person's ability to cope. If a person has gone their whole life thinking he or she will not get a disease because of some misconception, the ability to cope with seemingly contradictory test results can be difficult. One woman assumed her sister had the Huntington's gene, but her sister ended up not having the gene. As a result this woman had many concerns now especially since she had a child already. A person's ability to cope with bad news can depend on their perceptions. Third, misunderstandings can also have an impact on reproductive decisions. The woman in the previous example falsely assumed she would not get HD so she did not even consider her reproductive options. Misconceptions can have an impact on a family for reproductive options as well.[89]

[85] Robert Klitzman, "Misunderstandings Concerning Genetics Among Patients Confronting Genetic Disease," 437–439.

[86] Susan Michie, John Weinman, Julie Miller, et al., "Predictive Genetic Testing: High Risk Expectations in the Face of Low Risk Information," 36.

[87] Robert Klitzman, "Misunderstandings Concerning Genetics Among Patients Confronting Genetic Disease," 440.

[88] Robert Klitzman, "Misunderstandings Concerning Genetics Among Patients Confronting Genetic Disease," 440.

[89] Klitzman, Robert, "Misunderstandings Concerning Genetics Among Patients Confronting Genetic Disease," 439–441.

3. Education

A study in "Public Perceptions of Ethical Issues Regarding Adult Predictive Genetic Testing" in *Health Care Analysis* by Douglas Martin and Heather Greenwood concluded that there needs to be more public education about PGT. Douglas Martin and Heather Greenwood say that there was anxiety due to the minimal public education about the BRCA genetic mutation. One person in this study said "it's an important issue that people need to know about, especially because it affects people of my heritage but beyond that. It's information that women can get to prevent them from passing away from disease."[90] Some people said there should be some government-sponsored education programs for PGT. Other people said it is "important that public education not overemphasize the genetic component of disease to the detriment of the investigation into other contributing factors to illness, such as "socio-economic or environmental conditions", as well as causing the public to neglect the possibility of non-genetic preventative measures, or to be overly worried about a disease for which they are not at high risk."[91] Also included in the discussion on public education was the physician's education and knowledge of PGT. Douglas Martin and Heather Greenwood said that some people feared that inadequate information of PGT especially BRCA testing would cause physicians to have fear of talking with their patients about the subject. As a result, this fear would lead physicians to have limited discussions concerning patient education. Maxwell Mehlman in "Predictive Genetic Testing in Urology: Ethical and Social Issues," said that physicians might lack appropriate education in order to interpret these test results.[92]

In order for physicians to encourage patient understanding, physicians should have adequate knowledge about the disease, understanding of the patient's test results, and a practical understanding of absolute and relative risks.[93] In a patient discussion about the risk of BRCA mutations, one physician tried to describe it in terms the patient might understand more easily. The doctor said the following:

> In explaining testing to patients, I find it useful to describe a gene as a building and to point out that just as a building has many rooms, so a gene has many chemicals. If even one of the thousands of chemicals in a gene is missing or changed, the product the gene makes will be a little "off," leading to increased cell growth and increased cancer risk. In the course of genetic testing, the laboratory will be "walking" through the BRCA1 and the BRCA2 buildings, looking for a damaged room (a mutation). If they find such damage in a gene, it will mean the individual has an increased risk of both breast and ovarian cancer.[94]

---

[90] Douglas Martin and Heather Greenwood, "Public Perceptions of Ethical Issues Regarding Adult Predictive Genetic Testing," 106.

[91] Douglas Martin and Heather Greenwood, "Public Perceptions of Ethical Issues Regarding Adult Predictive Genetic Testing," 106.

[92] Maxwell Mehlman, "Predictive Genetic Testing in Urology: Ethical and Social Issues," 433.

[93] Neil Sharpe and Ronald Carter, *Genetic Testing: Care, Consent, and Liability*, 381.

[94] Patricia Kelly, "Cancer Risks in Perspective: Information and Approaches for Clinicians," 387.

This physician encouraged a practical discussion about risks in terms of construction. Many times physicians have a significant impact on how patients will interpret risk and probabilities of PGT. The Self Regulatory Theory says that people recognize risk "influenced by factors such as identity, consequences, cause, control, and timeline."[95] Sometimes personal experiences can hurt physicians or patients in understanding risk probabilities, but other times using a patient's values and experiences can encourage greater understanding.

C. Treatment Options for Diagnosed Genetic Traits

PGT often has complicated treatment options for diagnosed genetic traits, because sometimes there are no treatments available for certain diseases. As a result, the disclosure of possible options is crucial in order to make appropriate decisions for PGT. The beginning of this section will look at disclosure and analyze standards and consent guidelines of disclosure. The second area, treatment options, will focus on possible treatment options for some diseases. Then the third area will conclude with specific recommended treatment plans and options for hereditary breast and ovarian cancer (HBOC).

1. Disclosure

Generally information that is material to a person's decision should be discussed, especially potential treatment options.[96] Part of this section will look at the standards of establishing adequate disclosure of treatment options for diagnosed genetic traits.[97] There are three general standards: a reasonable physician standard, reasonable patient standard, and a subjective standard. By adhering to the reasonable physician standard which is typically the most popular, physicians should disclosure all information that a reasonable physician would disclose in that situation to his or her patients. The only problem with this standard is that some patients might want more information. The reasonable patient standard requires disclosure of information that patients typically would want to know about a disease or treatment. The last standard is the subjective or specific patient standard.[98] This standard really depends on what information an individual patient would want.[99] This standard is typically not

---

[95] Robert Klitzman, "Misunderstandings Concerning Genetics Among Patients Confronting Genetic Disease," 431.

[96] Janet Dolgin and Lois Shepherd, *Bioethics and the Law*, 56.

[97] Neil F. Sharpe and Ronald Carter, *Genetic Testing: Care, Consent, and Liability*, 131.

[98] Lewis Vaughn, *Bioethics: Principles, Issues, and Cases*, 146; Janet Dolgin and Lois Shepherd, *Bioethics and the Law*, 55, 59; Bernard Lo, *Resolving Ethical Dilemmas*, 22.

[99] Bernard Lo, *Resolving Ethical Dilemmas*, 22.

used very often. The next chapter will discuss in depth some additional details of the standards of disclosure.

Doctors often ask how much information is needed for patients to be informed, and Howard Brody responds with two things in the book *Taking Sides: Clashing Views on Bioethical Issues*. First the doctor has to disclose the "basis on which the proposed treatment or the alternative possible treatments have been chosen," and second the patient should be able to ask questions about the physician's proposed treatment and reasoning to the patient's approval and satisfaction.[100] Also it has been argued that some procedures require stronger, specific consent than others, because the treatment or procedure is more risky and serious. The difference in consent of a low risk versus high risk procedure is important to discuss in relation to the distinguishing characteristics of PGT. Overall there is not a specific formula for knowing how much information a patient needs to be informed, but this section addresses disclosure of treatment options for PGT.[101]

2. Treatment Options

One potential benefit to PGT is the availability of treatment options for many diseases. If the test comes back with a positive result, then ideally the person can take preventive or prophylactic measures and/or prepare for the future. Sometimes there are treatments that could prevent the disease or lessen the severity of the disease.[102] Another general treatment option is continued surveillance.[103] Douglas Martin and Heather Greenwood in "Public Perceptions of Ethical Issues Regarding Adult Predictive Genetic Testing" also emphasize the importance of identifying treatment options. One of the audience members said it is "absolutely essential that they [women at high risk] know so that they can make sorts of choices in their lives that will permit them to live their lives in a more, I guess, more knowledgeable, and certainly a more planned fashion."[104] Many times the appropriate treatment option does not stick out at the beginning, and additional discussions need to take place before all the treatment options are realized and fully appreciated.[105] Also it is important to "ascertain how the client anticipates test results will affect his/her medical manage-

---

[100] Neil C. Manson and Onora O'Neill, *Rethinking Informed Consent in Bioethics*, 82.

[101] Robert M. Arnold and Charles W. Lidz, "Informed Consent: Clinical Aspects of Consent in Health Care," 11.

[102] Anita Silvers and Michael Ashley Stein, "An Equality Paradigm for Preventing Genetic Discrimination," 1348.

[103] Marion Harris, Ingrid Winship, and Merle Spriggs, "Controversies and Ethical Issues in Cancer-Genetics Clinics," 301.

[104] Douglas Martin and Heather Greenwood, "Public Perceptions of Ethical Issues Regarding Adult Predictive Genetic Testing," 106.

[105] Marion Harris, Ingrid Winship, and Merle Spriggs, "Controversies and Ethical Issues in Cancer-Genetics Clinics," 301.

ment and health behaviors."[106] Treatment options might be available, but sometimes patients might not want to participate in those treatments or prevention method.

3. Hereditary Breast and Ovarian Cancer

The following section is an example of potential treatment options for hereditary breast and ovarian cancer (HBOC). Sometimes treatment options are difficult to discuss for PGT, because often there are few curable diseases. This is often the case for HBOC, which has no specific treatment guidelines for those at risk. Research is still being done to determine general guidelines for medical staff. General treatment guidelines include more screening, chemotherapy and chemoprevention, surgery to prevent and/or slow the progression of cancer, and possibly changing diet or other aspects of life.

When combining an MRI, ultrasound, mammography, and clinical breast exams, about 95% of breast cancers were found. The National Society of Genetic Counselors (NSGC) recommends surveillance for women at high or moderate risk for breast cancer starting with a semiannual clinical breast examination at 25, self-exams monthly at 18, and yearly mammograms starting at 25. Women at low risk should do monthly self exams at 18, annual clinical breast exams between 25 to 35, and annual mammograms at 40. Chemotherapy includes therapy like tamoxifen, which has been shown to decrease risk by 50% for at-risk women. One study by M. C. King, S. Wieand, K. Hale, et al. concluded that the disease risk went down 62% for BRCA2 carriers when treated with tamoxifen, but there was not much affect on BRCA1 carriers. However, many other studies demonstrate a 50% decrease for both mutations. Tamoxifen is recommended up to 5 years for those at high risk and optional for women at moderate risk. After a prophylactic mastectomy, the risk typically decreases 90%. However there is still a small risk, since many people opt for a subcutaneous mastectomy, leaving more of the tissue intact, and not a total or simple mastectomy. Ovarian cancer on the other hand has fewer treatment options than breast cancer. Additional surveillance is harder and often does not result in early diagnosis. The screening also has many false positives, and sometimes those can lead to potentially harmful procedures like surgery. Surveillance for those at high risk of ovarian cancer should start with an annual or semiannual transvaginal ultrasound, pelvic exam, and testing at 25 or 10 years younger than when the first person was diagnosed in the family. Those with a family history of ovarian cancer (a moderate risk) should have annual or semiannual ultrasounds, pelvic exams, and testing between 30 and 35 or 10 years younger than the earliest diagnosis. Without BCRA and ovarian cancer in the family, surveillance and screening is not necessary. One chemoprevention for ovarian cancer might be oral contraceptives. At-risk women taking oral contraceptives for six plus years decreased their ovarian cancer

---

[106] Angela Trepanier, Mary Ahrens, Wendy McKinnon, et al., "Genetic Cancer Risk Assessment and Counseling: Recommendations of the National Society of Genetic Counselors," 107.

risk by about 60%. This treatment has been shown to have an impact on high risk women up to 15 years following the discontinuation of treatment. The NSGC says that women with a family history of ovarian cancer could use oral contraceptives for 5 years, but this form of prevention is still under debate. Prophylactic bilateral salpingo-oophorectomy (BSO) can reduce ovarian cancer by about 80–96% for those at high risk with the BRCA mutations. The BSO can be done either with or without a hysterectomy, but after a BSO women cannot have children. The NSGC says "the earlier a pre-menopausal woman has BSO, the more risk reduction there is for development of a future breast cancer."[107] While it can reduce HBOC, there is about a 4% risk of developing peritoneal cancer from the remaining tissue in the abdominal cavity. A paradox of this procedure is that often hormone replacement therapy (HRT) is needed after surgery, because women undergo an instant surgical menopause. While a BSO decreases the risk of breast cancer by 50%, the HRT is often said to increase the incidence of breast cancer. Recently, studies concluded that short-term HRT after a BSO does not impact the risk of breast cancer as much as once thought. A BSO could help substantially with those at high risk for ovarian cancer. A BSO is not always encouraged for a medium risk, and it is not recommended for low risk. Males with BRCA mutations should also undergo continued surveillance including clinical breast exams and an as needed mammography. Men at high risk are encouraged to have annual clinical breast exams and monthly self-exams. Prostate cancer screening includes digital rectal exams and prostate specific antigen (PSA) tests. No chemoprevention or prophylactic surgery options for men at high risk for HBOC exist. Sometimes research studies for people with variants of unknown significance (VUS) and a family history of cancer try to identify other susceptibility genes that might be involved with HBOC.[108]

One study found that women who thought their "susceptibility to breast cancer as very likely to extremely likely engaged in fewer detective health behaviors than did those with lower risk perceptions."[109] Overall, there is not a consensus on perceived risks and health promotion behaviors, and this can be problematic at times. While there are surgeries and treatments for HBOC, these treatments are not guaranteed to eliminate and/or prevent the cancer nor is it guaranteed to significantly improve a person's quality of life. With surgery, there are a lot of issues to discuss with the physician. Discussions about these potential treatment options are necessary for all involved.

---

[107] Janice Berliner and Angela Fay, "Risk Assessment and Genetic Counseling for Hereditary Breast and Ovarian Cancer: Recommendations of the National Society of Genetic Counselors," 255.

[108] Janice Berliner and Angela Fay, "Risk Assessment and Genetic Counseling for Hereditary Breast and Ovarian Cancer: Recommendations of the National Society of Genetic Counselors," 252–256.

[109] Shoshana Shiloh and Shiri Ilan, "To Test or Not To Test? Moderators of the Relationship Between Risk Perceptions and Interest in Predictive Genetic Testing," 467.

D. Family-Related Genetic Information

Genetic testing information can be different than other types of medical information, because testing results also have an impact on the entire family. Results have the potential to "yield information about another person."[110] Sometimes testing involves testing of family members in order to identify the genetic mutation in the family. This type of testing procedure can cause contention to emerge in the field. Often in the case of genetic testing, people cite the problem of the right to know versus the right not to know one's genetic makeup. Should family members have a right to know or a right not to know? This is the question that often arises in the debate. Another question that arises is how does genetic testing typically deal with one person wanting to know while another family member does not want to know. Anita Silvers and Michael Ashley Stein in the *Vanderbilt Law Review* say "The individual-consent mechanism ill fits a technology that is based on the relational nature of genetic information."[111] This issue will be addressed further in future chapters.

Many times genetic mutations can be hereditary.[112] If a specific mutation and variant is found, then sometimes that test can also be used to diagnose a symptomatic relative.[113] The symptomatic individual can be tested to see if he or she has the same genetic mutation. If so then other members of the family might want to have PGT in order to see if he or she is at an increased risk for developing that disease. This section will look at the concern of family-related genetic information. Because genetic information can relate to the entire family, often there are problems that can arise as a consequence.[114] Possessing genetic information can result in discrimination, privacy concerns, a burden of knowledge, and coercion.[115] Confidentiality and discrimination can be a concern with genetics, but since the passing of the Genetic Information Non-discriminatory Act (GINA) in 2003, genetic discrimination has not been as prevalent. However discrimination can still be an unintended consequence for the patient and the patient's family and can play a role in informed

---

[110] Regina E. Ensenauer, Virginia V. Michels, and Shanda S. Reinke, "Genetic Testing: Practical, Ethical, and Counseling Considerations," 64.

[111] Anita Silvers and Michael Ashley Stein, "An Equality Paradigm for Preventing Genetic Discrimination," 1357.

[112] Abigail L. Rose, Nikki Peters, Judy A. Shea, et al., "Attitudes and Misconceptions about Predictive Genetic Testing for Cancer Risk," 146.

[113] Anita Silvers and Michael Ashley Stein. "An Equality Paradigm for Preventing Genetic Discrimination," 1347.

[114] Regina E. Ensenauer, Virginia V. Michels, and Shanda S. Reinke, "Genetic Testing: Practical, Ethical, and Counseling Considerations," 69.

[115] Regina Ensenauer M.D., Virginia Michels M.D., and Shanda Reinke M.S., "Genetic Testing: Practical, Ethical, and Counseling Considerations," 63; Bert Heinrichs, "What Should We Want to Know About Our Future? A Kantian View on Predictive Genetic Testing. Medicine," 29; Michael Burgess PhD, Claude Lanberg, MD, PhD, and Bartha Maria Knoppers, LLD, "Bioethics for Clinicians: 14. Ethics and Genetics in Medicine," 1309; Brita Arver, Aina Haegermark, Ulla Platten, et al., "Evaluation of Psychosocial Effects of Pre-Symptomatic Testing for Breast/Ovarian and Colon Cancer Pre-Disposing Genes: a 12-Month Follow-Up," 109.

consent and PGT. The Vanderbilt Law Review says "fear of discrimination thus has the potential to block benefits that otherwise might be gained from genomic knowledge."[116] Even though this article by Anita Silvers and Michael Ashley Stein is talking about disability and employment discrimination, this statement is also true of other types of discrimination including familial discrimination or stigmatization. Part of the problem with genetic information is that "Once discovered, it has the potential to affect many biological family members through time, rendering them vulnerable to the same genetic prediction."[117]

This section will look at communication, disclosure and non-disclosure of information to relatives, genetic exceptionalism, and coercion. The first area will specifically look at some communication patterns within families in order to analyze the impact of genetic information on families. The second area looks at the issue of disclosing test results to families versus not disclosing information. The third area focuses on the debate of whether genetic information is exceptional information or just normal medical information. The fourth and last area is a discussion on coercion of families and patients from possible influences of genetic information.

1. Communication Patterns

There have been some studies looking into communication patterns of families. One study by S. H. Chaffee and J. M. McLeod in the 1970s divided family communication into two approaches. Communication was grouped by socio-oriented or concept-oriented styles. The socio-oriented people wanted to keep peace and unity in the family, and so information that could cause division or problems within the family would not be discussed typically. The concept-oriented families were more concerned with open communication. This type of pattern lends itself to more communication within families especially in the context of genetic testing. In 1991, L. D. Ritchie made some changes to these communication patterns. The revised patterns were conformity or conversation oriented. The conformity oriented pattern typically emphasized the children's responsibility to conform to the parents' expectations and viewpoints. There are appropriate topics and then there are inappropriate topics for family discussions, and the goal of this view is to stay away from conflict with the parents. The conformity view does not encourage showing emotions. The conversation oriented view is equivalent to the concept-oriented view, and the goal of this view is open communication among family members. There are also some additional communication patterns. Studies by M. R. Bury have looked at communication styles for chronic diseases and have identified two patterns of communication: accommodation and active denial. Accommodation typically involves open communication about the disease; while active denial generally limits the discussion that occurs in regards to the disease and the implications. A study done by R.

---

[116] Anita Silvers and Michael Ashley Stein, "An Equality Paradigm for Preventing Genetic Discrimination," 1351.

[117] Susan Wolf and Jeffrey Kahn, "Genetic Testing and the Future of Disability Insurance: Ethics, Law & Policy," 9.

Kenen, A. Ardern-Jones, and R. Eeles in 2004 looked at disclosure patterns for genetic testing results, specifically hereditary breast and ovarian cancer (HBOC). This study found five approaches to communication. The first, open/supportive, allowed patients and those tested to disclose and talk about any aspect of the disease and testing process with family. Second, directly blocked openly establishes limitations for the suitable and unsuitable aspects of discussion among the family and those tested. The third style, blocked indirectly, also establishes boundaries for discussion, but most often uses non-verbal communication to set the boundaries. Fourth, self-censored discloses information on a case-by-case basis depending on the individual's comfort level. This study divides the self-censored style into two categories: reactive and proactive self-censored. The reactive self-censored style discusses information while gauging an individual's reactions, and then limiting disclosure if a person is uncomfortable with the topic of discussion. A person using the proactive self-censored approach would not discuss certain information to family members if the person tested thought it might cause additional concern and division among the family. The fifth, third party, uses another person to disclose information to a family member on his or her behalf.[118]

Communication about genetic testing results among family members is often not a simple straightforward procedure. One study by Clara Gaff, Veronica Collins, Tiffany Symes, and Jane Halliday concluded that there are different trends between men and women, carriers and non-carriers, and the type of information being disclosed. Many times people disclose information to their families because they believe their family has a right to know the genetic information.[119] A study by B. J. Wilson, K. Forrest, E. R. van Teijlingen, et al. said that communication of genetic testing results was influenced by complex family dynamics. This study demonstrated that the process could be influenced by "the nature of the disease, whether or not preventive measures were available, the overall pattern of family communication, and the individual coping styles of family members."[120] The study also said that feelings of "guilt, denial, rationalization, and/or the desire to protect others" could have a significant impact on communication and disclosure to family members.[121] While a typical diagnostic blood test generally has medical information for that specific patient, a positive or negative predictive genet test can impact the entire family.[122] Hereditary cancers can only be identified when more than one person in the family is tested.[123]

---

[118] Kathryn Holt, "What Do We Tell the Children? Contrasting the Disclosure Choices of Two HD Families Regarding Risk Status and Predictive Genetic Testing," 254–255.

[119] Clara L. Gaff, Veronica Collins, Tiffany Symes, et al., "Facilitating Family Communication about Predictive Genetic Testing: Probands' Perceptions," 134.

[120] Kathryn Holt, "What Do We Tell the Children? Contrasting the Disclosure Choices of Two HD Families Regarding Risk Status and Predictive Genetic Testing," 255.

[121] Kathryn Holt, "What Do We Tell the Children? Contrasting the Disclosure Choices of Two HD Families Regarding Risk Status and Predictive Genetic Testing," 255.

[122] Marion Harris, Ingrid Winship, and Merle Spriggs, "Controversies and Ethical Issues in Cancer-Genetics Clinics," 301; Maxwell Mehlman, "Predictive Genetic Testing in Urology: Ethical and Social Issues," 435; James Evans, Cecile Skrzynia, and Wylie Burke, "The Complexities of Predictive Genetic Testing," 1053.

[123] Maxwell Mehlman, "Predictive Genetic Testing in Urology: Ethical and Social Issues," 435.

2. Disclosure & Non-Disclosure of Test Results to Relatives

Generally people are encouraged to tell family members if the test came back with an increased risk and there are relatives that could be at-risk. The family might appreciate the information or might not want to know anything about that information. Either relatives will find out or the family will be ignorant of a person's test results. However, both of those situations can have consequences for the family. James Evans, Cecile Skrzynia, and Wylie Burke in "The Complexities of Predictive Genetic Testing," from the *British Medical Journal* say "the utility of a predictive genetic test will therefore depend on whose point of view is considered."[124] The article by Clara Gaff, Veronica Collins, Tiffany Symes, et al., said that disclosure can be difficult sometimes, and the authors suggested having additional support from the genetics staff. Clara Gaff, Veronica Collins, Tiffany Symes, et al., also concludes that most of the people with the HNPCC mutation generally had good reactions after disclosing genetic information with at-risk relatives. This study concluded that men typically had more difficulties in disclosing genetic information to family than women.[125] Disclosure of test results is encouraged so that family members might be able to participate in genetic testing as well to see if they are at an increased risk or not. The at-risk family members could also participate in surveillance and/or preventative measures if available. Also sometimes at-risk family members might want to take this information into account for family planning and reproductive purposes.[126]

On the other side, some family members might not want to know in order to avoid worry, mental and emotional damage, and/or discrimination.[127] One study on genetic information said that many times there are more "psychological and social risks rather than physical risks."[128] Often people are hesitant to tell this information, because of the implications. Sometimes disclosing this information to relatives can put a strain on the family relationships. Generally pressure can come from both sides. The person tested can encourage or pressure the family to get tested or the family with a known risk could encourage additional members of the family to get tested. Either way this type of information brings an additional layer of anxiety and concern for all those involved.[129]

---

[124] James Evans, Cecile Skrzynia, and Wylie Burke, "The Complexities of Predictive Genetic Testing," 1053.

[125] Clara L. Gaff, Veronica Collins, Tiffany Symes, et al., "Facilitating Family Communication about Predictive Genetic Testing: Probans' Perceptions," 134, 137.

[126] Marion Harris, Ingrid Winship, and Merle Spriggs, "Controversies and Ethical Issues in Cancer-Genetics Clinics," 301–302; James Evans, Cecile Skrzynia, and Wylie Burke, "The Complexities of Predictive Genetic Testing," 1053.

[127] Marion Harris, Ingrid Winship, and Merle Spriggs, "Controversies and Ethical Issues in Cancer-Genetics Clinics," 301; Regina E. Ensenauer, Virginia V. Michels, and Shanda S. Reinke, "Genetic Testing: Practical, Ethical, and Counseling Considerations," 69.

[128] Janet Dolgin and Lois Shepherd, *Bioethics and the Law*, 69.

[129] Linda Farber Post, Jeffrey Blustein, and Nancy Neveloff Dubler, *Handbook for Health Care Ethics Committees*, 42–43; Marion Harris, Ingrid Winship, and Merle Spriggs, "Controversies and

Non-disclosure is not recommended, because then the family is not aware of their potential increased risks for disease. In a study about non-disclosure, 206 geneticists out of 800 responded to a survey. In this study, 60% said that they had encountered people who would not disclose test results to his or her family. Some of the diseases that were not disclosed to families include Huntington's disease, familial translocations, and familial cancer syndromes. In this study, the reasons included concern about discrimination, fear about future relationships after disclosure, and already fractured family relationships. In this study, some of the geneticists thought about disclosing information to the families, but most did not disclose anything. There were four geneticists though that did present increased risk results to families in seven cases. The American Society of Human Genetics gave a statement on disclosing family-related genetic information in 1998. The patient's confidentiality needs to be respected. The ASHG document says that "In the context of medical information, privacy rights translate into protection of personal data, affirmation of confidentiality, and freedom of choice."[130] For most cases, disclosure cannot come from the physician. However, the statement went on to say that only in exceptional cases can a patient's confidentiality be overridden. These conditions are the same for breaching confidentiality in many other instances as well. Harris, Winship, and Spriggs explain that the stipulations include "that attempts to encourage disclosure have failed, that harm is serious and foreseeable, that at-risk individuals can be identified, and that the disease is preventable or treatable, or early monitoring is medically accepted to reduce risk or avert harm."[131] The goal of disclosure is to inform relatives so that he or she can make informed decisions concerning their health. The risks of disclosing this information without permission should be less than the risks that could result from telling the family.[132]

These recommendations are generally accepted by many groups including the President's Commission for the Study of Ethical Problems in Medicine and Biomedical and Behavioral Research, the Nuffield Council on Bioethics, and the World Health Organization (WHO). The American Medical Association (AMA) goes further than recommending disclosure when the group says that patients should be informed before testing occurs that disclosing test results to relatives is typically expected. As a result, physicians should help with this process of disclosing information to at-risk relatives. Disclosure to third parties without permission is protected under the Health Insurance Portability and Accountability Act (HIPAA) of 1996. Before confidentiality and privacy can be breached, HIPAA requires that the incident is a "serious and imminent threat to the health or safety of a person or the

---

Ethical Issues in Cancer-Genetics Clinics," 302–303.

[130] The American Society of Human Genetics Social Issues Subcommittee on Familial Disclosure, "ASHG Statement: Professional Disclosure of Familial Genetic Information," 474.

[131] Marion Harris, Ingrid Winship, and Merle Spriggs, "Controversies and Ethical Issues in Cancer-Genetics Clinics," 303.

[132] Regina E. Ensenauer, Virginia V. Michels, and Shanda S. Reinke, "Genetic Testing: Practical, Ethical, and Counseling Considerations," 70.

public and the physician has the capacity to avert substantial harm."[133] Even though there is a potential harm to the at-risk relatives, it is not established right now that a possible genetic disease qualifies under this criteria.

3. Genetic Exceptionalism

Because of the complexity of genetic information, there are family concerns that are raised by the right to know or not to know. The foundation of this argument can stem from the debate on genetic exceptionalism versus normal medical information. Genetic exceptionalism is the idea that genetic information is "special," distinctive, and different than other types of medical information. Those who argue in favor of genetic exceptionalism due so from the facts that it has to do with the entire family, it has predictive value, there is the potential for discrimination and psychological harm, and currently the full potential of extracting information from samples is unknown.[134] While the predictive nature of PGT is not necessarily enough to differentiate it from nongenetic testing, some predictive genetic tests have the ability to predict with a high degree of certainty such as tests for Huntington's disease. While nongenetic tests can predict risks, nongenetic tests cannot predict with a high degree of certainty, and so PGT has in some situations has a greater level of predicting diseases than nongenetic tests. Another important aspect of PGT is perception. Genetic information is often seen as more personal and important than other medical information. Michael J. Green and Jeffrey R. Botkin in "Genetic Exceptionalism in Medicine: Clarifying the Differences between Genetic and Nongenetic Tests," say "Right or wrong, genetic information is believed to reveal who we "really" are, so information from genetic testing is often seen as more consequential than that from other sources."[135] This idea of revealing who you "really" are can lead to an extreme form of genetic exceptionalism, which is genetic determinism. This often arises when a person or society focuses solely on the role of genetics to the exclusion of other factors. The basis of genetic determinism lies in the idea that a person's genes determine who he is, and some believe that each new genetic development brings us closer to this idea of unlocking the key to life. In response Leon Kass says, "Precisely because we have been taught by these very scientists that genes hold the secret of life, and that our genotype is our essence if not quite our destiny, we are made nervous by those whose expert knowledge and technique touch our very being."[136]

---

[133] Marion Harris, Ingrid Winship, and Merle Spriggs, "Controversies and Ethical Issues in Cancer-Genetics Clinics," 303–304.

[134] Elizabeth Chapman, "Ethical Dilemmas in Testing for Late Onset Conditions: Reactions to Testing and Perceived Impact on Other Family Members," 351; Neil C. Manson and Onora O'Neill, *Rethinking Informed Consent in Bioethics*, 134; Michael J. Green and Jeffrey R. Botkin, "Genetic Exceptionalism" in Medicine: Clarifying the Differences between Genetic and Nongenetic Tests," 572.

[135] Michael J. Green and Jeffrey R. Botkin, "'Genetic Exceptionalism" in Medicine: Clarifying the Differences between Genetic and Nongenetic Tests," 571–573.

[136] Leon Kass, *Life, Liberty and the Defense of Dignity*, 57, 126.

Another concern of PGT is the fact that the information can influence a person's entire family. Michael J. Green and Jeffrey R. Botkin in "Genetic Exceptionalism in Medicine: Clarifying the Differences between Genetic and Nongenetic Tests," say genetic tests "identify predispositions that are exclusively transmitted vertically (from parent to child), while nongenetic tests identify predispositions transmitted in a variety of ways (exposure to common environmental risk factors or person-to-person contact)."[137] The difference between PGT and nongenetic predictive testing is transmission and diagnosis. If a mother has a positive test result for HD, then her children automatically have a 50% chance of developing HD as well. When she decides to get tested, those results have a significant impact for her children, and could even result in a diagnosis for one of them. Also, in the case of identical twins, a diagnosis of HD could be made for the twin that was not even tested. The authors explain that with genetic information, people can be diagnosed with a condition even without specifically participating in the test. While nongenetic testing has implications for the family, PGT can have a considerably higher level of risk to families. There are also people against the idea of genetic exceptionalism. Green and Botkin say that there are three common aspects of genetic and nongenetic predictive tests. First, the tests both try to predict future illnesses whether it is testing for BRCA or testing cholesterol for a potential stroke. Second, the general procedures for both are comparable; there is a family history discussion and an exam. Sometimes for PGT, there is additional blood work. Third, whether the records are kept electronically or in print, both involve the same procedures. Green and Botkin suggest that genetic and nongenetic information have the same risks and benefits when it comes to medical records. Authors like Neil Manson and Onora O'Neill say that most things said about genetic information can also be said of other non-genetic information and both can be acquired through observation without the person's knowledge. Also, genetic information requires a lot of interpretation, and specific information about an individual that might not be evident at the beginning.[138] Green and Botkin suggest that even though PGT has the ability to predict disease, nongenetic tests can also predict future illnesses, giving examples of testing for HIV, TB, and cholesterol. After getting results of HIV, this nongenetic test can have a significant impact on a person's medical future and his or her family. Many tests have the ability to predict future medical problems, and as a result, the predictive nature of the test is not distinctive enough to separate it from nongenetic information. Questions about disclosure and confidentiality of family members would arise from both PGT and nongenetic predictive testing. In regards to discrimination, there are many types of nongenetic medical information that can cause social and legal discrimination; however, discrimination in both instances should be discouraged. Psychological risks are not exclusive to PGT, and often times there can be significant psychological harms when having a positive HIV test. Instead of differentiating tests by genetic or nongenetic, Green and Botkin suggest analyzing tests by looking at four areas.

---

[137] Michael J. Green and Jeffrey R. Botkin, "'Genetic Exceptionalism' in Medicine: Clarifying the Differences between Genetic and Nongenetic Tests," 572.

[138] Neil C. Manson and Onora O'Neill, *Rethinking Informed Consent in Bioethics*, 136.

Those areas include: "(1) the degree to which information learned from the test can be stigmatizing, (2) the effect of the test results on others, (3) the availability of effective interventions to alter the natural course predicted by the information, and (4) the complexity involved in interpreting test results."[139] The authors argue that genetics has a limited effect on gaining additional analysis or protections for a test, because genetics is only one of the aspects involved. The authors suggest that the clinical consequences are more important than the genetic foundations of the test.[140]

The idea behind genetic determinism can be damaging since it elevates genetics and generally excludes other factors. One extreme example of genetic determinism focuses on the eugenics movement of sterilization laws and Nazi concentration camps, which was started by people who focused solely on scientific knowledge and genetic attributes.[141] Having a singular focus on a person's genes can cause some problems for both the patient and the patient's family. In their article, Michael Green and Jeffrey Botkin conclude by saying, "practitioners and patients must consider the consequences of any predictive testing before an asymptomatic person learns what he or she might not want to know."[142] While this work does not argue for genetic exceptionalism, it should be noted that genetic information does possess a unique value to individuals and their family. This area demonstrates the importance genetic information has on consent for the patient and the patient's family. As a result, appropriate measures are needed to ensure the responsibility of genetic information especially in areas that can have potential side effects on others.[143]

4. Coercion

Douglas Martin and Heather Greenwood in "Public Perceptions of Ethical Issues Regarding Adult Predictive Genetic Testing," also look at external pressures of PGT. The public who were involved in the study were concerned that "external pressures may affect the capacity for free choice, such as pressure from family members, either to be tested or not to be tested, because of the impact of the resulting knowledge."[144] The public was also concerned about the possible implications of this testing such as reproductive decisions. One person said "there may be an ethical obligation on the part of women primarily, men too I guess, who test posi-

---

[139] Michael J. Green and Jeffrey R. Botkin, "'Genetic Exceptionalism' in Medicine: Clarifying the Differences between Genetic and Nongenetic Tests," 573.

[140] Michael J. Green and Jeffrey R. Botkin, "'Genetic Exceptionalism' in Medicine: Clarifying the Differences between Genetic and Nongenetic Tests," 571–573.

[141] Barry S Coller, "The Physician-Scientist, the State, and the Oath: Thoughts for our Times," 2567.

[142] Michael J. Green and Jeffrey R. Botkin, "'Genetic Exceptionalism' in Medicine: Clarifying the Differences between Genetic and Nongenetic Tests," 573.

[143] Neil C. Manson and Onora O'Neill, *Rethinking Informed Consent in Bioethics*, 144.

[144] Douglas Martin and Heather Greenwood, "Public Perceptions of Ethical Issues Regarding Adult Predictive Genetic Testing," 107.

tive, not to have children."[145] Coercion can be a strong influence in family members and patient's decisions about PGT.

E. Conclusion

This chapter focused on PGT in general, and it analyzed four main areas including the science of PGT, understanding genetic risks, disclosing possible treatment options, and identifying the influence genetic information has on families. First, the science of PGT is important to understand, because it is the foundation of all the other aspects of testing. PGT is the analysis of risk predictions for diseases. The science of PGT should help people understand and be aware of the uncertainties that go into this type of testing. Because the science of PGT is still relatively new, scientists are still trying to understand how certain genes interact and know which genes are involved in diseases.[146] Also knowing the science of PGT can help people to have a basic knowledge of the potential risks and benefits of testing.[147] The reasons that are generally given for participating in PGT include detecting and preventing disease, reducing the severity of disease through treatment, planning for the future, and eliminating uncertainty or anxiety about possible diseases.Sometimes these reasons can be broken into categories like motivational or emotional. Some of the potential risks of testing include anxiety, feelings of powerlessness, discrimination, and/or discrimination.[148]

The second section discussed was genetic risks and probabilities. Understanding genetic risks can be extremely complicated, but this section tries to address the basic test interpretations and possible misunderstandings that can accompany testing. Sometimes tests can have confusing, vague results which can be difficult to interpret.[149] Positive test results mean that the test identified a variation that put the individual at an increased risk of disease.[150] Negative results mean that there was no

---

[145] Douglas Martin and Heather Greenwood, "Public Perceptions of Ethical Issues Regarding Adult Predictive Genetic Testing," 107.

[146] Anita Silvers and Michael Ashley Stein, "An Equality Paradigm for Preventing Genetic Discrimination," 1347–1348, 1385; Susan Wolf and Jeffrey Kahn, "Genetic Testing and the Future of Disability Insurance: Ethics, Law & Policy," 8.

[147] Anita Silvers and Michael Ashley Stein, "An Equality Paradigm for Preventing Genetic Discrimination," 1346; James Evans, Cecile Skrzynia, and Wylie Burke, "The Complexities of Predictive Genetic Testing," 1053.

[148] Shoshana Shiloh and Shiri Ilan, "To Test or Not To Test? Moderators of the Relationship Between Risk Perceptions and Interest in Predictive Genetic Testing," 469; Neil Sharpe and Ronald Carter, Genetic Testing: Care, Consent, and Liability, 269–270; Douglas Martin and Heather Greenwood, "Public Perceptions of Ethical Issues Regarding Adult Predictive Genetic Testing," 107.

[149] Chris Berdik, "Genetic Tests Give Consumers Hints About Disease Risk; Critics Have Misgivings," Special; Maxwell Mehlman, "Predictive Genetic Testing in Urology: Ethical and Social Issues," 433.

[150] AMA, "Direct-to-Consumer Genetic Testing;" Regina E. Ensenauer, Virginia V. Michels, and Shanda S. Reinke, "Genetic Testing: Practical, Ethical, and Counseling Considerations," 66.

variation found, but there could still be false assurances.[151] A negative test means that a person has the same level of risk for disease as the general population.[152] When interpreting results, it is important to understand that diseases are multifactorial, taking into account many different variables that determine the amount of risk such as environmental and physical factors.[153] Also different genes affect people differently, and there is no way to know how people will be affected in the future.[154] Since understanding test results can be complicated, it is important to try to eliminate as many misunderstandings as possible. The three main categories of misunderstandings include genetic tests, genetic mechanisms, and statistics. Perceptions can make a significant impact on people, and if those perceptions prove to be faulty, then the people who held those beliefs are often confused and have even higher anxiety levels. Education can also help with understanding genetic risks and eliminating some of the misconceptions that are common.[155] Having increased public education can help patients with future communications with their doctors. In addition, physicians can have more education about how to communicate these concepts to patients in order to encourage meaningful discussions.[156]

The third section looks at potential treatment options. Sometimes people think this testing will help with future treatments, but sometimes there are no treatment options for certain diseases. Some thought that if a gene was found that "treatment existed, or would soon be developed—that prevention and treatment were possible, as is generally the case with other clinical tests that have been developed and used."[157] PGT is different than other medical tests, because sometimes testing does not lead to a cure or treatment. This area looks at possible disclosure standards for identifying options of PGT.[158] Disclosure is an important aspect, especially when identifying the possible treatment options for a particular disease.[159] Possible treatment options include preventive or prophylactic measures, measures to lessen or

---

[151] AMA, "Direct-to-Consumer Genetic Testing;" Cynthia Marietta and Amy McGuire, "Direct-to-Consumer Genetic Testing: Is It the Practice of Medicine?" 370.

[152] Marion Harris, Ingrid Winship, and Merle Spriggs, "Controversies and Ethical Issues in Cancer-Genetics Clinics," 302.

[153] Cynthia Marietta and Amy McGuire, "Direct-to-Consumer Genetic Testing: Is It the Practice of Medicine?" 370.

[154] AMA, "Direct-to-Consumer Genetic Testing;" Regina E. Ensenauer, Virginia V. Michels, and Shanda S. Reinke, "Genetic Testing: Practical, Ethical, and Counseling Considerations," 67.

[155] Robert Klitzman, "Misunderstandings Concerning Genetics Among Patients Confronting Genetic Disease," 433–434.

[156] Douglas Martin and Heather Greenwood, "Public Perceptions of Ethical Issues Regarding Adult Predictive Genetic Testing," 106; Neil Sharpe and Ronald Carter, Genetic Testing: Care, Consent, and Liability, 381.

[157] Robert Klitzman, "Misunderstandings Concerning Genetics Among Patients Confronting Genetic Disease," 434.

[158] Neil F. Sharpe and Ronald Carter, Genetic Testing: Care, Consent, and Liability, 131.

[159] Robert M. Arnold and Charles W. Lidz, "Informed Consent: Clinical Aspects of Consent in Health Care," 11.

prevent the disease, and/or just surveillance with no treatment.[160] Specific treatment options were discussed for HBOC, which demonstrate the importance of identifying and disclosing possible options for PGT.[161]

Since this testing relates to the entire family, the fourth part of this chapter discusses the importance of family-related genetic information in relation to PGT. This section emphasizes the impact a family can have on a person being tested and the impact a person being tested can have on the whole family.[162] Sometimes it can be difficult for people to tell his or her family about testing results, because those results have implications for the family as well.[163] Several family members have to be tested before a hereditary condition can be identified, but sometimes disclosure can be difficult.[164] This section offers some help when recommending additional support from genetics staff help patients disclose information to families.[165] Ideally patients should disclose test results to those that could be affected by the results in order to prepare for the future. If patients do not disclose that information, the families are not aware of the risk and cannot participate in PGT.[166] The issue of genetic exceptionalism also arises when discussing family-related information, because genetic exceptionalism recognizes that genetic information affects more than just the individual patient. Genetic exceptionalism focuses on the special nature of genetics, while recognizing the implications for the entire family.[167] While some argue for genetic exceptionalism, some argue against this idea saying that both genetic and non-genetic information can help to predict certain illnesses.[168] Since PGT has many implications for families, sometimes these external pressures can culminate

---

[160] Anita Silvers and Michael Ashley Stein, "An Equality Paradigm for Preventing Genetic Discrimination," 1348; Marion Harris, Ingrid Winship, and Merle Spriggs, "Controversies and Ethical Issues in Cancer-Genetics Clinics," 301.

[161] Janice Berliner and Angela Fay, "Risk Assessment and Genetic Counseling for Hereditary Breast and Ovarian Cancer: Recommendations of the National Society of Genetic Counselors," 252–255.

[162] Anita Silvers and Michael Ashley Stein, "An Equality Paradigm for Preventing Genetic Discrimination," 1357; Abigail L. Rose, Nikki Peters, Judy A. Shea, et al., "Attitudes and Misconceptions about Predictive Genetic Testing for Cancer Risk," 146.

[163] Kathryn Holt, "What Do We Tell the Children? Contrasting the Disclosure Choices of Two HD Families Regarding Risk Status and Predictive Genetic Testing," 254.

[164] Maxwell Mehlman, "Predictive Genetic Testing in Urology: Ethical and Social Issues," 435; Marion Harris, Ingrid Winship, and Merle Spriggs, "Controversies and Ethical Issues in Cancer-Genetics Clinics," 302.

[165] Clara L. Gaff, Veronica Collins, Tiffany Symes, et al., "Facilitating Family Communication about Predictive Genetic Testing: Probands' Perceptions," 134.

[166] Marion Harris, Ingrid Winship, and Merle Spriggs, "Controversies and Ethical Issues in Cancer-Genetics Clinics," 302–303.

[167] Leon Kass, Life, Liberty and the Defense of Dignity, 57; Michael J. Green and Jeffrey R. Botkin, "'Genetic Exceptionalism' in Medicine: Clarifying the Differences between Genetic and Nongenetic Tests," 571–572.

[168] Michael J. Green and Jeffrey R. Botkin, "'Genetic Exceptionalism' in Medicine: Clarifying the Differences between Genetic and Nongenetic Tests," 571–573; Neil C. Manson and Onora O'Neill, Rethinking Informed Consent in Bioethics, 136.

in coercion of the patient or the family.[169] This last section discusses the importance of eliminating coercion and/or controlling external pressures.

This chapter gives an overview of the factors that are important in PGT. The science of PGT is important in order to understand the rest of PGT. Genetic risks and probabilities are central to a person's decision about whether or not to participate in PGT. It is also crucial for people to know the possible treatment options or the lack of treatment options for a disease before deciding to go any further in their testing. Since PGT can impact both the patient and the patient's family, knowing the possible family implications can help to strengthen a person's informed consent for PGT. All of these aspects are central to the discussion of informed consent and PGT and help in understanding the concepts of the future chapters.

References

American Medical Association. "Direct-to-Consumer Genetic Testing." Accessed May 3, 2010. http://www.ama-assn.org/ama1/pub/upload/mm/464/dtc-genetic-test.pdf.

American Society of Human Genetics Social Issues Subcommittee on Familial Disclosure. "ASHG Statement: Professional Disclosure of Familial Genetic Information." *The American Journal of Human Genetics* 62: 2(February 1998): 474–483.

Arnold, Robert M. and Charles W. Lidz. "Informed Consent: Clinical Aspects of Consent in Health Care." In *Taking Sides: Clashing Views on Bioethical Issues*, edited by Carol Levine, 4–14. Boston: McGraw Hill Higher Education, 2010.

Arver, Brita, Aina Haegermark, Ulla Platten, et al. "Evaluation of Psychosocial Effects of Pre-Symptomatic Testing for Breast/Ovarian and Colon Cancer Pre-Disposing Genes: a 12-Month Follow-Up." *Familial Cancers* 3:2 (2004): 109–116.

Berdik, Chris. "Genetic Tests Give Consumers Hints About Disease Risk; Critics Have Misgivings." *Washington Post.* (January 26, 2010): Special, 1–2.

Berliner, Janice and Angela Fay. "Risk Assessment and Genetic Counseling for Hereditary Breast and Ovarian Cancer: Recommendations of the National Society of Genetic Counselors." *Journal of Genetic Counseling* 16:3 (2007): 241–260.

Broadstock, Marita, Susan Michie, Theresa Marteau. "Psychological Consequences of Predictive Genetic Testing: A Systematic Review." *European Journal of Human Genetics* 8 (2000): 731–738.

Burgess, Michael, PhD, Claude Lanberg, MD, PhD, Bartha Maria Knoppers, LLD. "Bioethics for Clinicians: 14. Ethics and Genetics in Medicine." *Canadian Medical Association Journal* 158:10 (1998): 1309–1313.

Chapman, Elizabeth. "Ethical Dilemmas in Testing for Late Onset Conditions: Reactions to Testing and Perceived Impact on Other Family Members." *Journal of Genetic Counseling* 11:5 (2002): 351–367.

Chial, Heidi. "Mendelian Genetics: Patterns of Inheritance and Single-Gene Disorders." *Nature Education* 1:1 (2008). Accessed November 10, 2012. http://www.nature.com/scitable/topicpage/mendelian-genetics-patterns-of-inheritance-and-single-966.

Coller, Barry S. "The Physician-Scientist, the State, and the Oath: Thoughts for our Times." *Journal of Clinical Investigation* 116: 10(October 2006): 2567–2570.

Collins, Francis. *The Language of Life.* New York: Harper Collins Publishers, 2010.

---

[169] Douglas Martin and Heather Greenwood, "Public Perceptions of Ethical Issues Regarding Adult Predictive Genetic Testing," 107.

Cox, Susan M. "Stories in Decisions: How At-Risk Individuals Decide to Request Predictive Testing for Huntington Disease," *Qualitative Sociology* 26: 2(Summer 2003): 257–280.

Dolgin, Janet and Lois Shepherd. *Bioethics and the Law.* New York: Aspen Publishers, 2005.

Emery, Jon, Kristine Barlow-Stewart, and Sylvia A. Metcalfe. "There's Cancer in the Family." *Australian Family Physician* 38: 4(April 2009): 194–198.

Ensenauer, Regina E., Virginia V. Michels, and Shanda S. Reinke. "Genetic Testing: Practical, Ethical, and Counseling Considerations." *Mayo Clinic Proceedings* 80: 1(January 2005): 63–73.

Evans, James, Cecile Skrzynia, and Wylie Burke. "The Complexities of Predictive Genetic Testing." *British Medical Journal* 322 (April 28, 2001): 1052–1056.

Gaff, Clara L., Veronica Collins, Tiffany Symes, and Jane Halliday. "Facilitating Family Communication about Predictive Genetic Testing: Probands' Perceptions." *Journal of Genetic Counseling* 14: 2(April 2005): 133–140.

Green, Michael J. and Jeffrey R. Botkin. "Genetic Exceptionalism" in Medicine: Clarifying the Differences between Genetic and Nongenetic Tests. *Annals of Internal Medicine* 138:7 (April 1, 2003): 571–575.

Harris, Marion, Ingrid Winship, Merle Spriggs. "Controversies and Ethical Issues in Cancer-Genetics Clinics." *Lancet Oncology* 6 (2005): 301–310.

Heinrichs, Bert. "What Should We Want to Know About Our Future? A Kantian View on Predictive Genetic Testing. Medicine." *Health Care and Philosophy* 8:1 (2005): 29–37.

Holt, Kathryn. "What Do We Tell the Children? Contrasting the Disclosure Choices of Two HD Families Regarding Risk Status and Predictive Genetic Testing." *Journal of Genetic Counseling* 15: 4(August 2006): 253–265.

Kass, Leon. *Life, Liberty and the Defense of Dignity.* San Francisco, CA: Encounter Books, 2002.

Kelly, Patricia. "Cancer Risks in Perspective: Information and Approaches for Clinicians." In *Genetic Testing: Care, Consent, and Liability,* edited by Neil Sharpe and Ronald Carter, 382–397. Hoboken, New Jersey: John Wiley & Sons, Inc., 2006.

Klitzman, Robert. "Misunderstandings Concerning Genetics Among Patients Confronting Genetic Disease," *Journal of Genetic Counseling* 19: 5(October 2010): 430–446.

Kraft, Peter, Ph.D., David Hunter. "Genetic Risk Prediction—Are We There Yet?" *The New England Journal of Medicine.* 360: 17 (April 23, 2009): 1701–1703.

Lo, Bernard. *Resolving Ethical Dilemmas.* Philadelphia, PA: Lippincott Williams and Wilkins, 2005.

Manson, Neil C. and Onora O'Neill. *Rethinking Informed Consent in Bioethics.* New York: Cambridge University Press, 2007.

Marietta, Cynthia and Amy McGuire. "Direct-to-Consumer Genetic Testing: Is It the Practice of Medicine?" *Journal of Law, Medicine & Ethics* 37: 2(Summer 2009): 369–374.

Martin, Douglas and Heather Greenwood. "Public Perceptions of Ethical Issues Regarding Adult Predictive Genetic Testing." *Health Care Analysis* 18: 2 (2010): 103–112.

Mehlman, Maxwell. "Predictive Genetic Testing in Urology: Ethical and Social Issues." *World Journal of Urology* 21 (2004): 433–437.

Michie, S., M. Bobrow, and T. M. Marteau, on behalf of the FAP Collaborative Research Group. "Predictive Genetic Testing in Children and Adults: A Study of Emotional Impact," *Journal of Medical Genetics* 38: 8(August 2001): 519–526.

Michie, Susan, John Weinman, Julie Miller, et al. "Predictive Genetic Testing: High Risk Expectations in the Face of Low Risk Information." *Journal of Behavioral Medicine* 25: 1(February 2002): 33–50.

Mitchell, Philip, Bettina Meiser, Alex Wilde, et al. "Predictive and Diagnostic Genetic Testing in Psychiatry." *Psychiatric Clinics of North America* 33: 1(March 2010): 225–243.

Ng, Pauline C., Sarah S. Murray, Samuel Levy, and J. Craig Venter. "An Agenda for Personalized Medicine." *Nature.* 461 (October 8, 2009): 724–726.

Post, Linda Farber, Jeffrey Blustein, and Nancy Neveloff Dubler. *Handbook for Health Care Ethics Committees.* Baltimore: The John Hopkins University Press, 2007.

Rose, Abigail L., Nikki Peters, Judy A. Shea, et al. "Attitudes and Misconceptions about Predictive Genetic Testing for Cancer Risk." *Community Genetics* 8 (2005): 145–151.

Sharpe, Neil F. and Ronald Carter. *Genetic Testing: Care, Consent, and Liability*. Hoboken, New Jersey: John Wiley & Sons, Inc., 2006.

Shiloh, Shoshana and Shiri Ilan. "To Test or Not To Test? Moderators of the Relationship Between Risk Perceptions and Interest in Predictive Genetic Testing." *Journal of Behavioral Medicine* 28: 5(October 2005): 467–479.

Silvers, Anita and Michael Ashley Stein. "An Equality Paradigm for Preventing Genetic Discrimination." *Vanderbilt Law Review* 55: 1341 (2002): 1340–1395.

Trepanier, Angela, Mary Ahrens, Wendy McKinnon, et al. "Genetic Cancer Risk Assessment and Counseling: Recommendations of the National Society of Genetic Counselors." *Journal of Genetic Counseling* 13: 2(April 2004): 83–114.

Vaughn, Lewis. *Bioethics: Principles, Issues, and Cases*. New York: Oxford University Press, 2009.

Wolf, Susan and Jeffrey Kahn. "Genetic Testing and the Future of Disability Insurance: Ethics, Law & Policy," *The Journal of Law, Medicine & Ethics* 35: 2 supplement (Summer 2007): 6–32.

Chapter 3
The History and Components of Informed Consent

The third chapter explores the history of consent to identify the widely recognized components of consent (understanding, disclosure, and voluntariness) that represent the current model. This first part will analyze the clinical and research history of informed consent and discuss specific cases. Then, the second part will look at the emergence of the components of informed consent which are comprehension, disclosure, and voluntariness. This section will discuss the components of consent that have influenced the current model.

The ethics of science and medicine is often discussed within the realm of bioethics. Bioethics discussions first started with the scientific and medical communities, and then theologians and philosophers entered the discussions. The study of bioethics promotes the identification and prevention of ethical concerns. One of the most important and foundational areas of bioethics is informed consent.[1] H. Tristram Engelhardt, Jr. suggests that an action involving another person is not ethically justifiable without that person's permission or consent. Thus, informed consent originated from the idea that individuals should have the right to make decisions themselves. In order for a medical treatment or research study to be morally acceptable, a person's consent is required before treatment or participation in research.[2]

Tom Beauchamp and James Childress note that there are often two interpretations of informed consent. Subsequently, these two interpretations need to be distinguished so that it is clear adequate consent has been given. The first interpretation deals with an autonomous authorization. This interpretation is demonstrated when a person actively and voluntarily gives permission for a procedure and/or treatment without coercion. This is most often seen as the ethical ideal for consent, because mere agreement with a recommendation for treatment is not enough to satisfy this first interpretation. The second interpretation deals with effective consent. This interpretation is generally identified as the legal and typical hospital approach before

---

[1] Albert Jonsen, *The Birth of Bioethics*, 352–353; George Annas, *American Bioethics: Crossing Human Rights and Health Law Boundaries,* 112; Nancy Press and C. H. Browner, "Risk, Autonomy, and Responsibility: Informed Consent for Prenatal Testing," S10.

[2] H. Tristram Engelhardt Jr., *The Foundations of Bioethics*, 288–289; James Childress, *Who Should Decide? Paternalism in Health Care,* 77.

© Springer International Publishing Switzerland 2015
J. Minor, *Informed Consent in Predictive Genetic Testing,*
DOI 10.1007/978-3-319-17416-7_3

a treatment can occur. This interpretation of consent looks at social and legal guidelines and does not emphasize autonomy. Because the second interpretation does not focus on the individual actively authorizing an action, sometimes the second interpretation falls short of the ethical ideal. However, that does not diminish the importance of the second interpretation, because hospitals need to have consent guidelines that can be applied easily without overwhelming the patient or physician. The mature minor doctrine is a helpful illustration for identifying the differences in these interpretations. A minor can understand and authorize a treatment under the definition of an autonomous authorization, but the minor cannot give effective consent without being recognized legally as a mature minor with all the rights of an adult. Thus, a person can authorize an action, while not being able to give effective consent.[3] While these interpretations are distinct, the prerequisites of effective consent are needed to make sure that the autonomous authorization can be upheld and implemented. In order for consent to be practical, both interpretations of consent are needed. If there is an autonomous authorization without fulfilling the requirements of effective consent, then consent has not taken place like the case of the mature minor doctrine. On the other hand, if there is an effective consent without an autonomous authorization, adequate consent has not taken place either. Combining the two interpretations can give a greater depth to consent. When looking at the history of consent, both of these concepts are utilized. A better understanding of consent history ensues when an individual is able to recognize which interpretation is being used at the time. Thus, it is important to differentiate between these two interpretations before discussing the background of consent.

A. The Background of Informed Consent

The first section of this chapter will give an overview of the history of informed consent in both the clinical and research fields. The background of consent analyzes the cases that helped to shape consent in history. The first part will look at the clinical history of consent and will focus on the patient treatment model. The second part will look at the history of consent in research and will focus on the research subject model of consent. The third section will summarize the history and look at the two models of consent.

1. Clinical History

The first section will divide the clinical history into three sections: the early history of consent, the cases during the1950s and 1960s, and then the cases in the late 1900s. Each will analyze the important cases that arose during that time.

---

[3] Tom Beauchamp and James Childress, *Principles of Biomedical Ethics*, 78; Ruth Faden and Tom Beauchamp, "The Concept of Informed Consent," 155–157.

a. Early History

In Hippocratic times, patients were typically not informed about their health.[4] In the Hippocratic tradition, there was no discussion of treatment options or the reasoning behind the physician's recommendations.[5] Instead of including patients in discussions of their health to encourage patient participation, the patients were only to obey the doctor. The responsibility of the physician was to protect the patients.[6] While the physician was to act in the patient's best interest, some type of permission was required before the physician started. As clarified by Albert Jonsen permission was either implied or explicit. This idea comes from the fifteenth century English common law, which required permission before touching. Even in the fifteenth century, if permission was not obtained, touching was considered an offense.[7]

In 1674, in some cultures, doctors and patients would agree on treatments; however, that was not the norm for the day. In the Mediterranean area, that emphasis on agreement evolved in 1756. During this time, detailed information was given to patients regarding their conditions and the proposed treatments. Since medical education was incomplete and physicians had limited experience at the time, Christopoulos, Falagas, Gourzis, and Trompoukis clarify that this level of understanding was unexpected. In one instance on April 1756, a father had signed a form saying that he understood his son's diagnosis and treatment, hired a doctor to carry out the treatment, and acknowledged that if anything went wrong he would not hold the doctor responsible. Even if the document was written to protect the doctor or the patient, this example demonstrates the considerable amount of understanding the father had towards his son's disease and treatment.[8]

One of the first legal cases for consent, *Slater v. Baker and Stapleton,* occurred in 1767. The court ruled that since requiring simple consent was typical during that time, the physician should be held responsible for failing to meet that standard.[9] In this case, getting consent from the patient was a means to encourage better cooperation after the operation and not to demonstrate autonomy or authority.[10] It was a means to an ends.

---

[4] Bonnie Steinbock, John Arras, and Alex John London, eds., *Ethical Issues in Modern Medicine,* 61.

[5] Jay Katz, "Physicians and Patients: A History of Silence," 135.

[6] Bonnie Steinbock, John Arras, and Alex John London, eds., *Ethical Issues in Modern Medicine,* 61; H. Tristram, Engelhardt Jr., *The Foundations of Bioethics,* 291; Robert Veatch, "Abandoning Informed Consent," 5.

[7] Albert Jonsen, *The Birth of Bioethics,* 355.

[8] Platon Christopoulos, Matthew E. Falagas, Philippos Gourzis, and Constantinos Trompoukis, "Aspects of Informed Consent in Medical Practice in the Eastern Mediterranean Region During the 17th and 18th Centuries," 1588–89, 1591.

[9] Jessica W. Berg, Paul S. Applebaum, Charles W. Lidz, and Lisa S. Parker, *Informed Consent: Legal Theory and Clinical Practice,* 42; Wouter Leclercq, Bram J. Keulers. Marc R. M. Scheltinga, et al., "A Review of Surgical Informed Consent: Past, Present, and Future. A Quest to Help Patients Make Better Decisions," 1408; Thomas Grisso and Paul S. Applebaum, *Assessing Competence to Consent to Treatment,* 4–5.

[10] H. Tristram, Engelhardt Jr., *The Foundations of Bioethics,* 303–304.

Beauchamp explains that Thomas Percival's book, *Medical Ethics,* in 1803 asserted that the patient's beneficence was more important than truth-telling. The book also suggested that this dishonesty was charitable.[11] Deception for the good of the patient was accepted, because the physician knew what was best for the patient at the time.[12] As a result, many physicians did not see the point of informed consent, and many times decisions were made without consulting the patients.[13] During this time in history, the physician's benevolent intentions were emphasized more than patient consent. Thus consent regulations were not seen to be a necessity.

The principles of informed consent originated around 1905 with *Mohr v. Williams.*[14] Anna Mohr gave consent for an operation on her right ear, but noticing she needed surgery on the left instead, the physician performed surgery without her consent for that side. The court said the physician should have gotten consent for that as well.[15] Another case in 1905, *Pratt v. Dams,* ruled that consent from the specific individual needed to take place before surgery. Dr. Pratt only told Mr. Davis about the need for his wife's surgery. Mrs. Davis did not consent to or know about the surgery to remove her uterus and ovaries. Thinking Mrs. Davis did not warrant additional information, Dr. Pratt did not tell her, because he did not want her to worry or be hostile.[16]

The *Schloendorff v. the Society of the New York Hospitals* case in 1914 established the nature of the consent discussion. After complaining of stomach problems, a woman consented to an examination in New York in 1908. She did not consent to surgery, but the doctor operated anyway. As a result, the operation led to gangrene and the loss of fingers.[17] With this case Justice Cardozo ruled that all competent adults should be able to make medical decisions for him- or herself.[18] Since doctors can be liable for surgeries done without consent· the physician in this case was liable for damages he caused.[19] In his work on informed consent, Beauchamp explains that the case illustrates patient self-determination and supports the fifteenth century principle that protected against unwanted touching.[20] However, Lewis Vaughn notes

---

[11] Tom Beauchamp, "Informed Consent," 186–187; Willard Gaylin and Bruce Jennings, *The Perversion of Autonomy,* 49.

[12] Carol Levine ed., *Taking Sides: Clashing Views on Bioethical Issues,* 2.

[13] Janet Dolgin and Lois Shepherd, *Bioethics and the Law,* 5.

[14] Wouter Leclercq, Bram J. Keulers. Marc R. M. Scheltinga, et al., "A Review of Surgical Informed Consent: Past, Present, and Future. A Quest to Help Patients Make Better Decisions," 1408.

[15] Tom Beauchamp and James Childress, *Principles of Biomedical Ethics,* 78.

[16] Margaret Swain, "A Brief History of Informed Consent," 19–20.

[17] Jerry Menikoff, *Law and Bioethics: An Introduction,* 155–156; Janet Dolgin and Lois Shepherd, *Bioethics and the Law,* 58–59; H. Tristram Engelhardt Jr., *The Foundations of Bioethics,* 304; Wouter Leclercq, Bram J. Keulers. Marc R. M. Scheltinga, et al., "A Review of Surgical Informed Consent: Past, Present, and Future. A Quest to Help Patients Make Better Decisions," 1408.

[18] James Childress, *Who Should Decide? Paternalism in Health Care,* 133.

[19] Albert Jonsen, *The Birth of Bioethics,* 355; Jerry Menikoff, *Law and Bioethics: An Introduction,* 156.

[20] Tom Beauchamp, "Informed Consent," 187–188; Alfred Tauber, *Patient Autonomy and the Ethics of Responsibility,* 75.

that while the case emphasized self-determination, the ruling did not combine being informed with being able to consent.[21] Another way of demonstrating this point is made by Alfred Tauber when he explains that a simple "yes" or "no" answer was acceptable for consent at that time. Later in the 1920s and 30s, consent started to demonstrate more of an emphasis on patient participation with the *Haskins v. Howard* case in 1929.[22] However there were also exceptions to that; one being an emphasis on consent in order to protect doctors against malpractice suits.[23] During this time, some cases focused more on patient participation and authorization, while others emphasized more of an effective consent to protect against litigation.

b. Mid 1900s

In 1955, judges in the *Hunt v. Bradshaw* case ruled that failure to disclose information about potential paralysis after surgery was enough for liability.[24] In 1957, *Salgo v. Leland Stanford Junior University Board of Trustees* focused on the duty of physicians to disclose material information.[25] Martin Salgo was paralyzed after having a translumbar aortography. Because the physician did not tell him of the risk for paralysis, the court ruled in favor of Mr. Salgo.[26] During the ruling, the California Supreme Court said there was a duty for physicians to disclose relevant information in order to make an intelligent decision.[27] This was the first case that used the phrase "informed consent," which was coined by Justice Bray.[28] This case was also one of the first to link disclosure to patient consent.[29]

Several cases in the 1960s develop the concepts of disclosure. As a result of the *Natanson v. Kline* case of 1960, Hana Osman suggests that the consequences of not informing patients changed from battery to negligence.[30] Mrs. Natanson, claiming her doctor did not inform her of the risks of cobalt therapy, suffered serious burns.[31]

---

[21] Lewis Vaughn, *Bioethics: Principles, Issues, and Cases*, 144.

[22] Alfred Tauber, *Patient Autonomy and the Ethics of Responsibility*, 75.

[23] Hana Osman, "History and Development of the Doctrine of Informed Consent," 42.

[24] Margaret Swain, "A Brief History of Informed Consent," 19–20.

[25] Janet L. Dolgin, "The Legal Development of the Informed Consent Doctrine: Past and Present," 98–99.

[26] Albert Jonsen, *The Birth of Bioethics*, 355.

[27] Jessica W. Berg, Paul S. Applebaum, Charles W. Lidz, and Lisa S. Parker, *Informed Consent: Legal Theory and Clinical Practice*, 44; Roberta M. Berry, "Informed Consent Law, Ethics, and Practice: From Infancy to Reflective Adolescence," 65–66.

[28] Alfred Tauber, *Patient Autonomy and the Ethics of Responsibility*, 254; Tom Beauchamp, "Informed Consent," 188.

[29] Lewis Vaughn, *Bioethics: Principles, Issues, and Cases*, 144.

[30] Hana Osman, "History and Development of the Doctrine of Informed Consent," 42, 43; Carol Levine ed., *Taking Sides: Clashing Views on Bioethical Issues*, 3.

[31] Albert Jonsen, *The Birth of Bioethics*, 355.

The case determined that the risks, benefits, and alternatives of a proposed treatment needed to be disclosed.[32] If one of those areas is left out of the discussion, then negligence can occur.[33] This case emphasizes the three general types of information that should be disclosed. Another case takes that information further. In the *Mitchell* case, the court suggested that physicians should inform patients about some of the more severe risks as well.[34] Then in a Kansas case dealing with patient paralysis after a sodium urokan injection, disclosure of the risks, benefits, and alternatives was proven not to be enough. In this case, Justice Schroeder said that doctors needed to inform patients in easy to understand language about the disease, treatment options, possible risks, and the likelihood of a positive outcome.[35] Thus, disclosure was beginning to be linked with understanding. As a result, doctors were required to give patients suitable information before getting consent.

Albert Jonsen explains that the 1960s brought about the professional duty of the physician to disclose material information to patients. There were a couple of transplantation cases that demonstrated the importance of disclosure especially when evaluating the risks and benefits to a healthy donor. A transplant case in 1969 in Kentucky looked into transplantation involving identical twins at the Peter Bent Brigham Hospital. One twin needed a transplant, but the other was healthy and theoretically able to donate to the other twin. Since the twins were minors, this caused debate about the risks and benefits of transplantation in minors. Generally medical procedures for minors were acceptable if there was a medical benefit, but questions arose about what the benefit was to the healthy twin donating the organ. After looking at three cases, the judges said surgery was acceptable if certain conditions were met including consent of the parents and donor and proof that the healthy twin profited even psychiatrically from the procedure. In one of the cases, the potential kidney donor, Jerry Strunk, was mentally retarded and living in the state mental hospital. Approving the transplant, the court ruled that Jerry would actually benefit by having his brother live. Thus the court adhered to the principle of benefit for both the donor and the recipient.[36] While these cases bring up many issues, the important aspect for consent was the evaluation of the available information. In order for the healthy twin to consent to transplantation, the physician needed to provide adequate information of the risks and benefits for each party involved.

---

[32] Lewis Vaughn, *Bioethics: Principles, Issues, and Cases*, 148.

[33] Alfred Tauber, *Patient Autonomy and the Ethics of Responsibility*, 135.

[34] Jessica W. Berg, Paul S. Applebaum, Charles W. Lidz, and Lisa S. Parker, *Informed Consent: Legal Theory and Clinical Practice*, 45.

[35] Jay Katz, "Informed Consent- Must It Remain a Fairy Tale?" In, Lewis Vaughn, *Bioethics: Principles, Issues, and Cases*, 162.

[36] Albert Jonsen, *The Birth of Bioethics*, 197–198, 355.

c. Late 1900s to early 2000

In 1972, the California Supreme Court in the *Cobb v. Grant* case ruled that all the information material to decision making should be disclosed to patients by physicians.[37] Also in 1972, the *Canterbury v. Spence* case in Washington D.C. added another dimension to disclosure. In 1958 Mr. Canterbury had a laminectomy due to shoulder pain and possibly a ruptured disc, and a day after surgery fell and became paralyzed. Dr. Spence then did a second surgery, but Mr. Canterbury was unable to recover fully and suffered from incontinence and partial paralysis. He sued claiming that the doctor never told him of the risk for paralysis. The court ruled the risk of paralysis was material to his decision, and thus was needed for consent.[38] Post, Blustein, and Dubler clarify this point further when explaining that enough information was needed so that a rational person could make a decision about a treatment.[39] However, because patients do not have a complete understanding of medicine and only have the doctor to help him or her reach an appropriate choice, the court ruled that physician disclosure was required.[40] The court ruled in favor of Mr. Canterbury, which demonstrated the importance of patient decision making. As a result of this case, Judge Robinson said that disclosure guidelines should be based off of the patient rather than the physician.[41] Because this case encouraged the reasonable patient standard, many states implemented that view instead of the reasonable physician standard.[42] However, the reasonable physician standard was still the most widely held view.

The 1980 case, *Truman v. Thomas*, concerned a woman named Rena Truman who died at the age of 30. Dr. Thomas was Rena Truman's doctor from 1963 until 1969. During that time, Dr. Thomas never did a pap smear. In 1969 she was diagnosed with advanced cervical cancer after going to another doctor. Her children sued Dr. Thomas, and said that if he had done a pap smear, their mother could still be alive or at least could have had a better chance of survival. Dr. Thomas said that he had told her she should get a pap smear, but Rena always rejected the idea, either because it was too costly or she did not feel like having it done. The ruling said that just because a patient does not agree to a procedure does not mean that the requirement for disclosure should be any less. The ruling suggests that the decision to reject a procedure does not change the doctor-patient relationship, because both de-

---

[37] Lewis Vaughn, *Bioethics: Principles, Issues, and Cases*, 148.

[38] Jerry Menikoff, *Law and Bioethics: An Introduction*, 189.

[39] Linda Farber Post, Jeffrey Blustein, and Nancy Neveloff Dubler, *Handbook for Health Care Ethics Committees*, 286; Janet L. Dolgin, "The Legal Development of the Informed Consent Doctrine: Past and Present," 101.

[40] Spottswood W. Robinson, "United States Court of Appeals Canterbury v. Spence," 133.

[41] Lewis Vaughn, *Bioethics: Principles, Issues, and Cases*, 145, 148, 150; Carol Levine ed., *Taking Sides: Clashing Views on Bioethical Issues*, 3; Linda Farber Post, Jeffrey Blustein, and Nancy Neveloff Dubler, *Handbook for Health Care Ethics Committees*, 286.

[42] Jerry Menikoff, *Law and Bioethics: An Introduction*, 167.

cisions require physician assistance and input.[43] The court originally ruled that Dr. Thomas was not negligent for not specifically informing Rena about the possible risks of not having a pap smear. But later an appeal tested his duty of care in not fully explaining the consequences of rejecting a pap smear. Dolgin and Shepherd suggest that this case illustrates the need for explaining both the risks and benefits whether the patient consents or not to a medical procedure.[44]

The case in California in 1990, *Moore v. Regents of the University of California* analyzed potential conflicts of interests. After diagnosing Mr. Moore with hairy-cell leukemia, the physician withheld information about his plans for Mr. Moore's unique samples. Since there was not a lot of research done on this leukemia, the doctor used his tissue to get a patent on the cells. Deliberately withholding this information, the doctor received the patent before proceeding to remove Mr. Moore's spleen. The court ruled the physicians also had to disclose personal, non-medical information if that information could affect the patient's decision-making capabilities. Because the physician's judgment could have been impaired by financial conflicts of interests and the patient was not informed about this research or the patent, the court determined that Mr. Moore did not give informed consent.[45]

The *Arato v. Avedon* case in California in 1993 evaluated the duty of a physician to give the life expectancy of a patient. This case involved a patient undergoing experimental chemotherapy and radiation for an advanced stage of cancer. While the physician told the patient and family the risks and benefits and his poor prognosis, statistics were not given for his chance of survival. The case stated that the patient would not have consented to chemotherapy if he knew the low success rates and life expectancy.[46] However, the ruling determined adequate information was given to make an informed decision. Because statistics are not always dependable, the court said the statistics were not necessary.[47] Another case looking at disclosure of additional information was the *Johnson v. Kokemoor* case in 1996. As clarified by Janet Dolgin, the case was based on a physician's failure to report his inexperience with the proposed surgery.[48] The court determined that a physician's lack of experience can change the risks for surgery. As a result, the ruling explained that general risks could significantly increase if an inexperienced doctor performs the procedure.[49]

---

[43] Edward P. Richards, III, JD, MPH, "Consent and Informed Consent. Case Compliments of Versuslaw. Truman v. Thomas, 611 P.2d 902 (Cal.1980)."

[44] Janet Dolgin and Lois Shepherd, *Bioethics and the Law*, 61; Jerry Menikoff, *Law and Bioethics: An Introduction,* 168.

[45] Tom Beauchamp and James Childress, *Principles of Biomedical Ethics*, 81; Linda Farber Post, Jeffrey Blustein, and Nancy Neveloff Dubler, *Handbook for Health Care Ethics Committees*, 286–287.

[46] Carol Levine ed., *Taking Sides: Clashing Views on Bioethical Issues*, 21.

[47] Linda Farber Post, Jeffrey Blustein, and Nancy Neveloff Dubler, *Handbook for Health Care Ethics Committees*, 286–287.

[48] Janet L. Dolgin, "The Legal Development of the Informed Consent Doctrine: Past and Present," 103–104.

[49] Janet Dolgin and Lois Shepherd, *Bioethics and the Law*, 62–63; Jerry Menikoff, *Law and Bioethics: An Introduction,* 186–188.

Another way of noting this point is made by B. Sonny Bal and Theodore Choma when explaining that presenting patients with general statistics and ignoring other statistics that could yield material information is not recommended and could be misleading. In the end however, the patient dropped the claim. Both the *Arato v. Avedon* and the *Johnson v. Kokemoor* case demonstrate some additional information that might be material to a patient's decision.[50]

All of these initial cases formulate the principles and ideas of the informed consent procedures of today. The next area will focus on the history of research cases for informed consent.

2. Research History

While the clinical aspects of informed consent were being established, the morality of human subject research was being formed and analyzed. Jonsen illuminates this point further. Because there are only future benefits and no individual therapeutic purpose to research, the ethics of human subject research was questioned.[51] This section looks at the early history, the mid 1900s, and then the late 1900s to early 2000s.

a. Early History

Engelhardt explains that in 1538 in the *Summa Armilla,* Bartolomaeus Fumus said doctors err when substituting accepted procedures for experimental measures, because the physicians are experimenting with patients and exposing them to harm. A Jesuit moral theologian John Ford argued that if research was to take place, then consent was essential for experimental studies that did not heal but evaluated side effects. If consent was ignored, then the research was immoral, unethical, and illegal. Jonsen notes that another important aspect of research consent was suggested by Dr. Otto Guttentag. In order for research consent to be ethical, the differences between physician and physician experimenter had to be recognized. To reduce confusion about research and medical treatment, people need to be aware of the different goals of the two positions.[52] This is often one of the most important aspects of research consent. This section will discuss the major cases that shaped consent for human subject research.

The Walter Reed yellow fever experiments in the 1880s helped to establish procedures for informed consent.[53] Dr. Reed and Drs. James Carroll, Jesse Lazear,

---

[50] B. Sonny Bal and Theodore J. Choma, "What to Disclose? Revisiting Informed Consent," 1346.

[51] Albert Jonsen, *The Birth of Bioethics*, 355–356.

[52] H. Tristram, Engelhardt Jr., *The Foundations of Bioethics*, 330–331; Albert Jonsen, *The Birth of Bioethics*, 138, 149, 152, 356.

[53] Tom Beauchamp, "Informed Consent," 187.

and Aristide Agramonte tested their hypothesis of yellow fever transmission from mosquitoes. Since Dr. Lazear and some staff died from self-experimentation, the researchers sought volunteers and created a form that described the purpose and risks of the experiment. The forms said that the people volunteered freely. Reimbursement would be given to survivors or relatives if the subject died. In the end, 25 got sick but none died. Proving beneficial, the results demonstrated the mode of transmission and proved mosquitoes were the source. The yellow fever experiments made it possible for healthy volunteers to freely consent. As a result, in 1886 Dr. Charles Francis Withington, receiving an award for his dissertation *The Relation of Hospitals to Medical Education*, said that in-patients were more than biological samples and nobody should participate against their will especially if the research had no clear medical purpose. Then later in 1900, the Prussian Ministry of Religious, Educational and Medical Affairs said that research with no clear benefit to the individual should not be conducted unless he or she explicitly consents after the risks and benefits were explained. Later the guidelines were strengthened to include regulations for vulnerable populations and documentation procedures. Looking at vulnerable populations and documentation, in 1912, the research of Dr. Hideyo Noguchi with the Rockefeller Institute was questioned, because he infected 400 people from mental hospitals, orphanages, or hospitals with syphilis without obtaining their consent. As a result, Walter Cannon, a Harvard physiologist, argued that before being published in a research journal which this case was, the articles should ensure and document that both research subjects and their families are informed of the experimental procedure and given a chance to give consent. Even though there were regulations being developed for research consent, research studies in general were still novel and sometimes premature. In 1935, since researchers were using a live polio vaccine during testing, 9 children died, and as a result, research was discontinued for 20 years.[54]

During the 1940s, vaccines were developed for shigella, research was done with military using mustard gas without their consent, and pregnant women were given radioactive iron for an experimental program. In 1941 research was conducted at the Ohio Soldiers and Sailors Orphanage, New Jersey State Colony for the Feeble-Minded, and a mental hospital in Dixon, Illinois. Radiation experiments with several thousand individuals were also conducted during this time, and many times the exposed area had to be removed. Research during the war generally had very low consent standards, and as a result war time experiments were seen differently than patient experiments. Gregory Pence compared consent of research subjects to the selective service which did not require consent for being drafted. Pence conveys that some people went to war, while others were ordered to participate in research for things like vaccines. These views led up to the time of Nazi research, which involved some of the most appalling experimentation against humanity. During this time, there were numerous experiments conducted on unwilling individuals or prisoners like observational studies for differing altitudes, vaccination experiments, and

---

[54] Albert Jonsen, *A Short History of Medical Ethics*, 88–89; Albert Jonsen, *The Birth of Bioethics*, 130–133.

sterilization techniques. At Buchenwald in 1943–1945, prisoners, Jews, and other people involuntarily received trial typhus vaccines. Out of the 1000 injected, 158 individuals died from that experiment.[55]

Dr. Ernst Grawitz studied staphylococci by putting samples in women's legs, and then tried to identify drugs that would eliminate it. Dr. Sigmund Rascher studied hypothermia at Ravensbruck by subjecting naked prisoners to freezing water in order to identify revival procedures for pilots who crashed. Some of the worst research was with the "angel of death," Dr. Josef Mengele. Needing revolutionary research to become a Professor, Mengele started experimenting at Auschwitz in 1943. Pence expresses that his experiments tried to circumvent genetics by changing the individual's environment to create the perfect blonde hair, blue eyed person without disease. To cut down on the variables, he used about 150–200 twins from concentration camps. He tried to produce blue eyes by shooting dye in the eyes, transplant organs among twins, create twins by making them reproduce, and even surgically conjoin twins which resulted in gangrene. He used his twins to study the differences by infecting one and using the other as a control, after he had killed both. His research, based on eugenics, was responsible for approximately 400,000 deaths. Although he was never caught, the Nuremberg Tribunal tried 20 physicians and 3 medical administrators, charged with subjecting people involuntarily to research. In the end, nine of the accused got life prison sentences and seven were sentenced to death.[56]

As noted by Miller and Wertheimer, the Nuremberg Code was established in 1946 to protect against the harms and atrocities committed in the name of science.[57] The Code is typically recognized as the beginning of informed consent.[58] Requiring voluntary and free consent, the Code says that the individual needs enough information and understanding in order to make an informed decision.[59] These guidelines tried to provide increased attention on the dignity of research subjects when making decisions, but Dolgin and Shepherd suggest that the patient's decisions and consent will not be protected appropriately unless researchers adopt these obligations.[60] Jonsen articulates that the Code set forth the idea that research should benefit humanity while eliminating needless pain and promoting the responsibility to withdraw from dangerous research trials. Then later, the AMA House of Delegates approved regulations for the ethical use of human subject research on December 28, 1947 that were based on the Code. On July 14, 1949, Dr. Leo Alexander, a psychia-

---

[55] Gregory Pence, *Medical Ethics: Accounts of the Cases that Shaped and Define Medical Ethics*, 216; Michelle Byrne, "The Concept of Informed Consent in Qualitative Research," 401.

[56] Albert Jonsen, *The Birth of Bioethics*, 134–135; Gregory Pence, *Medical Ethics: Accounts of the Cases that Shaped and Define Medical Ethics*, 216–219, 232.

[57] Franklin Miller and Alan Wertheimer, *The Ethics of Consent*, 375; Albert Jonsen, *The Birth of Bioethics*, 134.

[58] Jose Miola, "The Need for Informed Consent: Lessons from the Ancient Greeks," 152.

[59] The Nuremberg Tribunal, "The Nuremberg Code (1947)," 433; Robert Levine, "Informed Consent: Some Challenges to the Universal Validity of the Western Model," 143; Paul Root Wolpe and Jon F. Merz, "Hospital ERs on Front Line in Informed-Consent Debate," 127.

[60] Janet Dolgin and Lois Shepherd, *Bioethics and the Law*, 411.

trist who had helped with the Tribunal, said that the Nazi experiments arose from both the pursuit of scientific knowledge and unsettling political and personal motivations. During this time, many people thought Americans were being polluted by utilitarianism which focused on the greater good and often ignored the individual's good. As a result of this, many did not grasp what happened in Germany. Several thought it was applicable only for savages and not the United States.[61] However, the next several years brought equally appalling research cases which occurred in the United States.

b. Mid 1900s

After the war, in the 1950s and 60s investigators were highly motivated to eliminate disease and sickness.[62] Charles McCarthy suggests that if there was no benefit to volunteers, then it was wrong to knowingly subject a person to an unauthorized assault on privacy without adequate consent.[63] One case that demonstrates this further was the Porton Down research. Ulf Schmidt describes the Porton Down research of 1953 in which gas and toxic smoke inhalation was studied. In this study, Professor Pulvertaft said that some soldiers might be getting persuaded to participate in research without adequate disclosure.[64] The NIH made policies in 1953 emphasizing the difference between healthy volunteers and patients.[65] One of the cases that demonstrate these ideas further is the Willowbrook study. In 1956 the Willowbrook case arose in New York at a hospital where most were mentally retarded. Drs. Saul Krugman, Joan Giles, and Jack Hammond, studying the effects and natural history of hepatitis, infected some of the new patients with hepatitis in hopes of developing a vaccine. Because the hospital let researchers experiment on many of the patients for the good of society, David and Sheila Rothman noted that the lines of treatment and research were blurred in this hospital.[66] Since most children would get hepatitis anyway by living there, the hospital considered this study to be acceptable. As clarified by Beauchamp and Childress, this research was justified by citing the immunity after and the safety of the children since they were away from others. But, the resulting immunity would also occur in others who recovered from the disease. Not being the main goal, immunity was an inadvertent side effect; albeit it was a positive side effect. However, the end result did not justify this experiment, because as stated by Jonsen, a research trial has to be ethical at the beginning. One problem with this study was the fact that there were other alternatives to decrease hepatitis such

---

[61] Albert Jonsen, *The Birth of Bioethics*, 134–137.

[62] Gregory Pence, *Medical Ethics: Accounts of the Cases that Shaped and Define Medical Ethics*, 219; Tom Beauchamp, "Informed Consent," 188.

[63] Charles McCarthy, "The Evolving Story of Justice in Federal Research Policy," 13.

[64] Ulf Schmidt, "Cold War at Porton Down: Informed Consent in Britain's Biological and Chemical Warfare Experiments," 371–372.

[65] Charles McCarthy, "The Evolving Story of Justice in Federal Research Policy," 13.

[66] David J. Rothman and Sheila M. Rothman, "The Willowbrook Hepatitis Studies," 750–752.

as a gamma-globulin vaccine, which had already been used to successfully lower the disease frequency at this institution. Opponents argue that the children should not be used to further scientific research, but that doctors have a responsibility to help the children. In regards to consent, one of the biggest problems with this study was the therapeutic misconception. The patients were confused as research subjects and vice versa. Another problem with consent was the way in which consent was obtained. At the beginning parents were sent letters or had private discussions with the physician, but towards the end, parents were grouped together to discuss the protocol. Researchers argued that this method of consent allowed them to have better consent, but all the risks might not have been given like cirrhosis or other deadly liver problems. Thus, it was not clear whether the parents actually understood what the study was and what the risks and benefits were.[67]

Then in the late 1950s, the area of placebos was brought up. There were a couple of studies that looked at procedures to treat angina. The experiment included consent of surgery for an internal mammary artery ligation, but it did not cover the fact that not everyone would have this procedure done. Some patients had a fake surgery, a placebo surgery, while others had the real procedure. Because researchers thought simple consent was acceptable at this time, this case was not questioned in the beginning. Thus in the beginning, obtaining simple consent was enough to conduct trials without disclosing what research was being done.[68] However, in time, other principles were added to consent that encouraged additional disclosure.

In the 1960s some ideas about research were starting to change, including the idea that the sole requirement for physician-investigators was to be responsible and truthful. On March 8, 1962, Merrell Pharmaceuticals had to withdraw its drug and tell people of the possible consequences of taking this medication. The Kefauver-Harris amendment, established by the FDA to regulate new medications, required proof of efficacy and voluntary consent of subjects in drug trials.[69] As clarified by Beauchamp, this amendment required doctors to tell people it was an experimental drug. During this time, the government was more involved in regulations for human subject research and protection. Another case that demonstrates there is more to evaluating an experiment than the researcher's beneficence and truthfulness was the Jewish Chronic Disease study. In July 1963, the Jewish Chronic Disease Hospital in Brooklyn conducted a research experiment involving older hospital patients with unclear competence levels. Dr. Chester Southam with Sloan-Kettering Institute for Cancer Research and Dr. Emmanuel Mandel with the Jewish Chronic Disease Hospital injected patients with cancer cells without their consent. Consenting to a skin test, the patients were not told about the cancer cells and research, because often mentioning cancer caused patients to be concerned and suspicious.[70] Since risk

---

[67] Tom Beauchamp and James Childress, *Principles of Biomedical Ethics*, 428–429; Albert Jonsen, *The Birth of Bioethics*, 153–154.

[68] Franklin Miller and Alan Wertheimer, *The Ethics of Consent*, 376–377.

[69] Albert Jonsen, *The Birth of Bioethics*, 141–142.

[70] Tom Beauchamp, "Informed Consent," 189; Barron H. Lerner, "Sins of Omission- Cancer Research without Informed Consent," 628–629.

was very low, the doctors did not mention cancer for the patient's best interest. Dr. Southam said that injecting cancer cells was not risky, but he was also hesitant to inject himself since there were a limited amount of cancer researchers. By stating it was a skin test and not research, confusion occurred which led people to assume it was treatment when it was not.[71] Miller and Wertheimer argue that Dr. Southam did not comprehend the important distinction of research and medical care.[72] Before consent is obtained, people need to know the differences between the research and typical medical care. In this case, both doctors' licenses were suspended, because they obtained consent through coercion and deception. The court said that passion and enthusiasm for research cannot disregard certain protections.[73]

In June 1964, the World Medical Association's guidelines for good research, "Principles for Those in Research and Experimentation," were updated and became the Helsinki Declaration. Jose Miola explains that the Helsinki Declaration, which was stronger than the Nuremberg Code, addressed the human dignity of all individuals and argued against the idea of deadly human experimentation. The Declaration also defined the difference of patient treatment research and nonclinical research, saying that trials without therapeutic benefit required additional safeguards.[74] While nonclinical research typically does not benefit the patient, the goal of clinical treatment research should solely be for the patient's benefit.[75] Another result of the Declaration was the ability of relatives or surrogates decision makers to give consent for those who are not able to make decisions for themselves.[76] While the Helsinki Declaration was very helpful to research safeguards, the Declaration discussed issues of consent together with being a good, trustworthy physician-investigator. As a result, Jonsen suggests that the implied decline in the significance of consent was due to many people thinking the only important aspect of research was the character and dependability of the researcher.[77]

Around the same time as the debates about research safeguards, Charles McCarthy explains that the NIH established a committee led by Robert Livingston to look into human subject research. Also at this time, Dr. Henry Beecher wrote an article which gave many examples of blatantly unethical research cases. Because of the many corrupt research cases, the committee went against the prevailing idea of that day and said there was more to decision making than just the views of the physician and researcher. As a result, the committee suggested the need for a regula-

---

[71] John D. Arras, "The Jewish Chronic Disease Hospital Case," 744.

[72] Franklin Miller and Alan Wertheimer, *The Ethics of Consent*, 377–379.

[73] Barron H. Lerner, "Sins of Omission- Cancer Research without Informed Consent," 629.

[74] Jose Miola, "The Need for Informed Consent: Lessons from the Ancient Greeks," 157; Paul Root Wolpe and Jon F. Merz, "Hospital ERs on Front Line in Informed-Consent Debate," 128.

[75] Tom Beauchamp and LeRoy Walters eds., *Contemporary Issues in Bioethics*, 431.

[76] Jessica W. Berg, Paul S. Applebaum, Charles W. Lidz, and Lisa S. Parker, *Informed Consent: Legal Theory and Clinical Practice*, 252–253; Debra Pinals and Paul Applebaum, "The History and Current Status of Competence and Informed Consent in Psychiatric Research," 86.

[77] Albert Jonsen, *The Birth of Bioethics*, 136; Nigel Cameron, *The New Medicine: Life and Death After Hippocrates*, 112.

tory body and oversight committee for human subject research.[78] Thus, Institutional Review Boards (IRBs) were established in 1966. IRBs try to eliminate unnecessary risk by analyzing the risks and benefits of a trial and encouraging consent before participation.[79] Consent during this time was especially important, because the line between research and medicine was continually being distorted.[80] As a result of the many challenging cases, the first written informed consent for research started at the NIH Clinical Center in Bethesda, MD in 1966, and other places implemented this towards the end of the 1970s.[81]

c. Late 1900s to early 2000

On July 26, 1972 the *New York Times* described one of the most appalling research cases in the United States, the Tuskegee Syphilis study. Lasting 40 years, the study involved approximately 600 black men from Tuskegee, Alabama who were un-knowingly given syphilis in order to study the effects on the body.[82] In the begin-ning the men were given free transportation, food, and medicine, but towards the middle in order to get them back to the hospital, the researchers sent letters saying that they had "bad blood" and needed medical care including spinal taps.[83] At the end, only 74 of the 400 men with diagnosed syphilis were alive. After Peter Buxtun complained about the study in 1966, the researchers reviewing the study decided to secretly continue, but in 1972 Buxtun told the story to a medical reporter. After the story broke, the Tuskegee Syphilis Study Ad Hoc Panel in 1972 had different conclusions, saying that the study should have never started and the study should be discontinued. This nightmare was made worse by the fact that the government regu-lated this project and never treated any of the individuals even after penicillin was readily available by 1948.[84] Dr. Wenger, head of a venereal disease clinic, said that the only way to get the men for autopsy was to put them in a government hospital to instill more confidence.[85] Because there were very limited policies for consent

---

[78] Charles McCarthy, "The Evolving Story of Justice in Federal Research Policy," 18–20; Albert Jonsen, *The Birth of Bioethics*, 142–143; Paul Root Wolpe and Jon F. Merz, "Hospital ERs on Front Line in Informed-Consent Debate," 128.

[79] Dale Whittington, "Ethical Issues with Contingent Valuation Surveys in Developing Countries: A Note on Informed Consent and Other Concerns," 507; Kenneth Getz and Deborah Borfitz, *Informed Consent: The Consumer's Guide to the Risks and Benefits of Volunteering for Clinical Trials*, 106.

[80] M. Sara Rosenthal, "Informed Consent in the Nuclear Medicine Setting," 2.

[81] Jeffrey Kahn, "Informed Consent in the Context of Communities," 918.

[82] Charles McCarthy, "The Evolving Story of Justice in Federal Research Policy," 21; Patricia King, "Race, Justice, and Research," 89.

[83] Albert Jonsen, *The Birth of Bioethics*, 147–148.

[84] Albert Jonsen, *The Birth of Bioethics*, 147–148; Gregory Pence, *Medical Ethics: Accounts of the Cases that Shaped and Define Medical Ethics*, 226.

[85] Allan M. Brandt, "Racism and Research: The Case of the Tuskegee Syphilis Study," 758.

procedures or for oversight committees in this study, IRBs became more popular and influential after this.[86] Jonsen notes that this case was the most significant for the public's view of ethics. A class-action suit against the government was settled in 1974 which gave compensation and free medical care for subjects and relatives of the deceased. However, it is unclear whether the people trusted the government for medical care after this. This case promulgated the many questions and concerns of research ethics and highlighted the importance race had during that time.[87]

Miller and Wertheimer explain that in 1974 the National Commission for the Protection of Human Subjects of Biomedical and Behavioral Research was created to establish ethical research guidelines.[88] Recognizing the need for consent of both healthy and sick volunteers, the Commission agreed on surrogate decision making for nontherapeutic research if there was lower than average risk. Looking at levels of risk, the Commission established some levels of protection. The Office for Protection from Research Risks (OPRR) was developed to analyze research guidelines and regulate compliance. In the 1970s, a discussion of research on prisoners started. Up until this point, a prisoner's sentence was reduced if he or she participated in research. However Jessica Mitford in her book, *Kind and Usual Punishment: The Prison Business*, said that prisons put unnecessary burdens and intimidation on individuals which created an intrinsic coercion. Originally thinking voluntary consent did not apply to prisoners, the Commission re-evaluated and concluded that research was permissible in some instances when risks and benefits were equitable, prisoners wanted to participate, and research would help the quality of medical care for prisoners. But since there was not enough emphasis on changing the prison system, prisoner research gradually decreased after March 1976 when the Justice Department eliminated the availability of most of those programs.[89] In 1977, some prisoners were given the option of being released from Newgate Prison if they participated in a smallpox vaccine trial. Since the standard sentence there was death by hanging, many considered themselves lucky since no one died during the trial.[90] When the National Commission put together their recommendations for patient protection and research, the organized guidelines became known as "The

---

[86] Tom Beauchamp, "Informed Consent," 189; Dale Whittington, "Ethical Issues with Contingent Valuation Surveys in Developing Countries: A Note on Informed Consent and Other Concerns," 508.

[87] Albert Jonsen, *The Birth of Bioethics*, 147–148; Gregory Pence, *Medical Ethics: Accounts of the Cases that Shaped and Define Medical Ethics*, 226; Allan M. Brandt, "Racism and Research: The Case of the Tuskegee Syphilis Study," 762.

[88] Franklin Miller and Alan Wertheimer, *The Ethics of Consent*, 59; Janet Dolgin and Lois Shepherd, *Bioethics and the Law*, 6; Robert Levine, "Informed Consent: Some Challenges to the Universal Validity of the Western Model," 143–144.

[89] Albert Jonsen, *The Birth of Bioethics*, 136, 151–157; Jessica W. Berg, Paul S. Applebaum, Charles W. Lidz, and Lisa S. Parker, *Informed Consent: Legal Theory and Clinical Practice*, 268–269.

[90] Tom Beauchamp and James Childress, *Principles of Biomedical Ethics*, 96.

Belmont Report" in 1979.[91] The Report emphasized the importance of autonomy and beneficence in order to protect the research subjects.[92]

Then the Common Rule was adopted for research in 1991. This rule defined minimal risk as nothing more than an ordinary risk of everyday life. Minimal risk was used in evaluating whether or not an individual should participate in a research study.[93] One case that raised questions about minimal risk was a case at the University of California at Los Angeles (UCLA) in 1994. As described by Pinals and Applebaum, this case observed psychotic patients after withdrawing their medication in order to study the disorder relapse. One of the problems with this study was the fact that research said if a person is taken off a medication, then sometimes that person will not be able to respond as well the next time. This study also brought attention to the use of placebos for people already on beneficial medications.[94] Because there was a chance the individual could have residual effects from this study, it was not clear whether this was considered a minimal risk or not. In addition to minimal risk discussions, because this case studied psychotic patents with no medication, questions about competency and vulnerable populations arose as well.

In 1995, the Advisory Committee on Human Radiation Experiments (ACHRE) looked into human subject research in 1944 to 1974.[95]In about half of the cases, the committee found the disclosure of risks and other material information was lacking and there was little concern for those with limited decision-making capabilities. The National Bioethics Advisory Commission's (NBAC) analyzed these cases in their report, "Research Involving Persons with Mental Disorders That May Affect Decisionmaking Capacity." The report recommended having an independent professional analyze a person's capacity to consent to research if there was a greater than average risk.[96] Also the ACHRE recommended apologizing for some studies, because some of the worst cases led to a significant lack of trust in the medical system.[97] In 1997, President Clinton officially apologized for the Tuskegee Syphilis

---

[91] Janet Dolgin and Lois Shepherd, *Bioethics and the Law*, 6, 439; Tom Beauchamp, *Standing on Principles*, 3–4.

[92] The National Commission for the Protection of Human Subjects of Biomedical and Behavioral Research, "The Belmont Report: Ethical Principles and Guidelines for the Protection of Human Subjects of Research," 765–766; Kenneth Getz and Deborah Borfitz, *Informed Consent: The Consumer's Guide to the Risks and Benefits of Volunteering for Clinical Trials*, 103.

[93] Benjamin Freedman, Abraham Fuks, and Charles Weijer, "In Loco Parentis: Minimal Risk as an Ethical Threshold for Research upon Children," 829; Paul Root Wolpe and Jon F. Merz, "Hospital ERs on Front Line in Informed-Consent Debate," 128; Misha Angrist, "Eyes Wide Open: The Personal Genome Project, Citizen Science and Veracity in Informed Consent," 691.

[94] Debra Pinals and Paul Applebaum, "The History and Current Status of Competence and Informed Consent in Psychiatric Research," 82–83, 86.

[95] Advisory Committee on Human Radiation Experiments, "Final Report: Executive Summary (1995)," 479; Charles McCarthy, "The Evolving Story of Justice in Federal Research Policy," 27.

[96] Debra Pinals and Paul Applebaum, "The History and Current Status of Competence and Informed Consent in Psychiatric Research," 83–84.

[97] Advisory Committee on Human Radiation Experiments, "Final Report: Executive Summary (1995)," 482; Gregory Pence, *Medical Ethics: Accounts of the Cases that Shaped and Define Medical Ethics*, 226, 232–233; Albert Jonsen, *The Birth of Bioethics*, 139.

Study.[98] At that time, $10 million from the government went to the subjects and/or relatives of the Study.[99]

In 1999, 18 year-old Jesse Gelsinger died from complications of an experimental study looking at ornithine transcarbamylase deficiency (OTC) at the University of Pennsylvania. Andrew Thompson and Norman Temple note that while the study would not benefit him, Jesse understood it had a chance of helping others. But 4 days after the procedure, he died from multiple organ failure.[100] A wrongful death suit was brought against Dr. Wilson saying he was aware the virus had caused problems in the past for people with OTC. It was later identified that Dr. Wilson had financial conflicts of interests with the company responsible for the adenovirus. The claim argued that Dr. Wilson did not use clear language so that the family could understand plainly what was involved. Over the next several years, the NIH, having strict guidelines, suspended clinical research at several research universities.[101]

Then in the early 2000s, a couple of cases dealt with inadequate disclosure. The first case occurred in 2000 in Uganda. Enrolling about 15,000 people, this study looked at questions about HIV transmission. As clarified by Paul Farmer and Nicole Gastineau Campos, the report said that the participants were not told about treatment and spouses were not told about the other spouse's disease status.[102] The second case occurred in 2001 in the United States. In 2001, researchers of the Krieger lead paint study solicited people to move into houses with lead paint.[103] The Institute enrolled 108 lower economic families, but did not tell them of the risk of mental retardation from lead paint. Maryland Judge Dale Cathell held that the board had suggested researchers drew up forms circumventing regulations for risk disclosure. One critic compared the children to canaries used in mining.[104] As a result, there were several lawsuits from parents of children suffering from complications such as learning disabilities. The court argued that parents and researchers could not deliberately expose children to harmful situations where no benefit was expected.[105] This

---

[98] William J. Clinton, "In Apology for the Study Done in Tuskegee," 402–403.

[99] Patricia King, "Race, Justice, and Research," 101.

[100] Andrew Thompson and Norman J. Temple eds., *Ethics, Medical Research, and Medicine: Commercialism versus Environmentalism and Social Justice,* 158–160.

[101] Gregory Pence, *Medical Ethics: Accounts of the Cases that Shaped and Define Medical Ethics,* 233–235; Kenneth Getz and Deborah Borfitz, *Informed Consent: The Consumer's Guide to the Risks and Benefits of Volunteering for Clinical Trials,* 144.

[102] Paul Farmer and Nicole Gastineau Campos, "New Malaise: Bioethics and Human Rights in the Global Era," 294.

[103] Alex John London, "Children and "Minimal Risk" Research: The Kennedy-Krieger Lead Paint Study," 811–812; David Buchanan and Franklin G. Miller, "Justice in Research on Human Subjects," 386–387.

[104] Gregory Pence, *Medical Ethics: Accounts of the Cases that Shaped and Define Medical Ethics,* 233–235.

[105] Alex John London, "Children and "Minimal Risk" Research: The Kennedy-Krieger Lead Paint Study," 813.

was a major case for research involving children since there was no possibility of benefit. Both cases illustrate a lack of disclosure to research subjects.

In 2003, the Greenberg v. Miami Children's Hospital Research Institute case in Florida evaluated the research under Dr. Matalon. In 1987 Dr. Matalon joined Dr. Greenberg to identify the Canavan gene in order to create a genetic screening test. Dr. Greenberg and the Chicago Chapter of the National Tay-Sachs and Allied Diseases Association (NTSAD), Inc. asked the Canavan families to give some tissue samples and money to help their research progress. As a result of the information, Dr. Greenberg and the NTSAD created a registry with medical and social information about the families. After changing workplaces in 1990, Dr. Matalon continued his research and the families continued giving him their support. In 1993, Dr. Matalon found the gene, applied for a patent on September 1994, and became the sole inventor on the patent in October 1997. A year later, the families said that Miami Children's Hospital and Research Institute were pressuring testing centers with legal actions and royalty fees as a result of the patent. However, the families claimed that Dr. Matalon and Miami Children's breached the informed consent by not informing the families of the patent and the potential fees. Since the families thought the test would not be commercialized in order to lower the cost and find a cure, they said they might not have participated in the research if they knew otherwise. However, the court ruled against the families, because the families were seen more as contributors of money and samples.[106]

3. Conclusion

Consent is generally required to minimize harm to both the patient and research subject. However, when studying these two areas, the history illustrates some of the complexities of differentiating between clinical and research consent. In 1962 Walter Modell argued that a patient automatically consents to research when going to a doctor for help even if he or she did not explicitly give consent. Through the many cases that shaped consent requirements, clinical and research authorization were further delineated. The Jewish Chronic Disease Hospital case illustrates that differentiating between the clinical and research context is especially important for consent. If research enlists vulnerable populations where patients are confused with participants, then informed consent has not occurred adequately.[107] Thus, Laura Weiss Roberts suggests that people need to recognize the differences between clinical and research contexts and objectives before consent is given. If research participants do not realize the experiment has no medical benefit for them personally, then therapeutic misconception exists and consent should be questioned.[108]

---

[106] Janet Dolgin and Lois Shepherd, *Bioethics and the Law*, 65–66, 68.
[107] Franklin Miller and Alan Wertheimer, *The Ethics of Consent*, 58, 376, 382.
[108] Laura Weiss Roberts, "Informed Consent and the Capacity for Voluntarism," 708–709.

Because new developments in genetics have the opportunity for both research subject and patient treatment models of consent, this book will adopt both for PGT. Since genetic testing can reveal many different treatment options, consent for PGT should have a strong patient treatment focus. On the other hand, since PGT can perform research on the resulting information, consent should have an emphasis on a research subject model as well. While both approaches will be used in certain situations, the main focus of PGT for this work will be on the patient treatment model.

B. Emergence of the Components of Informed Consent

The second section discusses the emergence of the components of consent within the historical setting. By evaluating the historical, ethical, and legal aspects of consent, a greater view of consent is possible.[109] This section will analyze the current components of consent that have arisen from history. In order for there to be adequate consent, Tom Beauchamp suggests evaluating three aspects. First, there has to be an understanding of the information. Second, after evaluating the disclosed information and recommendations, a decision can be made and permission obtained. Third, consent has to be voluntary without undue sources of coercion.[110] After taking into account those aspects, an individual should be able to give a reasonably justified consent for a procedure or study. These three components will be looked at further in the proceeding sections.

The first area will look at comprehension. Specific examples and cases will be discussed in relation to the history. Then the concepts of autonomy, competence, and understanding will be discussed further. The second area will focus on disclosure looking at the history, the standards, and the information that is typically included in disclosure. The third and last area that will be discussed is voluntariness. This area will give specific examples of cases that demonstrated voluntariness or a lack of voluntariness. Then the concepts that arose from the historical examples of informed consent will be analyzed further in regards to voluntariness. Each category will discuss the questions that arise from the idea of what comprises informed consent.

---

[109] Susan Marr, "Protect Your Practice: Informed Consent," 180.

[110] Tom Beauchamp, "Informed Consent," 185–186; The National Commission for the Protection of Human Subjects of Biomedical and Behavioral Research, "The Belmont Report: Ethical Principles and Guidelines for the Protection of Human Subjects of Research," 767; Debra Pinals and Paul Applebaum, "The History and Current Status of Competence and Informed Consent in Psychiatric Research," 84; Bernard Gert, Charles Culver, and K. Clouser, *Bioethics: A Systematic Approach,* 213; Debbie Schachter, Sukirtha Tharmalingam, and Irwin Kleinman, "Informed Consent and Stimulant Medication: Adolescents' and Parents' Ability to Understand Information about Benefits and Risks of Stimulant Medication for the Treatment of Attention-Deficient/Hyperactivity Disorder," 139; Jeffrey Carlisle and Ann T. Neulicht, "The Necessity of Professional Disclosure and Informed Consent for Rehabilitation Counselors," 25; James Childress, *Who Should Decide? Paternalism in Health Care, 134.*

1. Comprehension

The first section deals with comprehension in relation to informed consent. The history of comprehension with specific examples will be analyzed at the beginning. Then the ideas which arose from the history of consent and comprehension are broken down and discussed further. Those ideas include autonomy, competence, and understanding.

a. History

The relationship between comprehension and autonomy has been formulated throughout history. Stephen Wear expresses that at the beginning, doctors assumed patients consented to treatment, because the patients sought the doctor out for a problem. Often the mere presence of the patient was enough to signal permission to the doctor, even if the patient did not understand everything involved in the treatment.[111] This practice supported the idea that physicians were in charge and that the autonomy of the patient did not matter. Paternalism was the overwhelming principle during that time. However, in the seventeenth century, De Sorbiere, a French doctor and philosopher, thought about full disclosure, but then said it was not practical and could lead to a lack of physician trust. He argued that this idea might make patients question whether or not he was able to practice medicine properly. In addition, he said that normally patients would not be able to understand enough to make an intelligent decision.[112] Even though he dismissed the idea, he did acknowledge that some people might be able to give consent for themselves. This idea would be developed later.

Albert Jonsen explains that the Walter Reed yellow fever experiments around 1880 encouraged the ideas of autonomy and comprehension in research consent. Following that case, Dr. Charles Francis Withington in 1886 argued that people should be able to consent to research themselves. Toward the twentieth century, Mark Twain suggested that faith and confidence in the doctor was all that was required at the time. Around 1903 Richard Cabot expressed that patients should be informed and physicians should disclose some information. However because paternalism was still prevalent at the time, Cabot was not arguing that patients should make decisions themselves. He was arguing for more information with simple consent. A little later Dr. Francis Moore supported the ideas of Cabot that physicians should discuss the dangers of treatment with the patients. But as he noted, since patients do not have adequate education or evaluation skills to make that decision, the patient should not be allowed to actually make the decision.[113] The *Schloendorff*

---

[111] Stephen Wear, *Informed Consent: Patient Autonomy and Clinician Beneficence within Health Care,* 34.

[112] Alfred Tauber, *Patient Autonomy and the Ethics of Responsibility,* 67.

[113] Albert Jonsen, *The Birth of Bioethics,* 131–132, 199; Alfred Tauber, *Patient Autonomy and the Ethics of Responsibility,* 74–75.

v. the Society of the New York Hospitals case in 1914 started the new emphasis on
patient autonomy. Justice Benjamin Cardozo's famous quote demonstrated a new
emphasis on patient self-determination.[114] Because the Nazi experiments lacked autonomy and comprehension of risks, the Nuremberg Code was needed to establish
the requirement of adequate understanding for research.[115] The Willowbrook study
in 1956 was another case illustrating insufficient consent and comprehension of
risks.[116] While autonomy was starting to progress, the idea of comprehension of
risks and benefits also started to arise. The 1957 case, *Salgo v. Leland Stanford
Junior University Board of Trustees,* concluded that some information needed to be
discussed with the patient in order to encourage understanding. However, if confusion exists about the differences between research and treatment, understanding
is not present. The Jewish Chronic Disease Hospital case in 1963 illustrates the
confusion that existed among comprehension and research consent. One witness
in Southam's defense said that consent was adequate, because there was no risk.
The witness suggested that a minimal level of risk was enough to satisfy consent.[117]
Also since the participants thought the research was for their benefit, the patients
evidently did not comprehend or understand the experiment. Then later the court in
the *Canterbury v. Spence* case took comprehension further and said that autonomy
depends on the amount of information that is needed for an enlightened decision.[118]
The Tuskegee Syphilis study demonstrated an alarming lack of autonomy and comprehension.[119]

One of the cases that illustrate many aspects of comprehension and consent was
the suicide of Dr. Chad Calland with the UCSF School of Medicine after having 5
kidney transplants. An article, "Iatrogenic Problems in End-Stage Renal Failure,"
published right after his death, said that his doctors, who were also his friends, did
not understand his goals of treatment and values concerning quality of life and
dialysis. He was concerned about the differences in viewpoints and suggested that
patients suffered unsympathetic treatment. In response to those events, there was
a conference. At the conference Albert Jonsen noted that sometimes there can be a
difference in how physicians and patients view success or failure. While a doctor
often looks at medical aspects to measure success, patients often look at values and
quality of life. This case emphasizes the autonomy and understanding of patients
when consenting to treatment. Later, Charles Fried's *Medical Experimentation:*

---

[114] Jerry Menikoff, *Law and Bioethics: An Introduction,* 306; Linda Farber Post, Jeffrey Blustein,
and Nancy Neveloff Dubler, *Handbook for Health Care Ethics Committees,* 286.

[115] Gregory Pence, *Medical Ethics: Accounts of the Cases that Shaped and Define Medical Ethics,*
218–219; Franklin Miller and Alan Wertheimer, *The Ethics of Consent,* 387; Nigel Cameron, The
New Medicine, 85.

[116] Stephen Wear, *Informed Consent: Patient Autonomy and Clinician Beneficence within Health
Care,* 31.

[117] Franklin Miller and Alan Wertheimer, *The Ethics of Consent,* 378–379.

[118] Tom Beauchamp, "Informed Consent," 190; Spottswood W. Robinson, "United States Court of
Appeals Canterbury v. Spence," 133–134; Susan Marr, "Protect Your Practice: Informed Consent,"
180.

[119] Stephen Wear, *Informed Consent: Patient Autonomy and Clinician Beneficence within Health
Care,* 30–31.

Personal Integrity and Social Policy put individual autonomy above the good of society.[120] The Belmont Report in 1979 based the justification of consent on autonomy.[121] As a result of these examples, autonomy began to be the primary concern for consent. Around 1981, the AMA supported consent as a key requirement to ensure the autonomy of patients, and this policy applied to even the reluctant physicians.[122] However, in order to promote autonomy, the patient has to have adequate information to make a decision. As a result, the competency of the patient or subject was linked to comprehension for consent. The AMA document said that competent individuals did not have to arrive at the same conclusions; consent did not have to result in similar decisions.[123] But then in 1994, the UCLA case came into question, because it was not clear the psychiatric patients were competent to make a decision about research participation. In 1995, NBAC gave guidelines for human subject research which included an area on competency. The report said that if risk is lower, sometimes surrogates can make decisions to let a person participate. While this report tried to establish guidelines to help protect vulnerable patients, some doctors thought the report categorized all patients with psychiatric problems as incompetent. However, Pinals and Applebaum point out that it is wrong to assume all mentally ill are unable to consent.[124] The risks involved in the Jesse Gelsinger case and the Krieger lead paint study were not clearly explained enough, and as a result comprehension was lacking and consent was questionable.[125]

Jay Katz concludes that many physicians thought patients were not educated enough to make appropriate choices. Thus, physicians assumed responsibility for their patients. Katz suggests that if the law of consent is to change, then judges have to have a practical vision for applying autonomy. Because the rules of autonomy were so new, sometimes doctors applied them more extensively than initially intended.[126] As a result, the emphasis of autonomy today is typically the most prevalent when looking at consent.

b. Autonomy

Autonomy is often cited as a major principle of informed consent.[127] Autonomy can encourage patients to make their own decisions, promote personal goals, and become more active in their health. Thus, an autonomous choice reflects the patient's

---

[120] Albert Jonsen, *The Birth of Bioethics*, 152–153, 199–200.

[121] Franklin Miller and Alan Wertheimer, *The Ethics of Consent*, 59; Tom Beauchamp, *Standing on Principles*, 7, 9.

[122] Tom Beauchamp, "Informed Consent," 190.

[123] Alfred Tauber, *Patient Autonomy and the Ethics of Responsibility*, 77.

[124] Debra Pinals and Paul Applebaum, "The History and Current Status of Competence and Informed Consent in Psychiatric Research," 89.

[125] Gregory Pence, *Medical Ethics: Accounts of the Cases that Shaped and Define Medical Ethics*, 233–235.

[126] Jay Katz, "Physicians and Patients: A History of Silence," 136, 138.

[127] Neil C. Manson and Onora O'Neill, *Rethinking Informed Consent in Bioethics*, 70; Clare M. Delany, "Respecting Patient Autonomy and Obtaining Their Informed Consent: Ethical Theory-

values and beliefs.[128] Since physicians do not always know how specific treatments will affect a patient's values or relationships, individual patients are in a better position to make their own decisions.[129] However, sometimes there are personal or external pressures like misunderstandings that can cause the individual's autonomy to be reduced.[130] As a result, the individual needs to be aware of the limitations of autonomy on decision making. In summary, Berg, Applebaum, Lidz, and Parker explain that it is the philosophical underpinnings of Mill's liberty principles to be free and Kant's moral obligations for independence that allows people to act autonomously.[131]

While the basis of autonomy is now firmly held, the ideas of autonomy have shifted throughout the history of consent.[132] In the beginning, there was a strong paternalistic view of patients and doctors.[133] Paternalism is linked back to Hippocrates who said that healing can be promoted by hiding certain medical facts.[134] During this time, physicians were told to instruct patients, to promote obedience, and to rebuke those not following orders.[135] Encouraging obedience was to protect the patient against his or her own emotions and fears so as not to make impulsive decisions. Paternalists did not see the point in causing patients pain with the possible uncertainties of treatment. If physicians did not follow those guidelines, then some equated this as abandoning the patient. The popular view for that time was that M.D. stood for "make decision," and if the physician was not able to make a decision, then he did not belong in medicine.[136] While paternalism was based on a strong view of beneficence towards the patient, paternalism was questioned in the twentieth century. After numerous cases brought the honesty and accountability of physicians and researchers under review, the emphasis of paternalism was

---

Missing in Action," 198–199; Howard Brody, *Ethical Decisions in Medicine,* 199; Bruce Jennings, "Autonomy," 77.

[128] John O. Beahrs and Thomas G. Gutheil, "Informed Consent in Psychotherapy," 4–5; Dan Brock, "Patient Competence and Surrogate Decision-Making," 133; Onora O'Neill, *Autonomy and Trust in Bioethics,* 28; John Williams, "Consent," 11; Willard Gaylin and Bruce Jennings, *The Perversion of Autonomy,* 4; M. Sara Rosenthal, "Informed Consent in the Nuclear Medicine Setting," 1, 3.

[129] Robert Veatch, "Abandoning Informed Consent," 7, 9.

[130] Tom Beauchamp and James Childress, *Principles of Biomedical Ethics,* 58.

[131] Jessica W. Berg, Paul S. Applebaum, Charles W. Lidz, and Lisa S. Parker, *Informed Consent: Legal Theory and Clinical Practice,* 16, 24.

[132] Roberta M. Berry, "Informed Consent Law, Ethics, and Practice: From Infancy to Reflective Adolescence," 70; Janet L. Dolgin, "The Legal Development of the Informed Consent Doctrine: Past and Present," 97.

[133] Tom L. Beauchamp, "Informed Consent: Its History, Meaning, and Present Challenges," 515; Barron H. Lerner, "Beyond Informed Consent: Did Cancer Patients Challenge Their Physicians in the Post-World War II Era?" 508–509.

[134] Alfred Tauber, *Patient Autonomy and the Ethics of Responsibility,* 66–67; Jay Katz, "Informed Consent- Must It Remain a Fairy Tale?" 159.

[135] Albert Jonsen, *The Birth of Bioethics,* 354.

[136] Stephen Wear, *Informed Consent: Patient Autonomy and Clinician Beneficence within Health Care,* 34, 38.

beginning to dwindle.[137] As a result, people started to endorse autonomy to promote their safety and beneficence. As clarified by Wear, the autonomy vs. paternalism debate is not between right or wrong, but between completely different goals for medicine.[138] A different way of explaining this point is made by Edmund Pellegrino who notes that a strong emphasis on beneficence will lead to promoting good, but sometimes the level of beneficence that is needed or wanted can be difficult to balance in medicine.[139] Even though physicians might know what the best option is, doing it without consent is a mistake.[140]

One area that often arises in autonomy is the question of application. Neil Manson and Onora O'Neill ask the questiondoes it matter that autonomous choices could be bad, right or wrong, or possibly detrimental? Some physicians and researchers argue that recommendations should only suggest those on an agreed upon list, because patients should not be able to ask for every type of treatment possible.[141] However, there is not just one acceptable option for each decision.[142] Katz expresses that while the law regulates people's actions to ensure a safe society for others, the law typically cannot regulate personal decisions. Since the majority of the risk is to the individual person agreeing to a procedure or trial, this area of consent is largely uncertain.[143] People have unsafe behaviors and actions all the time while knowing the consequences, such as eating too much or smoking.[144] While some decisions can seem irrational to some, other people might think the decisions are well thought out. Decisions do not always have to be uniform and standardized.[145] Another way of noting this was made by Katz explaining that since the opinions and beliefs of doctors and patients are typically not the same, a person's individual decision might not make sense to the doctor, but that does not mean the decision is wrong.[146] Choices of a competent, accountable person can be valid even if others view their decisions as faulty or mistaken and if their values are not the same as everyone else's.[147] In our

---

[137] Jessica W. Berg, Paul S. Applebaum, Charles W. Lidz, and Lisa S. Parker, *Informed Consent: Legal Theory and Clinical Practice*, 20; Robert Veatch, "Abandoning Informed Consent," 6; Jeffrey Carlisle and Ann T. Neulicht, "The Necessity of Professional Disclosure and Informed Consent for Rehabilitation Counselors," 28; Onora O'Neill, *Autonomy and Trust in Bioethics*, 2, 8,11; George Annas, *American Bioethics: Crossing Human Rights and Health Law Boundaries*, 95; Tom Beauchamp, "Informed Consent: Its History and Meaning," 59–60.

[138] Stephen Wear, *Informed Consent: Patient Autonomy and Clinician Beneficence within Health Care*, 33.

[139] Edmund Pellegrino, "Benefit and Harm," 102.

[140] Robert Veatch, "Abandoning Informed Consent," 7, 9.

[141] Neil C. Manson and Onora O'Neill, *Rethinking Informed Consent in Bioethics*, 70–71.

[142] Donald Evans, "Autonomy and Individual Responsibility," 119.

[143] Jay Katz, "Physicians and Patients: A History of Silence," 137.

[144] Alan Goldman, "The Refutation of Medical Paternalism," 68.

[145] Susan Marr, "Protect Your Practice: Informed Consent," 180.

[146] Jay Katz, "Physicians and Patients: A History of Silence," 137–138.

[147] H. Tristram Engelhardt Jr., *The Foundations of Bioethics*, 305; Willard Gaylin and Bruce Jennings, *The Perversion of Autonomy*, 4.

culture, individual autonomy is promoted even if others can make a better choice.[148] The application of individual autonomy on decision making is still being debated.[149]

In conclusion, the tensions between autonomy and the physician's responsibility to care for patients have led to regulations that can increase a patient's rights to choose but decrease liberty.[150] More is needed for consent than just a poor view of autonomy, which in the past has been promoted by selecting an option.[151] As clarified by Terrence Ackerman, autonomy is generally linked with noninterference, but sometimes noninterference does not respect a person's autonomy. If sickness impacts autonomy and a physician is neutral, then that noninterference can limit a person's decisions.[152] E. Haavi Morreim takes that idea further when explaining that by focusing solely on human freedom, the moral principle of responsibility can be overlooked. Thus noninterference should not be the ideal emphasis of autonomy.[153] Instead Engelhardt argues that autonomy should be viewed as an agreement so that even people with dissimilar values can respect other people's independence and choices.[154] While autonomy might be an illusion today, there can be approaches to encourage a deeper autonomy for the future.[155]

c. Competence

In order to have comprehension and autonomy, Leclercq, Keulers Scheltinga, et al. suggest that a patient must first be competent to make decisions for him- or herself.[156] Sometimes the terms competence and capacity are used interchangeably, but capacity is a legal term while competence is the general term used for decision-making ability. Because capacity cannot be determined without a legal assessment, this book focuses on competence for decision making.[157] Grisso and Applebaum suggest that competence is seen as having knowledge of the circumstances and

---

[148] Thomas Grisso and Paul S. Applebaum, *Assessing Competence to Consent to Treatment,* 12.

[149] Leon Eisenberg, "The Social Imperatives of Medical Research," 454.

[150] Jay Katz, "Physicians and Patients: A History of Silence," 136.

[151] Neil C. Manson and Onora O'Neill, *Rethinking Informed Consent in Bioethics*, 70.

[152] Terrence Ackerman, "Why Doctors Should Intervene," 75.

[153] E. H. Morreim, *Balancing Act: The New Medical Ethics of Medicine's New Economics*, 134–135; Roberta M. Berry, "Informed Consent Law, Ethics, and Practice: From Infancy to Reflective Adolescence," 69–70.

[154] H. Tristram Engelhardt Jr., *The Foundations of Bioethics*, 69, 102–103.

[155] Jay Katz, "Physicians and Patients: A History of Silence," 138.

[156] Wouter Leclercq, Bram J. Keulers, Marc R. M. Scheltinga, et al., "A Review of Surgical Informed Consent: Past, Present, and Future. A Quest to Help Patients Make Better Decisions," 1406.

[157] Debbie Schachter, Sukirtha Tharmalingam, and Irwin Kleinman, "Informed Consent and Stimulant Medication: Adolescents' and Parents' Ability to Understand Information about Benefits and Risks of Stimulant Medication for the Treatment of Attention-Deficient/Hyperactivity Disorder," 139.

demonstrating reasoning abilities.[158] But in order to show there is adequate knowledge and reasoning, people need to be able to communicate their ideas.[159] These three areas are the basis of the discussion on competence and will be analyzed further.

Competence for decision making generally looks at three areas: understanding the facts, evaluating the information, and communicating a choice. First, Berg, Applebaum, Lidz, and Parker explain that in order for an individual to be competent, the person should have the potential to understand.[160] People should understand the facts of disclosure and their circumstances. This area is often debated, because the level of understanding is not always straightforward. Sometimes the level of risk affects the level of understanding that is needed. If a treatment or research proposal is risky, then participants should generally have a higher level of understanding. One study by Benson et al. illustrates that with additional education and discussion, patients with some mental deficiencies could have an acceptable level of understanding in some areas. Also, because a person's beliefs about their condition can affect the level of understanding that is exhibited, the person should have a proper view of their disease. People who do not believe they are sick will have a harder time understanding and adequately consenting to treatment or research participation. Then specifically in regards to research participation, understanding also should include appreciating the fact that this research is not therapeutic in nature.[161] The individual should understand the disclosed information, the individual's condition, and the nature of the research study if applicable. Second, the person should be able to apply and evaluate the information. While the decision does not have to be the one accepted by everyone else, the person needs to be able to demonstrate reasoning capabilities. Sometimes people with and without mental deficiencies can have trouble with this. Demonstrating reasoning abilities is an important aspect of competence.[162] Being able to evaluate the information that was presented will help in reaching a decision. Third, after understanding and evaluating the information, a person has to be able to make and communicate a decision. An important aspect of this is that the decision should be consistent over time. If a person is constantly changing the decision, sometimes that can signal psychological problems caus-

---

[158] Thomas Grisso and Paul S. Applebaum, *Assessing Competence to Consent to Treatment*, 10–11; M. Sara Rosenthal, "Informed Consent in the Nuclear Medicine Setting," 2.

[159] Hana Osman, "History and Development of the Doctrine of Informed Consent," 45.

[160] Jessica W. Berg, Paul S. Applebaum, Charles W. Lidz, and Lisa S. Parker, *Informed Consent: Legal Theory and Clinical Practice*, 100–101; Thomas Grisso and Paul S. Applebaum, *Assessing Competence to Consent to Treatment*, 34–35.

[161] Debra Pinals and Paul Applebaum, "The History and Current Status of Competence and Informed Consent in Psychiatric Research," 85–87; Dan Brock, "Patient Competence and Surrogate Decision-Making," 130; Thomas Grisso and Paul S. Applebaum, *Assessing Competence to Consent to Treatment*, 10–11, 43, 51; H. Tristram, Engelhardt Jr., *The Foundations of Bioethics*, 306.

[162] Debra Pinals and Paul Applebaum, "The History and Current Status of Competence and Informed Consent in Psychiatric Research," 85–87; Dan Brock, "Patient Competence and Surrogate Decision-Making," 130.

ing competence to be questioned.[163] This last area should demonstrate a deliberate choice. Childress argues that approval is different than informed consent. A person may approve of the research, but that does not mean the individual has given his consent to participate in the research.[164] All three of these areas are generally analyzed when looking into the competence of an individual.

Even after assessing competence there is some debate about certain groups that might not be able to make decisions adequately like children or the mentally ill.[165] The debate around children looks at whether they are mature enough to analyze the information in relation to their goals.[166] This aspect is even more complicated while looking at research participation. When looking into justifications for research involving children, Paul Ramsey suggests that sometimes faulty motivations can be attributed to children. Often research participation is justified in adults, because the adults have an interest in promoting a certain medical cause; however, children are not the same, and most do not wish to promote a cause like a cancer walk. Ramsey concludes that parents should not be able to consent for their children to be entered into a non-therapeutic study.[167] Thus the competence and justifications of consent to research participation involving children is a very complex matter. Another group that might not be able to make decisions adequately is those with mental diseases. By looking at the MacArthur Treatment Competence study, Pinals and Appelbaum conclude that those with psychological problems should not automatically be assumed incompetent. If a certain group is presumed to be incompetent and left out of studies, then sometimes the results are not applicable to all groups. As a result, the authors suggest degrees of competence for decision making.[168] Often the more serious procedures or research studies require a higher level of assurance that the patient is competent.[169] Even when there are groups with limited abilities, assessments have to be made before assuming incompetence. Sometimes after additional time and education, competence can be encouraged.[170]

---

[163] Debra Pinals and Paul Applebaum, "The History and Current Status of Competence and Informed Consent in Psychiatric Research," 85–87.

[164] James Childress, *Who Should Decide? Paternalism in Health Care*, 78; Wouter Leclercq, Bram J. Keulers. Marc R. M. Scheltinga, et al., "A Review of Surgical Informed Consent: Past, Present, and Future. A Quest to Help Patients Make Better Decisions," 1410.

[165] Donald Evans, "Autonomy and Individual Responsibility," 119; Jason Karlawish, "Research on Cognitively Impaired Adults," 599, 602.

[166] Debbie Schachter, Sukirtha Tharmalingam, and Irwin Kleinman, "Informed Consent and Stimulant Medication: Adolescents' and Parents' Ability to Understand Information about Benefits and Risks of Stimulant Medication for the Treatment of Attention-Deficient/Hyperactivity Disorder," 139.

[167] Paul Ramsey, *The Patient as Person: Explorations in Medical Ethics*, 1, 5, 11–12; Thomas H. Murray, "Research on Children and the Scope of Responsible Parenthood," 819.

[168] Debra Pinals and Paul Applebaum, "The History and Current Status of Competence and Informed Consent in Psychiatric Research," 85–88, 90–91; Dan Brock, "Patient Competence and Surrogate Decision-Making," 130; Thomas Grisso and Paul S. Applebaum, *Assessing Competence to Consent to Treatment,* 10–11.

[169] M. Sara Rosenthal, "Informed Consent in the Nuclear Medicine Setting," 2.

[170] Jessica W. Berg, Paul S. Applebaum, Charles W. Lidz, and Lisa S. Parker, *Informed Consent: Legal Theory and Clinical Practice*, 99; Thomas Grisso and Paul S. Applebaum, *Assessing Com-*

d. Understanding

Informed consent can focus on information, understanding, or both.[171] Schachter, Tharmalingam, and Kleinman point out that understanding is not the same as remembering information.[172] In order to promote understanding, both information and education are needed.[173] Because understanding is typically more involved than merely presenting a list of facts, many times information is emphasized over understanding. Even though understanding is the ideal, understanding is not always present in medical and research cases.[174] Some people argue that medical information is too complex to understand or that the patient's decision-making skills are not adequate. Often the question asked is can sick patients understand and apply the medical information while handling the doubts and ambiguities that are common in medicine.[175] In response, Dan Brock notes that this cynicism is not necessary. He suggests that patients only need to understand what will happen if no treatment occurs and how the risks, benefits, and treatments will affect their quality of life. If doctors explain all of this, then patients should be able to make informed decisions.[176]

However, there are some aspects that can limit understanding as well. First, one of the problems discussed in a study on research protocols in Europe and the USA was the large amount of information on the consent forms. Difficulties can result when researchers assume the subjects understand everything on the form. Fitzgerald, Marotte, Verdier, et al. argue that even in less-developed countries, understanding could result if enough attention was given to education and communication.[177] Understanding can be negatively impacted if too many side effects are given in a short period of time.[178] Second, understanding can be limited if the language on

---

petence to Consent to Treatment, 101–102

[171] Jessica W. Berg, Paul S. Applebaum, Charles W. Lidz, and Lisa S. Parker, *Informed Consent: Legal Theory and Clinical Practice*, 66.

[172] Debbie Schachter, Sukirtha Tharmalingam, and Irwin Kleinman, "Informed Consent and Stimulant Medication: Adolescents' and Parents' Ability to Understand Information about Benefits and Risks of Stimulant Medication for the Treatment of Attention-Deficient/Hyperactivity Disorder," 140.

[173] Lewis Vaughn, *Bioethics: Principles, Issues, and Cases*, 146–7; Bernard Gert, Charles Culver, and K. Clouser, *Bioethics: A Systematic Approach*, 221–222; Regine Kollek, "Article 6: Consent," 123, 136; Martha Macintyre, "Informed Consent and Mining Projects: A View from Papua New Guinea," 61.

[174] Jessica W. Berg, Paul S. Applebaum, Charles W. Lidz, and Lisa S. Parker, *Informed Consent: Legal Theory and Clinical Practice*, 102.

[175] Stephen Wear, *Informed Consent: Patient Autonomy and Clinician Beneficence within Health Care*, 34.

[176] Dan Brock, "Patient Competence and Surrogate Decision-Making," 129.

[177] Daniel W. Fitzgerald, Cecile Marotte, Rose Irene Verdier, Warren D. Johnson, et al., "Comprehension during Informed Consent in a Less-Developed Country," 1301–1302.

[178] The National Commission for the Protection of Human Subjects of Biomedical and Behavioral Research, "The Belmont Report: Ethical Principles and Guidelines for the Protection of Human Subjects of Research," 768.

the form is confusing.[179] The information on consent forms is also being analyzed in terms of clarity.[180] Third, having an inadequate amount of time can limit understanding as well. One case that illustrates this is a dismissed malpractice case in Canada. A woman argued she had not given consent for the doctor to inject her eye with medication. Surprised when he did the procedure right after telling her about it, she said that she thought she would have had time to think about the procedure.[181] As clarified by the Belmont Report, the way information is given can be just as important as the actual information presented.[182] Fourth, not having enough physician involvement can limit understanding. Arnold and Lidz argue that informed consent should be a process involving continual communication with the physician to encourage patient participation.[183] However, instead of a strong doctor-patient relationship, Katz points out that history has illustrated a lack of physician attention and involvement.[184]

Consent is not just making sure the risks and benefits have been recited, but it should promote an understanding of the implications and goals of medical treatment and/or clinical research. If understanding is not present, then participants might not have truly made an informed consent. By having a greater level of understanding, the comprehension and autonomy of the individual will be encouraged as well.[185]

2. Disclosure

The second section looks at the emergence of the idea of disclosure in informed consent by analyzing the history, standards of disclosure, and necessary information to be disclosed. The history of disclosure will give specific examples and cases. The three main standards of disclosure will be analyzed in the second section. Then, the third section will look at the ideas of material information and therapeutic misconceptions.

---

[179] H.C. Howard, Y. Joly, D. Avard, et al., "Informed Consent in the Context of Pharmacogenomic Research: Ethical Considerations," 160.

[180] Edwin G. Belzer Jr., Lynn McIntryre, Catherine Simpson, et al., "A Method to Increase Informed Consent in School Health Research," 316.

[181] Bill Rogers, "Lawsuit a Reminder to be Certain of Informed Consent," 42.

[182] The National Commission for the Protection of Human Subjects of Biomedical and Behavioral Research, "The Belmont Report: Ethical Principles and Guidelines for the Protection of Human Subjects of Research," 768.

[183] Robert M. Arnold and Charles W. Lidz, "Informed Consent: Clinical Aspects of Consent in Health Care," 9–10.

[184] Jay Katz, "Physicians and Patients: A History of Silence," 136–137; Tom Beauchamp, "Informed Consent," 205; Onora O'Neill, *Autonomy and Trust in Bioethics,* 17–18.

[185] Edwin G. Belzer Jr., Lynn McIntryre, Catherine Simpson, et al., "A Method to Increase Informed Consent in School Health Research," 317; Franklin Miller and Alan Wertheimer, *The Ethics of Consent,* 388; Donald Evans, "Autonomy and Individual Responsibility," 118; Constance MacIntosh, "Indigenous Self-Determination and Research on Human Genetic Material: A Consideration of the Relevance of Debates on Patents and Informed Consent, and the Political Demands on Researchers," 237.

a. History

Katz explains that in the early history of consent, disclosure was really only important when unappreciative people did not follow what the physician said. With Hippocrates, physicians were not supposed to tell the patient anything about their health believing it might cause their health to decline.[186] Physicians believed that telling patients about their condition was insensitive and worse than withholding it. Thus, withholding information and extreme therapeutic privilege was justified, because the doctor knew what was best for the patient. However, some American doctors argued against this belief saying that the truth was more beneficial. One doctor, Dr. Samuel Johnson, did not appreciate the withholding of information, because he thought doctors had done it to him many times before. While truth-telling and disclosure would become a significant aspect of consent, the prevailing ideas of physician authority and therapeutic privilege were not easily swayed at the beginning.[187]

Issues of disclosure started being discussed as early as 1880 with the Walter Reed yellow fever experiments. Then in 1916, the discussion of patient decision making in research arose. Walter Cannon, Dr. Peabody, and the AMA debated back and forth on the importance of patient participation for research, but the prevailing view of physician authority won out at that time. In 1929, the *Haskins v. Howard* case sought to give patients more involvement in the decision-making process, but the case did not change the disclosure requirements.[188] Then the 1940s and 50s brought human subject research during war times in which there was limited or no disclosure to participants.[189] As a result of the research cases, the Nuremberg Code gave specific recommendations for disclosure including the risks, benefits, procedures, goals, and structure of the research study.[190] Disclosure became more important when patient rights began to arise in the late 1950s.[191] The *Salgo v. Leland, Natanson v. Kline,* and *Mitchell v. Robinson* cases focused mainly on disclosure of certain information. Tauber explains that during this time, courts were beginning to question whether patients had the right to accept as well as reject a procedure.[192] While rejecting a treatment was previously accepted, patients were now starting to accept treatments.[193] Because of this, patients needed more information in order to be able to accept a treatment. Thus, Arnold and Lidz suggest that informed consent and disclosure was emphasized even more due to societal trends.[194]

---

[186] Jay Katz, "Physicians and Patients: A History of Silence," 135.

[187] Albert Jonsen, *The Birth of Bioethics*, 354.

[188] Alfred Tauber, *Patient Autonomy and the Ethics of Responsibility*, 75; Albert Jonsen, *The Birth of Bioethics*, 130, 132–133.

[189] Gregory Pence, *Medical Ethics: Accounts of the Cases that Shaped and Define Medical Ethics*, 218–219, 232.

[190] The Nuremberg Tribunal, "The Nuremberg Code (1947)," 433.

[191] Carol Levine ed., *Taking Sides: Clashing Views on Bioethical Issues*, 3.

[192] Alfred Tauber, *Patient Autonomy and the Ethics of Responsibility*, 75–76.

[193] Thomas Grisso and Paul S. Applebaum, *Assessing Competence to Consent to Treatment*, 6.

[194] Robert M. Arnold and Charles W. Lidz, "Informed Consent: Clinical Aspects of Consent in Health Care," 4.

Since disclosure was now required, the main issue became what information was necessary to be disclosed. Miller and Wertheimer explain that the Jewish Chronic Disease Hospital case in 1963 did not disclose all necessary information to patients of the hospital.[195] Then in 1964, some of the prevailing beliefs about disclosure started to change when the popular view of physician authority came into question. In1965 the NIH established IRBs which would help with disclosure for human subject research. However even though there was more accountability, the Tuskegee Syphilis study illustrated a momentous lack of disclosure and truth-telling.[196] The *Cobb v. Grant* and *Canterbury v. Spence* cases in 1972 generally agreed that all information material to a decision including specific risks should be disclosed to the patient.[197] The 1980 case, *Truman v. Thomas*, asked how much disclosure was necessary. In response, some said that if the physician was required to explain everything to the patient, then the physician would spend too much time in education about tests. As a result of these discussions, Dolgin and Shepherd point out that two general categories of consent arose: the idealists and the realists. The idealists hold that physicians should seek quality conversations with the patients in order to encourage autonomy and understanding rather than the mere exchange of information. On the other hand, the realists, mostly physicians, suggest that many patients probably do not want this type of in-depth conversation. Because of that, the realists hold that the basic amount of information was enough.[198] These two categories help to explain the course of the discussion on disclosure. Then the 1990 case, *Moore v. Regents of the University of California*, deliberately withheld information from the patient due to a conflict of interest.[199] After that in 1996, the *Johnson v. Kokemoor* case discussed whether or not physician experience or inexperience should be disclosed to patients. However, the courts struggled with adding more to the disclosure rules at that time.[200] Then the Jesse Gelsinger case in 1999 and the Krieger lead paint study in 2001, which focused on the lack of disclosure for the procedure in general and the risks of the research.[201]

The attitudes and requirements of disclosure continued to evolve throughout history. Part of this change arose from public discussions of unimaginable clinical and

---

[195] Franklin Miller and Alan Wertheimer, *The Ethics of Consent*, 377–378.

[196] Albert Jonsen, *The Birth of Bioethics*, 143–144, 146–147, 356; Albert Jonsen, *A Short History of Medical Ethics*, 108; Gregory Pence, *Medical Ethics: Accounts of the Cases that Shaped and Define Medical Ethics*, 225.

[197] Lewis Vaughn, *Bioethics: Principles, Issues, and Cases*, 148, 150; Carol Levine ed., *Taking Sides: Clashing Views on Bioethical Issues*, 3; M. Sara Rosenthal, "Informed Consent in the Nuclear Medicine Setting," 1.

[198] Janet Dolgin and Lois Shepherd, *Bioethics and the Law*, 49–50, 61.

[199] Linda Farber Post, Jeffrey Blustein, and Nancy Neveloff Dubler, *Handbook for Health Care Ethics Committees*, 286; Beauchamp, Tom and James Childress, *Principles of Biomedical Ethics*, 81.

[200] Jerry Menikoff, *Law and Bioethics: An Introduction*, 186–187; B Sonny Bal and Theodore J. Choma, "What to Disclose? Revisiting Informed Consent," 1346.

[201] Gregory Pence, *Medical Ethics: Accounts of the Cases that Shaped and Define Medical Ethics*, 233–235.

research cases. Jonsen explains that in the beginning, doctors were encouraged not to have open discussions with their patients, but that changed over time. Now, disclosure and communication are required for adequate informed consent, and doctors recognize the patient's right to make medical decisions.[202]

b. Standards of Disclosure

Disclosure involves giving necessary information to patients who have a right to know.[203] Before a decision can be made, the risks and benefits of a particular procedure need to be addressed. As clarified by Beauchamp and Childress, disclosure is directly related to the decision-making process of the patient. The standards of disclosure are generally guided by the autonomy of the patient and the physician's duty to disclose certain information. There are three standards of disclosure which will be discussed further.[204]

First is the reasonable physician or physician based standard. This standard requires physicians to disclose information that a reasonable physician would disclose.[205] The standard arose in the beginning since physicians were the only ones able to inform patients about the risks and benefits. Since the physician does not know specifically what the patient believes to be important, this standard generally requires the physician to make value judgments. If information was left out that a reasonable physician would disclose, then the physician could be held accountable. Spottswood W. Robinson in the ruling for the *Canterbury* case expressed that holding strictly to a reasonable physician or professional standard is generally contradictory to the autonomy of the patient. Since medical groups and boards typically determine what information is necessary to provide in this standard, the patient's rights are not emphasized.[206] Instead, this standard demonstrates more of a paternalistic attitude. Second is the patient based or reasonable patient standard. This standard, promoted in the *Canterbury v. Spence* case, discloses the information that a normal or reasonable patient would like to know about a similar situation or procedure.[207] Because a patient's decision should be based on a certain level of information he or she has, Robinson suggests that the physician should be focused on what the patient wants to know.[208] Thus, the patient's need for certain information

---

[202] Albert Jonsen, *The Birth of Bioethics*, 357–358.

[203] Wouter Leclercq, Bram J. Keulers, Marc R. M. Scheltinga, et al., "A Review of Surgical Informed Consent: Past, Present, and Future. A Quest to Help Patients Make Better Decisions," 1408.

[204] Tom Beauchamp and James Childress, *Principles of Biomedical Ethics*, 121.

[205] Bernard Lo, *Resolving Ethical Dilemmas*, 22; Lewis Vaughn, *Bioethics: Principles, Issues, and Cases*, 146.

[206] Spottswood W. Robinson, "United States Court of Appeals Canterbury v. Spence," 133–134.

[207] James Childress, *Who Should Decide? Paternalism in Health Care*, 134–135; Lewis Vaughn, *Bioethics: Principles, Issues, and Cases*, 146.

[208] Spottswood W. Robinson, "United States Court of Appeals Canterbury v. Spence," 134.

was more important than what the physician might believe to be important. However, while this standard is accepted in several states, the physician based standard is generally more popular.[209] Third is the specific patient standard. This standard looks at what an individual patient would want to know about treatment or the disease.[210] The physician should look at the needs of the patient and then determine what information to present accordingly. Benjamin Freedman suggests that physicians should ask how much information the patients would like.[211] Because this standard is more in-depth, few states use it.[212]

These three standards are the main standards of disclosure for informed consent. While each standard is typically used individually, James Childress argues that the objective, reasonable patient standard should be used in conjunction with the subjective, specific patient standard. If a patient asks for specific information, that information should be given even if the reasonable patient standard is being used.[213] Taking those ideas further, Katz argues that it would be better if there were not objective and subjective labels for standards of disclosure. In reference to the *Canterbury* case, he says that the courts could have encouraged new guidelines. Rather than being bound to one standard, the new guidelines could promote communication with patients about disclosure needs and discuss any questions or fears the patient had in terms of treatments or other options.[214] Ideally, Katz's view of disclosure would help physicians broaden the meaning of disclosure and communication.

c. Information Disclosed

The disclosure of adequate information is essential to the consent process. Engelhardt argues that point further, because physicians and patients do not always share the same values and thoughts.[215] The goal of professional disclosure is giving information to encourage understanding and decision making.[216] Another way of noting this idea is made by John Beahrs and Thomas Gutheil when suggesting that patients should be familiar with the choices in order to evaluate and weigh the options before making an autonomous informed decision.[217] While there are no standardized

---

[209] Linda Farber Post, Jeffrey Blustein, and Nancy Neveloff Dubler, *Handbook for Health Care Ethics Committees*, 286.

[210] Lewis Vaughn, *Bioethics: Principles, Issues, and Cases*, 146; Bernard Lo, *Resolving Ethical Dilemmas*, 22.

[211] Benjamin Freedman, "Offering Truth: Once Ethical Approach to the Uninformed Cancer Patient," 113.

[212] Bernard Lo, *Resolving Ethical Dilemmas*, 22.

[213] James Childress, *Who Should Decide? Paternalism in Health Care*, 134–135.

[214] Jay Katz, "Physicians and Patients: A History of Silence," 138.

[215] H. Tristram Engelhardt Jr., *The Foundations of Bioethics*, 298.

[216] Jeffrey Carlisle and Ann T. Neulicht, "The Necessity of Professional Disclosure and Informed Consent for Rehabilitation Counselors," 26.

[217] John O. Beahrs and Thomas G. Gutheil, "Informed Consent in Psychotherapy," 8.

areas for disclosure, generally the risks, benefits, and alternatives need to be discussed for each potential procedure.[218] Some procedural areas to discuss include the length of procedure and hospitalization, recovery time, and what to expect after treatment or no treatment.[219] Some additional issues to consider about the treatment include issues such as the seriousness, likelihood, and timing of the risks and benefits.[220] While physicians need to disclose certain information to their patients, physicians also should know what is expected of them in order to identify possible conflicts with a proposed treatment.[221] In conclusion, all the material information of both the patient and physician should be disclosed to encourage adequate decision making.[222]

For medical treatment, there are three basic standards, but for human subject research, Regine Kollek suggests that the question of what should be disclosed is a little more complicated.[223] Disclosure still needs to address the nature, purpose, risks, and benefits of the study, but other areas need to be disclosed as well for human subject experimentation. Disclosure should also look at how to withdraw from the trial, who will get the results, how the results will be disclosed at the end, and what the compensation for injury is.[224] Also sometimes research experiments will need to keep some parts of the experiment hidden until the end of the project in order to keep the validity of the experiment. As clarified by the Belmont Report, these cases are justified if partial disclosure is required, if the undisclosed risks are minimal, and if there is a plan in place for disclosing the information after the study. It is important to differentiate between cases that require partial disclosure and cases where disclosure would be hard to obtain so partial disclosure is encouraged.[225] Another important aspect in research is the idea of therapeutic misconception. Laura Roberts analyzes this principle in relation to four areas: developmental factors like participation of minors, illness-related factors like mental disorders, psychological issues and religious values, and external pressures like institutional settings.[226] In

---

[218] Robert M. Arnold and Charles W. Lidz, "Informed Consent: Clinical Aspects of Consent in Health Care," 4; Spottswood W. Robinson, "United States Court of Appeals Canterbury v. Spence," 133; Lewis Vaughn, *Bioethics: Principles, Issues, and Cases*, 146; Bernard Gert, Charles Culver, and K. Clouser, *Bioethics: A Systematic Approach*, 202.

[219] M. Sara Rosenthal, "Informed Consent in the Nuclear Medicine Setting," 2.

[220] Linda Farber Post, Jeffrey Blustein, Nancy Neveloff Dubler, *Handbook for Health Care Ethics Committees*, 41; Bernard Gert, Charles Culver, and K. Clouser, *Bioethics: A Systematic Approach*, 214–215.

[221] H. Tristram, Engelhardt Jr., *The Foundations of Bioethics*, 299.

[222] Tom Beauchamp and James Childress, *Principles of Biomedical Ethics*, 81; Bernard Gert, Charles Culver, and K. Clouser, *Bioethics: A Systematic Approach*, 210.

[223] Regine Kollek, "Article 6: Consent," 132–133.

[224] Debra Pinals and Paul Applebaum, "The History and Current Status of Competence and Informed Consent in Psychiatric Research," 84–85; H.C. Howard, Y. Joly, D. Avard, et al., "Informed Consent in the Context of Pharmacogenomic Research: Ethical Considerations," 157.

[225] The National Commission for the Protection of Human Subjects of Biomedical and Behavioral Research, "The Belmont Report: Ethical Principles and Guidelines for the Protection of Human Subjects of Research," 767–768.

[226] Laura Weiss Roberts, "Informed Consent and the Capacity for Voluntarism," 707–709.

order to protect against therapeutic misconception, disclosure should identify the differences between research and medical treatment.[227] Since the UCLA case did not emphasize the difference between research and treatment, the consent forms most likely suffered from therapeutic misconception.[228] This is probably one of the most common problems with human subject research and disclosure.

There are some general exceptions to disclosure such as emergency situations, therapeutic privilege, and the patient waiver.[229] First, Ernst and Fish explain that in an emergency situation, there is not enough time for disclosure, because either disclosure is unreasonable or it is just not possible.[230] Second, therapeutic privilege is used in situations where disclosure would result in significant harm to the patient. By claiming therapeutic privilege, the doctor says that irreversible harm will come to the patient if certain information is disclosed. While many times irreversible harm is difficult to justify, sometimes there can be a debate on the application of therapeutic privilege, like in cases of disclosing news about an incurable disease to an elderly patient.[231] Third, if a person voluntarily waives his right to decide, then aspects of disclosure are not necessary.[232] However, Susan Marr argues that even when patients refuse care, he or she still should be informed of the risks, benefits, and alternatives of treatment.[233]

Also from the debate of disclosure comes another idea. Emphasized in the *Cobb v. Grant* case, the right not to be informed began to be addressed. Disclosure is not necessarily a right to know but an opportunity to know information. Press and Browner argue that if there was a right not to know, then sometimes that right could place more pressure and problems on others.[234] While there might not be a responsibility to know or not to know, there should still be the chance to learn more.[235]

While disclosing all the applicable information is helpful and necessary, disclosure by itself does not always encourage appropriate decision making.[236] Felt, Bister, Strassnig, et al. argue that more information does not always lead to a better

---

[227] Janet Dolgin and Lois Shepherd, *Bioethics and the Law*, 411.

[228] Debra Pinals and Paul Applebaum, "The History and Current Status of Competence and Informed Consent in Psychiatric Research," 84–85.

[229] Ruth R. Faden and Tom L., Beauchamp, *A History and Theory of Informed Consent*, 35–39.

[230] Amy A. Ernst and Susan Fish, "Exception from Informed Consent: Viewpoint of Institutional Review Boards—Balancing Risks to Subjects, Community Consultation, and Future Directions," 1050.

[231] John Williams, "Consent," 12; Spottswood W. Robinson, "United States Court of Appeals Canterbury v. Spence," 134–135.

[232] Lewis Vaughn, *Bioethics: Principles, Issues, and Cases*, 145–146; Hana Osman, "History and Development of the Doctrine of Informed Consent," 46.

[233] Susan Marr, "Protect Your Practice: Informed Consent," 180.

[234] Nancy Press and C. H. Browner, "Risk, Autonomy, and Responsibility: Informed Consent for Prenatal Testing," S12.

[235] H. Tristram Engelhardt Jr., *The Foundations of Bioethics*, 316.

[236] Neil C. Manson and Onora O'Neill, *Rethinking Informed Consent in Bioethics*, 69–70.

informed consent.[237] Informed consent is an ethical ideal.[238] Because of this, Manson and O'Neill suggest that even though consent forms are the legal requirement, the forms often do not satisfy ethical principles or indicate meaningful consent has occurred.[239] Rules and guidelines can promote a positive image for an institution, but focusing solely on the legal requirements for disclosure can lead to a narrow view of disclosure with little regard for understanding of that information.[240] The law cannot promote adequate discussions of consent or advance ethical communication.[241] One example is the consent for IRBs. As clarified by Levine, the actual process of informed consent and IRBs tend to focus solely on information being disclosed and the language used to disclose them. As a result, this view of consent and disclosure does not universally align with the ideas set forth in the Declaration of Helsinki which emphasize the importance of respect for persons.[242] Thus Engelhardt notes that increased bureaucracy can lead to a more ritualistic consent, which typically does not encourage appropriate decision making.[243]

3. Voluntariness

The third section looks at voluntariness in informed consent. The beginning looks at the history of voluntariness citing specific historical examples where patients consented either voluntarily or involuntarily to procedures or treatments. Then the second section analyzes the concepts behind voluntariness and freedom of choice including the concepts of eugenics, coercion, and vulnerable populations.

a. History

The voluntariness of consent is often a major principle for genetic testing. In research participation, there were many examples of coercive, manipulative, and involuntary consent. However, Jonsen explains that the Walter Reed yellow fever experiments in the 1880s demonstrated a strong focus on voluntary consent, saying that the subjects freely consented to participate. In 1886, Dr. Charles Francis Withington argued in his dissertation that people should be able to choose whether

---

[237] Ulrike Felt, Milena D. Bister, Michael Strassnig, et al., "Refusing the Information Paradigm: Informed Consent, Medical Research, and Patient Participation," 92.

[238] Lewis Vaughn, *Bioethics: Principles, Issues, and Cases*, 144.

[239] Neil C. Manson and Onora O'Neill, *Rethinking Informed Consent in Bioethics*, 192.

[240] H. Tristram, Engelhardt Jr., *The Foundations of Bioethics*, 300; Jeffrey Carlisle and Ann T. Neulicht, "The Necessity of Professional Disclosure and Informed Consent for Rehabilitation Counselors," 25–26.

[241] Tom L. Beauchamp, "Informed Consent: Its History, Meaning, and Present Challenges," 518.

[242] Robert Levine, "Informed Consent: Some Challenges to the Universal Validity of the Western Model," 144.

[243] H. Tristram Engelhardt Jr., *The Foundations of Bioethics*, 299.

or not to participate. In 1912, Dr. Hideyo Noguchi's research, using participants from mental hospitals and orphanages, was questioned on the grounds of voluntariness.[244] The physician, in *Schloendorff v. the Society of the New York Hospitals* in 1914, consented to surgery for the patient who did not want surgery.[245] In 1900 and 1931, the Prussian Ministry of Religious, Educational and Medical Affairs developed guidelines that recognized the importance of voluntary consent. However the Nazi experiments, some of the worst cases of involuntary research, came shortly after those guidelines. The Nazi experiments often took advantage of a cost-benefit analysis and had strong links to coercion.[246] The Nuremberg Code of 1946 sought to obtain consent without coercion, deceit, and/or force. In the Code, voluntary consent comes from the social contract tradition *volenti non fit iniuria,* meaning "no injury is done where the subject is willing."[247] The Code was a strong justification for the requirement of voluntariness in consent.

Sara Rosenthal explains that Susan M. Reverby found a government funded experiment done in 1946–1948 which gave Guatemalan people syphilis without their consent. The goal was to determine the appropriate dosage for penicillin.[248] In 1956, the Willowbrook study raised the issue of parents consenting for their children to enter research studies. Manipulation and coercion was evident when the researchers told parents the only room left in the hospital was on the experimental unit. In 1963, the Jewish Chronic Disease Hospital also had questions of voluntary consent, because the participants did not know they were being injected with cancer cells. The Helsinki Declaration in 1964 did not recognize the need to have outside help in ensuring the voluntariness of consent, because at that time, the burden of obtaining consent was up to the researchers alone. Then in 1972, the Tuskegee Syphilis study demonstrated that Americans could follow the unethical practices of the Nazis as well, with involuntary research and coercion.[249] In this study, the socioeconomic level of the individuals made it increasingly hard to resist signing up for the study, and that vulnerability led to increased manipulation and coercion of the subjects. Beauchamp and Childress point out that sometimes vulnerable people are in need of something so badly that it creates a situation in which manipulation flourishes naturally. In these situations, it appears that people are left without a significant decision. Research with children was discussed in 1974 with the National Commission.[250] During that time, Paul Ramsey argued that children should never be used

---

[244] Albert Jonsen, *The Birth of Bioethics*, 130–132; Tom Beauchamp and James Childress, *Principles of Biomedical Ethics*, 78

[245] Jerry Menikoff, *Law and Bioethics: An Introduction,* 306; Alfred Tauber, *Patient Autonomy and the Ethics of Responsibility*, 75; Linda Farber Post, Jeffrey Blustein, and Nancy Neveloff Dubler, *Handbook for Health Care Ethics Committees*, 286.

[246] John Kilner, Rebecca Pentz, and Frank Young, eds., *Genetic Ethics*, 33.

[247] Neil C. Manson and Onora O'Neill, *Rethinking Informed Consent in Bioethics*, 3.

[248] M. Sara Rosenthal, "Informed Consent in the Nuclear Medicine Setting," 2.

[249] Albert Jonsen, *The Birth of Bioethics*, 356.

[250] Tom Beauchamp and James Childress, *Principles of Biomedical Ethics*, 96, 428–430; Albert Jonsen, *The Birth of Bioethics*, 143, 154–155, 356.

for research.[251] However, Fr. Richard McCormick based parental consent on what the child should want to do and not on the actual desires of the child at the time.[252]

During World War 2, consent to research participation was even allowed in prisons. It was not until Jessica Mitford raised questions that the practice of research participation in prisons was investigated further. The case of *Kaimowitz vs Michigan Department of Mental Health* demonstrated that a prisoner was not able to make a voluntary choice about research participation, because of the coerciveness of the prison system.[253] Beauchamp explains that the Commission said the circumstances of the prison system led to questions about the voluntariness of consent. Thus, individuals should be protected from conditions that eliminate liberty.[254] Then, the 1996 version of the Declaration of Helsinki expressed that extra protection should be provided and encouraged if there is a relationship with the doctor that might infringe on the voluntariness of consent. If that is the case, then an independent physician should get the informed consent of the person.[255]

The beginning of consent emphasized the physician's authority and the lack of voluntary consent for the patient. At that time, each case involved some type of manipulation, coercion, and/or vulnerable population. However, over time the voluntariness of the individual was recognized as an important aspect of consent.

b. Freedom of Choice

One requirement for informed consent is voluntariness.[256] A person demonstrates voluntariness when he or she is allowed to make independent decisions without coercion. Rosenthal argues that voluntariness demonstrates the freedom of individuals to make decisions. [257] In order for valid consent to occur, the competent person should be free to choose and make decisions without undue pressures.[258] While there can be both external and internal pressures that might influence a person, not all influences will limit the freedom of choice.[259] Roberts takes the freedom to choose further and suggests that voluntariness has the opportunity to demonstrate

---

[251] Paul Ramsey, *The Patient as Person: Explorations in Medical Ethics*, 12–13.

[252] Richard McCormick, "Proxy Consent in the Experimentation Situation," 12–13.

[253] Debra Pinals and Paul Applebaum, "The History and Current Status of Competence and Informed Consent in Psychiatric Research," 84.

[254] Tom Beauchamp, "Informed Consent," 199.

[255] World Medical Association, "Declaration of Helsinki (1996) Recommendations Guiding Physicians in Biomedical Research Involving Human Subjects," 435.

[256] Wouter Leclercq, Bram J. Keulers, Marc R. M. Scheltinga, et al., "A Review of Surgical Informed Consent: Past, Present, and Future. A Quest to Help Patients Make Better Decisions," 1406; H. Tristram Engelhardt Jr., *The Foundations of Bioethics*, 289; Willard Gaylin and Bruce Jennings, *The Perversion of Autonomy*, 9.

[257] M. Sara Rosenthal, "Informed Consent in the Nuclear Medicine Setting," 3.

[258] H. Tristram Engelhardt Jr., *The Foundations of Bioethics*, 305–306.

[259] Alan Goldman, "The Refutation of Medical Paternalism," 65; Tom Beauchamp, "Informed Consent," in, Robert Veatch, *Medical Ethics*, 200–201.

respect for persons. A respect for persons is encouraged when the individual's values, morals, and rights are protected.[260]

Voluntariness needs to be exercised for both medical treatment and research participation. People have to be free to choose to participate in research or medical treatment.[261] Since there is not a duty but an opportunity to participate in research, Jonsen connects the choice to participate with autonomy and voluntariness. When participants volunteer for research experiments, those volunteers need adequate knowledge and understanding to demonstrate autonomy and appropriate decision making. True volunteering is actively recognizing that the researcher's goals are the same as that individual's. Thus a person actively engaged in the research experiment demonstrates a solid justification for participation.[262]

This section will analyze the freedom of choice further by addressing the ideas and principles of eugenics, coercion, and vulnerable populations.

1). Eugenics

In 1869, Francis Galton invented the word *eugenics*, meaning the study of improving genetics and natural characteristics of individuals.[263] Although originally having an amoral connotation, today eugenics most often has controversial, if not detrimental, positions associated with it. For example, Debora Spar explains that in early Greece, the ideas of eugenics led to abandoning deformed babies to die.[264] While trying to improve genetics can be voluntary, there are many examples in history of involuntary eugenics such as the sterilization programs in the United States. Because the ideas involved in the programs were not overtly unethical to people at the time, the programs led the way for increasingly harmful cases that would later lead to the killing of undeserving and unhealthy people in concentration camps.[265]

Eugenics was heightened with the establishment of involuntary sterilization programs. Philip Reilly suggested that the renewed interest in genetics stressed the idea that some people had more genetic defects and flawed genetic structures than others. In 1878, feeble-minded women were put into asylums in New York to limit reproduction. However, people started to realize in the 1890s that institutionalization was not automatically the solution. As a result, some groups wanted to put laws in place to prohibit feebleminded or flawed women from marrying, like Connecticut in 1895. However, since the state could not completely control the marriage and segregation of defective individuals, discussions about sterilization of criminals started.

---

[260] Laura Weiss Roberts, "Informed Consent and the Capacity for Voluntarism," 709.

[261] Debra Pinals and Paul Applebaum, "The History and Current Status of Competence and Informed Consent in Psychiatric Research," 84.

[262] Albert Jonsen, *The Birth of Bioethics*, 151–152.

[263] G. Whitney, "Reproduction Technology for a New Eugenics," 179.

[264] Debora Spar, *The Baby Business: How Money, Science, and Politics Drive the Commerce of Conception*, 101.

[265] Tom Beauchamp and LeRoy Walters, eds., *Contemporary Issues in Bioethics*, 511–512.

The state had more control over the prisoners. Performing the first vasectomy, Albert Ochsner expressed that it would help with criminals, the poor, and uneducated. By the beginning of the 1900s, sterilizations were common procedures supported by law. Laws went into place in 1907 in Indiana. The laws said that sterilizations would be performed on any recurrent criminals in a state facility if there was a limited chance of improvement. These laws were first aimed at males, because the procedures for women were still too risky. Because of that, segregation was still the norm for defective women. As clarified by Reilly, there were over 3000 sterilizations done on criminals, the uneducated, and mentally ill. While sterilization was generally accepted, one judge in Iowa questioned the procedure and said that sterilization was demeaning and caused mental and physical suffering. However, sterilizations did not decrease, and in fact, forced sterilizations were becoming more accepted in the 1920s. As a result, *Buck v. Bell* in 1927 ruled that forced sterilization should take place, because "Three generations of imbeciles are enough."[266] Also in the 1920s a major group, the American Eugenics Society, realized that positive eugenics would be better than sterilization laws, and as a result, the group turned to family planning. In the 1930s, the Germans implemented a eugenics law, and the Nazis sterilized over 50,000 people in a year of the new law. By 1950, involuntary sterilizations had dropped significantly. In the 1960s, legislatures thought about having voluntary sterilizations linked to welfare payments, but that did not occur. Then in 1973, DHEW funded several programs that provided involuntary sterilizations, but later, some sterilized individuals decided to sue. These cases led to the requirement of ensuring competency and having extensive consent measures before voluntary sterilization took place.[267]

Throughout the years, the arguments for sterilizations and eugenics have continually changed. However, even now the eugenics movement has principles that can threaten the voluntary nature of consent.

2). Coercion

Often medical testing and the staff have the ability to manipulate people into participating in research studies or treatment. But in order to be voluntary, a decision has to be free from pressures that could manipulate or coerce.[268] The Belmont Report expresses that coercion normally exhibits a power differential that causes one person to have control over another. Many times the threat is so strong that the individual succumbs to the pressure.[269]

---

[266] Stephen Jay Gould, "Carrie Buck's Daughter," 529.

[267] Philip Reilly, "Eugenic Sterilization in the United States," 517–520, 522–524.

[268] Albert Jonsen, "A History of Bioethics as Discipline and Discourse," 7; M. Sara Rosenthal, "Informed Consent in the Nuclear Medicine Setting," 2; Ruth Macklin, "The Inner Workings of an Ethics Committee: Latest Battle over Jehovah's Witnesses," 233.

[269] The National Commission for the Protection of Human Subjects of Biomedical and Behavioral Research, "The Belmont Report: Ethical Principles and Guidelines for the Protection of Human

There can be other influences like manipulation and persuasion, but often coercion is the most overtly detrimental to voluntariness.[270] Beauchamp points out that while all manipulation is not inevitably coercive, manipulation with deception is.[271] Sometimes offering rewards can be even more coercive, because it is an intentional act to influence or deceive another.[272] The Council for International Organizations of Medical Sciences (CIOMS) and the World Health Organization (WHO) developed guidelines to address the issue of payment for research. If a sum of money is large enough to influence an individual to make a different decision, then that money is a coercive incentive.[273] Since coercion can be hidden and not easily identified at times, Engelhardt cautions people against assuming manipulation is acceptable.[274] Another area is persuasion. There is a difference between using reason to persuade people and using intimidation. Reasoning by itself is not coercive, but if a person is persuaded by other pressures, then sometimes the individual's freedom to choose is reduced.[275] However, people make decisions all the time while being influenced by conflicting viewpoints. Sometimes differing views can be appreciated like recommendations by doctors, and other times conflicting views can encourage coercion and intimidation. Because there will always be certain underlying influences, Beauchamp suggests that the main question is whether people are free enough to choose.[276] Choices involving additional pressures raise concerns about the validity and voluntariness of the resulting consent.[277] Simply applying autonomy and giving consent does not get rid of coercion. There is still the opportunity for abuse through the distortion of facts and deceptive details about treatment possibilities like the eugenics programs.[278] If a person consents under intimidation or duress, the consent is actually rescinded, because it ignores the voluntariness of the individual.[279]

Subjects of Research," 768.

[270] Willard Gaylin and Bruce Jennings, *The Perversion of Autonomy,* 144, 149–150.

[271] Tom Beauchamp, "Informed Consent," 200–201.

[272] H. Tristram Engelhardt Jr., *The Foundations of Bioethics*, 309.

[273] Council for International Organizations of Medical Sciences (CIOMS) in collaboration with The World Health Organization (WHO), "International Ethical Guidelines for Biomedical Research Involving Human Subjects (1993)," 438.

[274] H. Tristram Engelhardt Jr., *The Foundations of Bioethics*, 309.

[275] Jessica W. Berg, Paul S. Applebaum, Charles W. Lidz, and Lisa S. Parker, *Informed Consent: Legal Theory and Clinical Practice*, 68.

[276] Tom Beauchamp, "Informed Consent," 200–201.

[277] Jessica W. Berg, Paul S. Applebaum, Charles W. Lidz, and Lisa S. Parker, *Informed Consent: Legal Theory and Clinical Practice*, 68.

[278] Maria Patrao Neves, "Respect for Human Vulnerability and Personal Integrity," 162; Tom Beauchamp and LeRoy Walters, eds., *Contemporary Issues in Bioethics*, 511; Cara Dunne and Catherine Warren, "Lethal Autonomy: The Malfunction of the Informed Consent Mechanism within the Context of Prenatal Diagnosis of Genetic Variants," 165–166; Linda Farber Post, Jeffrey Blustein, and Nancy Neveloff Dubler, *Handbook for Health Care Ethics Committees*, 42.

[279] James Childress, *Who Should Decide? Paternalism in Health Care,* 78; Jessica W. Berg, Paul S. Applebaum, Charles W. Lidz, and Lisa S. Parker, *Informed Consent: Legal Theory and Clinical Practice*, 68.

Since decisions often affect more than one person, decision making does not have to be isolated.[280] Post, Blustein, and Dubler note that independent decision making is different from isolated decision making. Isolated decision making would exclude recommendations from doctors and a patient's family, which is generally not ideal.[281] However while family support is important, sometimes the family could have coercive influences.[282] Since genetic information can have an impact on the patient and the patient's family, informed consent needs to take into account the patient and his or her family values and beliefs about genetic testing.[283] As a result, family coercion needs to be addressed as well with genetic testing. The CIOMS and the WHO developed recommendations that include obligations to eliminate coercion and influencing pressures.[284]

While coercion eliminates a person's freedom to choose, sometimes there can also be situations that eliminate freedom as well. The next section will look at vulnerable populations.

3). Vulnerable Populations

This last section deals with vulnerable populations and settings. As clarified by the Belmont Report, some incentives can put an undue amount of pressure on already vulnerable people.[285] Certain groups of people will be more influenced by and susceptible to coercion than other groups. Vulnerable populations are different because of the degree of coercion and exploitation that are put upon them.[286] Exploitation demonstrates the power discrepancy that can occur in medicine and research.[287] As a result, there are generally special protections for vulnerable populations. Some vulnerable populations include prisoners, pregnant women, children, disabled, and institutionalized individuals.[288] Ross, Sundberg, and Flint give the Tuskegee study

---

[280] Dan Brock, "Patient Competence and Surrogate Decision-Making," 128; Thomas Grisso and Paul S. Applebaum, *Assessing Competence to Consent to Treatment,* 9.

[281] Linda Farber Post, Jeffrey Blustein, and Nancy Neveloff Dubler, *Handbook for Health Care Ethics Committees,* 42.

[282] Dan Brock, "Patient Competence and Surrogate Decision-Making," 128; Thomas Grisso and Paul S. Applebaum, *Assessing Competence to Consent to Treatment,* 9.

[283] Neil Sharpe and Ronald Carter, *Genetic Testing: Care, Consent, and Liability,* 131.

[284] Council for International Organizations of Medical Sciences (CIOMS) in collaboration with The World Health Organization (WHO), "International Ethical Guidelines for Biomedical Research Involving Human Subjects (1993)," 438.

[285] The National Commission for the Protection of Human Subjects of Biomedical and Behavioral Research, "The Belmont Report: Ethical Principles and Guidelines for the Protection of Human Subjects of Research," 768.

[286] Jonathan Moreno, "Convenient and Captive Populations," 111.

[287] Ruth Macklin, "Justice in International Research," 134.

[288] Jeffrey Kahn, "Informed Consent in the Context of Communities," 919; Laura Weiss Roberts, "Informed Consent and the Capacity for Voluntarism," 705–706; Amy A. Ernst and Susan Fish,

as an example in history of vulnerable populations.[289] Even with some of the added protections, the NBAC explains that sometimes certain populations should not be sought for research involvement at all due to their vulnerable position.[290]

Sometimes there are also situations that can be inherently coercive such as prisons. Tom Beauchamp points out that prisons are naturally coercive, and it is generally unrealistic to try to eliminate the pressures that exist in that setting. Coercion is generally thought of as intentional, but sometimes there can be unintentional coercive situations where nobody is putting pressure on another person. In the case of prisons, the Commission was afraid prisoners would be coerced into participating in research. However, just because a situation might have more opportunity for undue influences, people should not assume there are no other options than the coercive pressures.[291] Even though populations can be vulnerable, it does not mean that informed consent cannot ever take place. Earlier the debate focused on protecting vulnerable populations, but now the debate focuses on encouraging equal opportunity to participate in research by balancing coercion and having safeguards.[292]

Consent is a way of protecting against coercion and threats.[293] When the voluntariness of an individual is not emphasized, the best interests of patients are ignored.[294] Even if the risks are minimal, the voluntary consent of the individual should not be overlooked, because true voluntariness strengthens informed consent.[295] Thus, if coercion is not controlled adequately, informed consent is suspect. According to Engelhardt, true voluntary consent has the possibility of promoting the dignity of the person while addressing the errors inherent in research participation and consent.[296] However, Berg, Applebaum, Lidz, and Parker note that even though courts have supported the idea of voluntariness, they have not specifically defined this idea. As a result, voluntariness will be even more problematic in the future if doctors have to deal with cost analysis of treatments.[297]

"Exception from Informed Consent: Viewpoint of Institutional Review Boards—Balancing Risks to Subjects, Community Consultation, and Future Directions," 1052.

[289] James Ross, Elizabeth Sundberg, and Katherine Flint, "Informed Consent in School Health Research: Why, How, and Making it Easy," 172.

[290] National Bioethics Advisory Commission, "Protecting Research Participants— A Time for Change," 374.

[291] Tom Beauchamp, "Informed Consent," 201–202.

[292] Baruch A. Brody, "Research on the Vulnerable Sick," 32.

[293] Neil C. Manson and Onora O'Neill, Rethinking Informed Consent in Bioethics, 82.

[294] Tom Beauchamp and James Childress, Principles of Biomedical Ethics 96; Albert Jonsen, The Birth of Bioethics, 147.

[295] National Bioethics Advisory Commission, "Protecting Research Participants— A Time for Change," 374; Laura Weiss Roberts, "Informed Consent and the Capacity for Voluntarism," 709.

[296] H. Tristram Engelhardt Jr., The Foundations of Bioethics, 330–331.

[297] Jessica W. Berg, Paul S. Applebaum, Charles W. Lidz, and Lisa S. Parker, Informed Consent: Legal Theory and Clinical Practice, 69–70; Thomas Grisso and Paul S. Applebaum, Assessing Competence to Consent to Treatment, 9; Laura Weiss Roberts, "Informed Consent and the Capacity for Voluntarism," 705.

C. Conclusion

The history of informed consent is extremely important when analyzing the current and revised models of consent for PGT. Jonsen explains that the philosophical, theological, and legal perspectives of some of the most esteemed individuals in society were analyzed in the discussion of consent. Because of that, the history illuminates the high expectations and goals for consent.[298] The background of informed consent analyzed both the clinical and research history looking at the patient treatment and research subject model of consent. After looking at the history, the main components of the current model of consent were identified and analyzed in the second part of this chapter.

The history has demonstrated a couple of points. First, history has shown that establishing policies can help to reduce potentially bad outcomes. Ross, Sundberg, and Flint note that the regulations surrounding consent arose from unfavorable cases like the Nazis experiments and eugenics movements.[299] Some bad outcomes have already been reduced since undesirable consequences are not standard. However, more work could be done to reduce negative outcomes.[300] Second, history has demonstrated some limitations to consent. The principles of voluntariness and autonomy cannot justify acts that go against ethical values, like murder.[301] Another limitation is the amount of information. Currently doctors and researchers are not able to inform the patient adequately concerning genetics. The last limitation concerns the gap between the legal aspects of consent and the ethical ideals of consent. According to Dolgin and Shepherd, this gap exists because of the limitations of the medical system and the doctor-patient relationship. Because of that, the gap can be difficult to reduce without significant change.[302]

Even though history has progressively shaped the concepts of informed consent, Katz argues that more work needs to be done integrating the reality of consent today with the legal aspects and ethical goals of consent.[303] An evaluation of the history of informed consent is necessary in order for the current model of consent to be identified and evaluated in the subsequent chapters.

---

[298] Albert Jonsen, *The Birth of Bioethics*, 357; Jeffrey Kahn, "Informed Consent in the Context of Communities," 918.

[299] James Ross, Elizabeth Sundberg, and Katherine Flint, "Informed Consent in School Health Research: Why, How, and Making it Easy," 172; Paul Root Wolpe and Jon F. Merz, "Hospital ERs on Front Line in Informed-Consent Debate," 127.

[300] Debra Pinals and Paul Applebaum, "The History and Current Status of Competence and Informed Consent in Psychiatric Research," 89.

[301] James Childress, *Who Should Decide? Paternalism in Health Care*, 78–79.

[302] Janet Dolgin and Lois Shepherd, *Bioethics and the Law*, 49–50, 61, 69.

[303] Jay Katz, "Reflections on Informed Consent: 40 Years after its Birth," 466.

References

Ackerman, Terrence. "Why Doctors Should Intervene." In *Ethical Issues in Modern Medicine*, edited by Bonnie Steinbock, John Arras, and Alex John London, 73–77. Boston: McGraw Hill Publishing, 2009.

Advisory Committee on Human Radiation Experiments. "Final Report: Executive Summary (1995)." In *Contemporary Issues in Bioethics*, edited by Tom Beauchamp and LeRoy Walters, 479–483. Belmont, CA: Wadsworth Publishing Company, 1999.

Angrist, Misha. "Eyes Wide Open: The Personal Genome Project, Citizen Science and Veracity in Informed Consent." *Personalized Medicine* 6:6 (2009): 691–699.

Annas, George. *American Bioethics: Crossing Human Rights and Health Law Boundaries*. New York: Oxford University Press, 2005.

Arnold, Robert M. and Charles W. Lidz. "Informed Consent: Clinical Aspects of Consent in Health Care." In *Taking Sides: Clashing Views on Bioethical Issues*, edited by Carol Levine, 4–14. Boston: McGraw Hill Higher Education, 2010.

Arras, John D. "The Jewish Chronic Disease Hospital Case." In *Ethical Issues in Modern Medicine*, edited by Bonnie Steinbock, John Arras, and Alex John London, 740–749. Boston: McGraw Hill Publishing, 2009.

Bal, B. Sonny and Theodore J. Choma. "What to Disclose? Revisiting Informed Consent." *Clinical Orthopaedics and Related Research* 470: 5(May 2012): 1346–1356.

Beahrs, John O. and Thomas G. Gutheil. "Informed Consent in Psychotherapy." *The American Journal of Psychiatry* 158: 1(January 2001): 4–10.

Beauchamp, Tom L. "Informed Consent." In *Medical Ethics*, edited by Robert Veatch, 185–208. Sudbury, MA: Jones and Bartlett Publishers, 1997.

Beauchamp, Tom. "Informed Consent: Its History and Meaning." In *Standing on Principles*, Tom Beauchamp, 50–78. New York: Oxford University Press, 2010.

Beauchamp, Tom. *Standing on Principles*. New York: Oxford University Press, 2010.

Beauchamp, Tom L. "Informed Consent: Its History, Meaning, and Present Challenges." *Cambridge Quarterly of Healthcare Ethics* 20 (2011): 515–523.

Beauchamp, Tom and James Childress. *Principles of Biomedical Ethics*. New York: Oxford University Press, 2001.

Beauchamp, Tom and LeRoy Walters eds. *Contemporary Issues in Bioethics*. Belmont, CA: Wadsworth Publishing Company, 1999.

Belzer, Edwin G., Jr., Lynn McIntryre, Catherine Simpson, et al. "A Method to Increase Informed Consent in School Health Research." *The Journal of School Health* 63: 7(September 1993): 316–317.

Berg, Jessica W., Paul S. Applebaum, Charles W. Lidz, and Lisa S. Parker. *Informed Consent: Legal Theory and Clinical Practice*. New York: Oxford University Press, 2001.

Berry, Roberta M. "Informed Consent Law, Ethics, and Practice: From Infancy to Reflective Adolescence." *HealthCare Ethics Committee Forum* 17: 1 (2005): 64–81.

Brandt, Allan M. "Racism and Research: The Case of the Tuskegee Syphilis Study." In *Ethical Issues in Modern Medicine*, edited by Bonnie Steinbock, John Arras, and Alex John London, 753–763. Boston: McGraw Hill Publishing, 2009.

Brock, Dan. "Patient Competence and Surrogate Decision-Making." In *The Blackwell Guide to Medical Ethics*, edited by Rosamond Rhodes, Leslie Francis, and Anita Silvers, 128–141. Malden, MA: Wiley-Blackwell Publishing, 2007.

Brody, Howard. *Ethical Decisions in Medicine*. Boston: Little, Brown, & Company, 1981.

Brody, Baruch A. "Research on the Vulnerable Sick." In *Beyond Consent: Seeking Justice in Research*, edited by Jeffrey Kahn, Anna Mastroianni, and Jeremy Sugarman, 32–46. New York: Oxford University Press, 1998.

Buchanan, David and Franklin G. Miller. "Justice in Research on Human Subjects." In *The Blackwell Guide to Medical Ethics*, edited by Rosamond Rhodes, Leslie Francis, and Anita Silvers, 373–392. Malden, MA: Wiley-Blackwell Publishing, 2007.

Byrne, Michelle. "The Concept of Informed Consent in Qualitative Research." *Association of Operating Room Nurses*. 74: 3(September 2001): 401–403.

Cameron, Nigel. *The New Medicine: Life and Death After Hippocrates*. Wheaton, IL: Crossway Books, 1991.

Carlisle, Jeffrey and Ann T. Neulicht. "The Necessity of Professional Disclosure and Informed Consent for Rehabilitation Counselors." *Journal of Applied Rehabilitation Counseling* 41: 2(Summer 2010): 25–31.

Childress, James. *Who Should Decide? Paternalism in Health Care*. New York: Oxford University Press, 1982.

Christopoulos, Platon, Matthew E. Falagas, Philippos Gourzis, and Constantinos Trompoukis. "Aspects of Informed Consent in Medical Practice in the Eastern Mediterranean Region During the 17th and 18th Centuries." *World Journal of Surgery* 31 (2007): 1587–1591.

Clinton, William J. "In Apology for the Study Done in Tuskegee." In *Contemporary Issues in Bioethics*, edited by Tom Beauchamp and LeRoy Walters, 402–403. Belmont, CA: Wadsworth Publishing Company, 2003.

Council for International Organizations of Medical Sciences (CIOMS) in collaboration with The World Health Organization (WHO). "International Ethical Guidelines for Biomedical Research Involving Human Subjects (1993)." In *Contemporary Issues in Bioethics*, edited by Tom Beauchamp and LeRoy Walters, 358–362. Belmont, CA: Wadsworth Publishing Company, 1999.

Delany, Clare M. "Respecting Patient Autonomy and Obtaining Their Informed Consent: Ethical Theory- Missing in Action." *Physiotherapy* 91:4 (2005): 197–203.

Dolgin, Janet L. "The Legal Development of the Informed Consent Doctrine: Past and Present." Special Section: Open Forum. *Cambridge Quarterly of Healthcare Ethics* 19 (2010): 97–109.

Dolgin, Janet and Lois Shepherd. *Bioethics and the Law*. New York: Aspen Publishers, 2005.

Dunne, Cara and Catherine Warren. "Lethal Autonomy: The Malfunction of the Informed Consent Mechanism within the Context of Prenatal Diagnosis of Genetic Variants." *Issues in Law & Medicine* 14: 2(Fall 1998): 165–202.

Eisenberg, Leon. "The Social Imperatives of Medical Research." In *Contemporary Issues in Bioethics*, edited by Tom Beauchamp and LeRoy Walters, 449–456. Belmont, CA: Wadsworth Publishing Company, 1999.

Engelhardt, H. Tristram, Jr *The Foundations of Bioethics*. New York: Oxford University Press, 1996.

Ernst, Amy A. and Susan Fish. "Exception from Informed Consent: Viewpoint of Institutional Review Boards—Balancing Risks to Subjects, Community Consultation, and Future Directions." *Academic Emergency Medicine* 12: 11(November 2005): 1050–1055.

Evans, Donald. "Autonomy and Individual Responsibility." In *The UNESCO Universal Declaration on Bioethics and Human Rights*, edited by Henk ten Have and Michele Jean, 111–122. Paris, France: UNESCO, 2009.

Faden, Ruth R. and Tom L. Beauchamp. *A History and Theory of Informed Consent*. New York: Oxford University Press, 1986.

Faden, Ruth and Tom Beauchamp. "The Concept of Informed Consent." In *Bioethics: Principles, Issues, and Cases*, edited by Lewis Vaughn, 154–58. New York: Oxford University Press, 2009.

Farmer, Paul and Nicole Gastineau Campos. "New Malaise: Bioethics and Human Rights in the Global Era." In *Bioethics: An Introduction to the History, Methods, and Practice*, edited by Nancy Jecker, Albert Jonsen, and Robert Pearlman, 293–306. Sudbury, MA: Jones and Bartlett Publishers, 2007.

Felt, Ulrike, Milena D. Bister, Michael Strassnig, and Ursula Wagner. "Refusing the Information Paradigm: Informed Consent, Medical Research, and Patient Participation." *Health: An Interdisciplinary Journal for the Social Study of Health, Illness and Medicine* 13: 1(October 2009): 87–106.

Fitzgerald, Daniel W., Cecile Marotte, Rose Irene Verdier, Warren D. Johnson, et al. "Comprehension during Informed Consent in a Less-Developed Country." *The Lancet* 360: 9342 (October 26, 2002): 1301–1302.

Freedman, Benjamin. "Offering Truth: Once Ethical Approach to the Uninformed Cancer Patient." In *Ethical Issues in Modern Medicine*, edited by Bonnie Steinbock, John Arras, and Alex John London, 110–116. Boston: McGraw Hill Publishing, 2009.

Freedman, Benjamin, Abraham Fuks, and Charles Weijer. "In Loco Parentis: Minimal Risk as an Ethical Threshold for Research upon Children." In *Ethical Issues in Modern Medicine*, edited by Bonnie Steinbock, John Arras, and Alex John London, 829–835. Boston: McGraw Hill Publishing, 2009.

Gaylin, Willard and Bruce Jennings. *The Perversion of Autonomy: Coercion and Constraints in a Liberal Society*. Washington, D.C.: Georgetown University Press, 2003.

Getz, Kenneth and Deborah Borfitz. *Informed Consent: The Consumer's Guide to the Risks and Benefits of Volunteering for Clinical Trials*. Boston: Thomson CenterWatch Corporation, 2002.

Gert, Bernard, Charles Culver, and K. Clouser. *Bioethics: A Systematic Approach*. New York: Oxford University Press, 2006.

Goldman, Alan. "The Refutation of Medical Paternalism." In *Ethical Issues in Modern Medicine*, edited by Bonnie Steinbock, John Arras, and Alex John London, 62–70. Boston: McGraw Hill Publishing, 2009.

Gould, Stephen Jay. "Carrie Buck's Daughter." In *Contemporary Issues in Bioethics*, edited by Tom Beauchamp and LeRoy Walters, 528–532. Belmont, CA: Wadsworth Publishing Company, 1999.

Grisso, Thomas and Paul S. Applebaum. *Assessing Competence to Consent to Treatment*. New York: Oxford University Press, 1998.

Howard, H.C., Y. Joly, D. Avard, et al. "Informed Consent in the Context of Pharmacogenomic Research: Ethical Considerations." *The Pharmacogenomics Journal* 11 (2011): 155–161.

Jonsen, Albert. *The Birth of Bioethics*. New York: Oxford University Press, 1998.

Jonsen, Albert. *A Short History of Medical Ethics*. New York: Oxford University Press, 2000.

Jonsen, Albert. "A History of Bioethics as Discipline and Discourse." In *Bioethics: An Introduction to the History, Methods, and Practice*, edited by Nancy Jecker, Albert Jonsen, and Robert Pearlman, 3–16. Sudbury, MA: Jones and Bartlett Publishers, 2007.

Kahn, Jeffrey. "Informed Consent in the Context of Communities." *The Journal of Nutrition* 135: 4(April 2005): 918–920.

Karlawish, Jason. "Research on Cognitively Impaired Adults." In *The Oxford Handbook of Bioethics*, edited by Bonnie Steinbock, 597–620. New York: Oxford University Press, 2007.

Katz, Jay. "Reflections on Informed Consent: 40 Years after its Birth." *Journal of the American College of Surgeons* 186: 4(April 1998): 466–74.

Katz, Jay. "Physicians and Patients: A History of Silence." In *Contemporary Issues in Bioethics*, edited by Tom Beauchamp and LeRoy Walters, 135–138. Belmont, CA: Wadsworth Publishing Company, 1999.

Katz, Jay. "Informed Consent- Must It Remain a Fairy Tale?" In *Bioethics: Principles, Issues, and Cases*, edited by Lewis Vaughn, 159–68. New York: Oxford University Press, 2010.

Kilner, John, Rebecca Pentz, Frank Young, eds. *Genetic Ethics*. Grand Rapids, MI: William B Eerdmans Publishing Company, 1997.

King, Patricia, "Race, Justice, and Research." In *Beyond Consent: Seeking Justice in Research*, edited by Jeffrey Kahn, Anna Mastroianni, and Jeremy Sugarman, 88–110. New York: Oxford University Press, 1998.

Kollek, Regine. "Article 6: Consent." In *The UNESCO Universal Declaration on Bioethics and Human Rights*, edited by Henk ten Have and Michele Jean, 123–138. Paris, France: UNESCO, 2009.

Leclercq, Wouter, Bram J. Keulers. Marc R. M. Scheltinga, et al. "A Review of Surgical Informed Consent: Past, Present, and Future. A Quest to Help Patients Make Better Decisions." *World Journal of Surgery* 34 (2010): 1406–1415.

Lerner, Barron H. "Beyond Informed Consent: Did Cancer Patients Challenge Their Physicians in the Post-World War II Era?" *Journal of the History of Medicine and Allied Sciences* 59: 4(October 2004): 507–21.

Lerner, Barron H. "Sins of Omission- Cancer Research without Informed Consent." *The New England Journal of Medicine* 351: 7 (August 12, 2004): 628–30.

Levine, Robert J. "Informed Consent: Some Challenges to the Universal Validity of the Western Model." In *Contemporary Issues in Bioethics*, edited by Tom Beauchamp and LeRoy Walters, 143–148. Belmont, CA: Wadsworth Publishing Company, 1999.

Levine, Carol ed. *Taking Sides: Clashing Views on Bioethical Issues.* Boston: McGraw Hill Higher Education, 2010.

Lo, Bernard. *Resolving Ethical Dilemmas.* Philadelphia, PA: Lippincott Williams and Wilkins, 2005.

London, Alex John. "Children and "Minimal Risk" Research: The Kennedy-Krieger Lead Paint Study." In *Ethical Issues in Modern Medicine*, edited by Bonnie Steinbock, John Arras, and Alex John London, 811–815. Boston: McGraw Hill Publishing, 2009.

MacIntosh, Constance. "Indigenous Self-Determination and Research on Human Genetic Material: A Consideration of the Relevance of Debates on Patents and Informed Consent, and the Political Demands on Researchers." *Health Law Journal* 13 (2005): 213–251.

Macintyre, Martha. "Informed Consent and Mining Projects: A View from Papua New Guinea." *Pacific Affairs* 80: 1(Spring 2007): 49–65.

Macklin, Ruth. "Justice in International Research." In *Beyond Consent: Seeking Justice in Research*, edited by Jeffrey Kahn, Anna Mastroianni, and Jeremy Sugarman, 131–146. New York: Oxford University Press, 1998.

Macklin, Ruth. "The Inner Workings of an Ethics Committee: Latest Battle over Jehovah's Witnesses." In *Bioethics: An Introduction to the History, Methods, and Practice*, edited by Nancy Jecker, Albert Jonsen, and Robert Pearlman, 232–235. Sudbury, MA: Jones and Bartlett Publishers, 2007.

Manson, Neil C. and Onora O'Neill. *Rethinking Informed Consent in Bioethics.* New York: Cambridge University Press, 2007.

Marr, Susan. "Protect Your Practice: Informed Consent." *Plastic Surgical Nursing* 22: 4(Winter 2002): 180–181.

McCarthy, Charles. "The Evolving Story of Justice in Federal Research Policy." In *Beyond Consent: Seeking Justice in Research*, edited by Jeffrey Kahn, Anna Mastroianni, and Jeremy Sugarman, 11–31. New York: Oxford University Press, 1998.

McCormick, Richard. "Proxy Consent in the Experimentation Situation." *Perspectives in Biology and Medicine* 18:1 (1974): 2–20.

Menikoff, Jerry. *Law and Bioethics: An Introduction.* Washington, D.C.: Georgetown University Press, 2001.

Miller, Franklin and Alan Wertheimer. *The Ethics of Consent.* New York: Oxford University Press, 2010.

Miola, Jose. "The Need for Informed Consent: Lessons from the Ancient Greeks." Special Section: The Power of Choice: Autonomy, Informed Consent, and the Right to Refuse. *Cambridge Quarterly of Healthcare Ethics* 15 (2006):152–160.

Morreim, E. H. *Balancing Act: The New Medical Ethics of Medicine's New Economics.* Washington, D.C.: Georgetown University Press, 1995.

Moreno, Jonathan. "Convenient and Captive Populations." In *Beyond Consent: Seeking Justice in Research*, edited by Jeffrey Kahn, Anna Mastroianni, and Jeremy Sugarman, 111–130. New York: Oxford University Press, 1998.

Murray, Thomas H. "Research on Children and the Scope of Responsible Parenthood." In *Ethical Issues in Modern Medicine*, edited by Bonnie Steinbock, John Arras, and Alex John London, 815–829. Boston: McGraw Hill Publishing, 2009.

National Bioethics Advisory Commission. "Protecting Research Participants—A Time for Change." In *Contemporary Issues in Bioethics*, edited by Tom Beauchamp and LeRoy Walters, 371–379. Belmont, CA: Wadsworth Publishing Company, 2003.

The National Commission for the Protection of Human Subjects of Biomedical and Behavioral Research. "The Belmont Report: Ethical Principles and Guidelines for the Protection of

Human Subjects of Research." In *Ethical Issues in Modern Medicine*, edited by Bonnie Steinbock, John Arras, and Alex John London, 764–770. Boston: McGraw Hill Publishing, 2009.

Neves, Maria Patrao. "Respect for Human Vulnerability and Personal Integrity." In *The UNESCO Universal Declaration on Bioethics and Human Rights*, edited by Henk ten Have and Michele Jean, 155–164. Paris, France: UNESCO, 2009.

The Nuremberg Tribunal. "The Nuremberg Code (1947)." In *Contemporary Issues in Bioethics*, edited by Tom Beauchamp and LeRoy Walters, 433. Belmont, CA: Wadsworth Publishing Company, 1999.

O'Neill, Onora. *Autonomy and Trust in Bioethics*. Cambridge, United Kingdom: Cambridge University Press, 2002.

Osman, Hana. "History and Development of the Doctrine of Informed Consent." *The International Electronic Journal of Health Education* 4 (2001): 41–47.

Pellegrino, Edmund. "Benefit and Harm." In *The UNESCO Universal Declaration on Bioethics and Human Rights*, edited by Henk ten Have and Michele Jean, 99–110. Paris, France: UNESCO, 2009.

Pence, Gregory. *Medical Ethics: Accounts of the Cases that Shaped and Define Medical Ethics*. Boston: McGraw Hill, 2008.

Pinals, Debra and Paul Appelbaum. "The History and Current Status of Competence and Informed Consent in Psychiatric Research." *The Israel Journal of Psychiatry and Related Sciences* 37:2 (2000): 82–94.

Post, Linda Farber, Jeffrey Blustein, and Nancy Neveloff Dubler. *Handbook for Health Care Ethics Committees*. Baltimore: The John Hopkins University Press, 2007.

Press, Nancy and C. H. Browner. "Risk, Autonomy, and Responsibility: Informed Consent for Prenatal Testing." *The Hastings Center Report* 25:3 (1995): S9–S12.

Ramsey, Paul. *The Patient as Person: Explorations in Medical Ethics*. New Haven, CT: Yale University Press, 2002.

Reilly, Philip. "Eugenic Sterilization in the United States." In *Contemporary Issues in Bioethics*, edited by Tom Beauchamp and LeRoy Walters, 516–525. Belmont, CA: Wadsworth Publishing Company, 1999.

Richards, Edward P., III, JD, MPH (Webmaster). "Consent and Informed Consent. Case Compliments of Versuslaw. *Truman v. Thomas*, 611 P.2d 902 (Cal.1980)." The Law, Science & Public Health Law Site. Accessed June 10, 2012. http://biotech.law.lsu.edu/cases/consent/Truman_v_Thomas.htm,

Roberts, Laura Weiss. "Informed Consent and the Capacity for Voluntarism." *The American Journal of Psychiatry* 159: 5(May 2002): 705–712.

Robinson, Spottswood W. "United States Court of Appeals Canterbury v. Spence." In *Contemporary Issues in Bioethics*, edited by Tom Beauchamp and LeRoy Walters, 133–135. Belmont, CA: Wadsworth Publishing Company, 1999.

Rogers, Bill. "Lawsuit a Reminder to be Certain of Informed Consent." *Medical Post* 47:17 (2011): 42.

Rosenthal, M. Sara. "Informed Consent in the Nuclear Medicine Setting." *Journal of Nuclear Medicine Technology* 39: 1(March 2011): 1–4.

Ross, James, Elizabeth Sundberg, and Katherine Flint. "Informed Consent in School Health Research: Why, How, and Making it Easy." *The Journal of School Health* 69:5 (1999): 171–176.

Rothman, David J. and Sheila M. Rothman. "The Willowbrook Hepatitis Studies." In *Ethical Issues in Modern Medicine*, edited by Bonnie Steinbock, John Arras, and Alex John London, 749–753. Boston: McGraw Hill Publishing, 2009.

Schachter, Debbie, Sukirtha Tharmalingam, and Irwin Kleinman. "Informed Consent and Stimulant Medication: Adolescents' and Parents' Ability to Understand Information about Benefits and Risks of Stimulant Medication for the Treatment of Attention-Deficient/Hyperactivity Disorder." *Journal of Child and Adolescent Psychopharmacology* 21:2 (2011): 139–148.

Schmidt, Ulf. "Cold War at Porton Down: Informed Consent in Britain's Biological and Chemical Warfare Experiments." Special Section: Bioethics and War. *Cambridge Quarterly of Healthcare Ethics* 15 (2006): 366–380.

Sharpe, Neil F. and Ronald Carter. *Genetic Testing: Care, Consent, and Liability*. Hoboken, New Jersey: John Wiley & Sons, Inc., 2006.

Spar, Debora. *The Baby Business: How Money, Science, and Politics Drive the Commerce of Conception*. Boston: Harvard Business School Press, 2006.

Steinbock, Bonnie, John Arras, and Alex John London, eds. *Ethical Issues in Modern Medicine*. Boston: McGraw Hill Publishing, 2009.

Swain, Margaret. "A Brief History of Informed Consent." *Family Advocate* 34:2 (2011): 19–22.

Tauber, Alfred. *Patient Autonomy and the Ethics of Responsibility*. Cambridge, MA: The MIT Press, 2005.

Thompson, Andrew and Normal J. Temple, eds. *Ethics, Medical Research, and Medicine: Commercialism versus Environmentalism and Social Justice*. Dordrecht, Netherlands: Kluwer Academic Publishers, 2001.

Vaughn, Lewis. *Bioethics: Principles, Issues, and Cases*. New York: Oxford University Press, 2009.

Veatch, Robert. "Abandoning Informed Consent." *The Hastings Center Report* 25:2 (1995): 5–12.

Wear, Stephen. *Informed Consent: Patient Autonomy and Clinician Beneficence within Health Care*. Washington, DC: Georgetown University Press, 1998.

Whitney, G. "Reproduction Technology for a New Eugenics." *The Mankind Quarterly* XL:2 (1999): 179–192.

Whittington, Dale. "Ethical Issues with Contingent Valuation Surveys in Developing Countries: A Note on Informed Consent and Other Concerns." *Environmental and Resource Economics* 28: 4(August 2004): 507–515.

Williams, John. "Consent." In *The Cambridge Textbook of Bioethics*, edited by Peter Singer and A. M. Viens, 11–16. Cambridge, United Kingdom: Cambridge University Press, 2008.

Wolpe, Paul Root and Jon F. Merz. "Hospital ERs on Front Line in Informed-Consent Debate." *Forum for Applied Research and Public Policy* 12: 3(Fall 1997): 127–131.

World Medical Association. "Declaration of Helsinki (1996) Recommendations Guiding Physicians in Biomedical Research Involving Human Subjects." In, Tom Beauchamp and LeRoy Walters eds., *Contemporary Issues in Bioethics* (Belmont, CA: Wadsworth Publishing Company: 1999), 434–436.

Chapter 4
Revised Model of Informed Consent

The fourth chapter explains the revised model by aligning the three distinguishing characteristics of PGT with the three widely recognized components in the current model. The practice of the current model of informed consent in matters related to genetics tends to be more of an event, disclosure model.[1] Tom Beauchamp explains that some technologies make it more difficult to encourage growth of both technological and patient rights.[2] The new genetic technologies being developed and implemented today have many implications for informed consent that are not being adequately addressed in the current model.

According to Ulrike Felt, Milena Bister, Michael Strassnig, and Ursula Wagner, if actual practices are different than what the ideal goals are, then some changes need to occur. As a result, the authors question if revising disclosure methods are the only necessary changes.[3] While one of the foundations of consent is disclosing information, the revised model seeks to go further. The revised model focuses on a process approach that promotes understanding over time with assessment mechanisms. The process of consent encourages respect for persons by supporting self-determination for decisions.[4]

To explain the significance of the revised model of consent, the following main categories of comprehension, disclosure, voluntariness, and patient safety are discussed. The first three categories will analyze both the current and revised model of informed consent for PGT, and the last category will discuss patient safety in the revised model.

---

[1] Stephen Wear, *Informed Consent: Patient Autonomy and Clinician Beneficence within Health Care*, 100; Neil C. Manson and Onora O'Neill, *Rethinking Informed Consent in Bioethics*, 69–71; Robert M. Arnold and Charles W. Lidz, "Informed Consent: Clinical Aspects of Consent in Health Care," 8.

[2] Tom L. Beauchamp, "Informed Consent: Its History, Meaning, and Present Challenges," 519–520.

[3] Ulrike Felt, Milena D. Bister, Michael Strassnig, and Ursula Wagner, "Refusing the Information Paradigm: Informed Consent, Medical Research, and Patient Participation," 103.

[4] Robert Levine, "Informed Consent: Some Challenges to the Universal Validity of the Western Model," 147.

© Springer International Publishing Switzerland 2015
J. Minor, *Informed Consent in Predictive Genetic Testing*,
DOI 10.1007/978-3-319-17416-7_4

A. Comprehension of Risk Assessment

The first area is the comprehension of risk assessment in informed consent for PGT. This section will look at how comprehension is applied in the current model. Then the second section will discuss how the revised model addresses some of the weaknesses of the current model and analyze how comprehension is applied in the revised model.

1. Current Model

First, PGT involves a risk analysis of the related probabilities that can be very complicated for patients to comprehend. Indeed a few diseases can be linked to specific genes. However, typically gene-related diseases involve probabilities that are difficult to calculate, including the interaction with the environment (epigenetics).[5] This point develops the importance of understanding in the current model of consent.

Risk assessment involves calculating probabilities to determine the likelihood of developing a disease. To accomplish this, the relation between autonomy and comprehension is crucial. Beauchamp and Childress note that understanding is related to the information that is disclosed about the circumstances and side effects of their decisions. The authors also suggest that full understanding about every detail is not required, but adequate understanding of the main concepts is needed. Sometimes not knowing a certain risk or detail about a test can reduce a person's understanding and can eliminate informed consent if that fact was material to the person's decision. Not only can disclosure influence decision-making, but communication has the ability to help and hinder comprehension.[6]

This section will analyze three main ideas involved with comprehension: autonomy, understanding genetic risks, and the doctor-patient relationship. Each idea will be evaluated in relation to the current model.

a. Autonomy

Informed consent focuses on the self-determination of people by requiring permission for doctors to start medical treatment or research.[7] The current model uses a standardized approach to consent that typically focuses on the autonomous patient signing a consent form without much discussion. This section will look at the degree of autonomy and paternalism and standardization of the current model.

---

[5] Robert Klitzman, "Misunderstandings Concerning Genetics Among Patients Confronting Genetic Disease," 444.

[6] Tom Beauchamp and James Childress, *Principles of Biomedical Ethics*, 127.

[7] Jessica W. Berg, Paul S. Applebaum, Charles W. Lidz, and Lisa S. Parker, *Informed Consent: Legal Theory and Clinical Practice*, 16.

1). Degree of Autonomy and Paternalism

Consent is often based on autonomy by respecting the individual's decision.[8] However, even if people consent, Robert Veatch points out that the consent might not be legitimate or encourage enough autonomy.[9] As a result, there are often differing levels of autonomy within consent. In America, autonomy and choice has always been promoted.[10] However in some cultures, presenting patients with options rather than a recommendation is viewed as a failure of the doctor for not having adequate abilities. As clarified by Michael Brannigan and Judith Boss, autonomy has an emphasis in individualism. However, that emphasis is not always true to people's actions, because many decisions and behaviors can affect others.[11] Thus, autonomous decisions can have an impact on the individual as well as consequences for others.

In a broad sense, autonomy often means accepting a patient's decision even if that decision does not make sense or ignores medical recommendations.[12] As a result, the consequences of a person's actions can also play a part in identifying the degree of autonomy, looking at whether autonomy is emphasized over beneficence or beneficence is emphasized over autonomy. Dan Brock argues that a patient's welfare should be protected if his or her autonomous decision results in negative consequences. Typically the emphasis on beneficence is higher if there is a higher risk to the patient, and as a result, the capacity of the patient is often analyzed more.[13] Thus, ideally the autonomy and beneficence of the patient should be comparable.[14]

However, Veatch explains that under examination, the current model of consent has "more of the traditional, authoritarian understanding of clinical decision-making than many people realize."[15] The history of consent has gone through two extremes from the excessive paternalism to excessive autonomy.[16] While the history of consent demonstrates the importance of autonomy that is free from eugenic thinking, sometimes autonomy is emphasized so much that the other principles and values are disregarded. Michael Burgess notes that if the decision of the participant is emphasized to the exclusion of some other values, then sometimes tests come out

---

[8] Lewis Vaughn, *Bioethics: Principles, Issues, and Cases*, 144.

[9] Robert Veatch, "Abandoning Informed Consent," 5.

[10] Jessica W. Berg, Paul S. Applebaum, Charles W. Lidz, and Lisa S. Parker, *Informed Consent: Legal Theory and Clinical Practice*, 21.

[11] Constance MacIntosh, "Indigenous Self-Determination and Research on Human Genetic Material: A Consideration of the Relevance of Debates on Patents and Informed Consent, and the Political Demands on Researchers," 236; Michael Brannigan and Judith Boss, *Healthcare Ethics in a Diverse Society*, 41.

[12] H. Tristram Engelhardt Jr., *The Foundations of Bioethics*, 301; Lewis Vaughn, *Bioethics: Principles, Issues, and Cases*, 144.

[13] Dan Brock, "Patient Competence and Surrogate Decision-Making," 134.

[14] Lewis Vaughn, *Bioethics: Principles, Issues, and Cases*, 144.

[15] Robert Veatch, "Abandoning Informed Consent," 6.

[16] Janet L. Dolgin, "The Legal Development of the Informed Consent Doctrine: Past and Present," 97; Alan Goldman, "The Refutation of Medical Paternalism," 62.

before the utility and benefit of the test is determined, like susceptibility testing.[17] Often there is little agreement about an appropriate degree of autonomy within the current model.

2). Standardization

In the current model, autonomy is emphasized by letting the patient decide whether or not to get tested. The current model uses an approach to autonomy that is standardized and generic, focusing on consent by providing a signature to accept or reject a test. Robert Arnold and Charles Lidz express that many doctors do not recognize the ability of consent to promote autonomy, but rather physicians see it as a legal doctrine that promotes a mechanical emphasis of disclosure and often leads to patient confusion or worry.[18] In this model, consent is generally given right before a treatment, or an event, is started. The current model uses a homogeneous approach to patients leading to standardization in the consent forms. However, not all information has the same meaning to each patient. Sometimes consent forms emphasize more of the legal ritualistic aspects of consent rather than the ethical, patient-centered approach.[19] Another way of noting this is made by Felt, Bister, Strassnig, and Wagner when suggesting that this "one-size-fits- all solution" can focus more on protocols and the law than ethics.[20] Standardization can decrease autonomy by implying all patients have the same basic needs, values, and informational requests.[21]

In conclusion, simple consent of accepting or rejecting a treatment demonstrates a nominal form of autonomy. Focusing solely on disclosure of information for a simple choice is not an adequate justification for consent.[22] Onora O'Neill states, "What is rather grandly called 'patient autonomy' often amounts simply to a right to choose or refuse treatments… and the corresponding obligations of practitioners not to proceed without patients' consent."[23] Hence, Katz argues that the ideas of making an informed decision and promoting patient respect are more make-believe. According to Katz, the current state of informed consent has encouraged an environment of autonomy and liberty, but has not given clear directions for applying autonomy to the current medical practice.[24] Without having an appropriate level of autonomy and emphasis on individual patients, informed consent with PGT will remain a legalistic tradition.

---

[17] Michael Burgess, "Beyond Consent: Ethical and Social Issues in Genetic Testing," 508; Michael Brannigan and Judith Boss, *Healthcare Ethics in a Diverse Society,* 41.

[18] Robert M. Arnold and Charles W. Lidz, "Informed Consent: Clinical Aspects of Consent in Health Care," 4–5.

[19] John O. Beahrs and Thomas G. Gutheil, "Informed Consent in Psychotherapy," 8.

[20] Ulrike Felt, Milena D. Bister, Michael Strassnig, and Ursula Wagner, "Refusing the Information Paradigm: Informed Consent, Medical Research, and Patient Participation," 103–104.

[21] Stephen Wear, *Informed Consent,* 94–96; Neil C. Manson and Onora O'Neill, *Rethinking Informed Consent in Bioethics,* 70, 80.

[22] Neil C. Manson and Onora O'Neill, *Rethinking Informed Consent in Bioethics,* 70, 185.

[23] Onora O'Neill, "Gaining Autonomy and Losing Trust?" 18.

[24] Jay Katz, "Physicians and Patients: A History of Silence," 138.

b. Understanding Genetic Risks

Since this model emphasizes the consent form, there is insufficient time and communication for understanding the meaning of PGT risk. Inadequate understanding and comprehension is demonstrated by the fact that people cannot remember important risks on the signed consent form. Stephen Wear explains that in one study by Morgan and Schwab, a small percentage of people actually remembered the risks that were involved with the study.[25] Since PGT is typically not diagnostic and has many influencing factors, risk assessments might encourage people to assume they will develop the disease while many people will not.[26] Both of these points illustrate the importance of understanding genetic risk assessments and probabilities. In this section, misunderstandings and education will be discussed further in order to understand the perspective of the current model.

1). Misunderstandings

Having a misunderstanding is to interpret something incorrectly or misconstrue something. From this definition Robert Klitzman suggests that there is a range or different degrees to understanding and misinterpreting. Misunderstandings in one area can cause misunderstandings in other areas as well. Misunderstandings for risk assessments can occur from statistics, the actual genetic test, and the mechanisms of the test.All three of those categories can be related to misconceptions for risk assessments with PGT. For example, one study suggested that testing for diseases like Huntington's disease (HD) involves a lower level of uncertainty than tests for the breast cancer gene (BRCA). Thus, the study concluded that understanding for the less ambiguous diseases was higher. On the other hand, misunderstandings for diseases with environmental factors led to more ambiguity and less understanding. In this study Klitzman noted that the misunderstanding in absolute and relative risks was higher for uncertain diseases like breast cancer than for diseases like HD.[27] Because PGT has many uncertainties, the predictive value for developing a specific disease is typically low. If the importance of uncertainty and the likelihood of false results are minimized and thus misunderstood, then understanding the genetic risks of PGT can be challenging for informed consent.[28]

---

[25] Stephen Wear, *Informed Consent*, 52–53; Bernard Lo, *Resolving Ethical Dilemmas*, 21.

[26] Svante Paabo, "The Human Genome and Our View of Ourselves," 497; AMA, "Direct-to-Consumer Genetic Testing;" Cynthia Marietta and Amy McGuire, "Direct-to-Consumer Genetic Testing: Is It the Practice of Medicine?" 370.

[27] Robert Klitzman, "Misunderstandings Concerning Genetics Among Patients Confronting Genetic Disease," 431–433, 441–442, 444.

[28] Cynthia James, Gail Geller, Barbara Bernhardt, et al., "Are Practicing and Future Physicians Prepared to Obtain Informed Consent? The Case of Genetic Testing for Susceptibility to Breast Cancer," 204, 206, 209; Tom Beauchamp and James Childress, *Principles of Biomedical Ethics*, 130.

2). Education and Time

Many studies conclude that, even after signing the consent form, research participants and patients do not have enough understanding of the information presented,
consent forms, and/or research trials and do not know the patient rights and responsibilities.[29] Thus it is important to recognize some barriers that can impact the
general comprehension of risk assessments.[30] One of the biggest barriers to understanding is an inadequate amount of time.[31] Because the current model emphasizes
a one-time event focusing on the consent form, this approach does not allow for
sufficient time to process and understand all of the information presented. If there
is not enough time for education and communication, then a patient and research
subject's understanding will be diminished.

Another barrier is an inadequate level of education. Often patients and research
subjects are not educated enough on PGT to understand the nuances of the testing
procedures and results. Even physicians can have differing levels of education on
PGT. James, Geller, Bernhardt, et al. evaluate one study that looks at physician
practices and the implications of PGT on informed consent. The study concluded
that fourth-year medical students had a better idea of how to calculate the predictive
value of a BRCA test than current physicians or first-year medical students. Studies
suggest that oncologists typically did well in interpreting the predictive value, but
gynecologists did not do as well. Since physicians often have varying levels of education concerning PGT, physicians can sometimes misinterpret and misrepresent
the predictive value of the testing. This study concluded that physicians did not take
into consideration the possibility of false-negative, and as a result, the test was misinterpreted and the patients had a lack of understanding.[32] However, simple education is not always enough either. Sometimes there are differing views of the natural
world that can result in a lack of understanding certain information.[33] Even after
appropriate education, there can also be emotional and/or family issues that can
impact a person's understanding as well. In this case, at times the faulty information
or long-held inaccurate assumptions take precedence over the appropriate views.[34]

According to Arnold and Lidz, as it is right now informed consent appears "either
to promote uninformed—and thus suboptimal—decisions, or to encourage patients

---

[29] Daniel W. Fitzgerald, Cecile Marotte, Rose Irene Verdier, et al., "Comprehension during Informed Consent in a Less-Developed Country," 1301; Jessica W. Berg, Paul S. Applebaum, Charles
W. Lidz, and Lisa S. Parker, *Informed Consent: Legal Theory and Clinical Practice*, 65, 102.

[30] Stephen Wear, *Informed Consent,* 61–62; Albert Jonsen, Mark Siegler, William Winslade, *Clinical Ethics: A Practical Approach to Ethical Decisions in Clinical Medicine,* 59.

[31] Stephen Wear, *Informed Consent,* 62.

[32] Cynthia James, Gail Geller, Barbara Bernhardt, et al., "Are Practicing and Future Physicians
Prepared to Obtain Informed Consent? The Case of Genetic Testing for Susceptibility to Breast
Cancer," 204, 206, 209.

[33] Martha Macintyre, "Informed Consent and Mining Projects: A View from Papua New Guinea,"
59.

[34] Robert Klitzman, "Misunderstandings Concerning Genetics Among Patients Confronting Genetic Disease," 441–442.

to blindly accept healthcare professionals' recommendations."[35] Without appropriate comprehension, risk probabilities have the potential to cause fear, confusion, and false assurances.[36] Hence, patients need more sophisticated consent approaches to ensure they understand the complexities of risk probabilities.

c. Doctor-Patient Relationship

The current doctor-patient relationship focuses upon the patient freely signing the consent form without sufficient education of the patient about the meaning of PGT. Currently patient risk assessments are discussed with a clinician. However Wear explains that the current model typically does not dedicate a significant amount of time to doctor-patient discussions of risk assessment of the related probabilities.[37] Because as Arnold and Lidz suggest, physicians often think informed consent is too time-consuming and ritualistic and leads to lower medical care.[38] Standard consent forms could diminish the relationship between the doctor and patient or researcher and subject.[39] Instead of having increased communication, often the consent forms assume understanding once signed.[40] Once the providers assume understanding, typically there is a silence between the doctors and patients and/or researchers and subjects.[41] This section will first explain the current interaction of the doctor and patient and then discuss the state of communication and education in the current model.

1). Current Doctor-Patient Interaction

In the mid 1970s, doctors viewed the requirements of consent as not practical and in some cases not aligned with appropriate medical care. The doctor-patient relationship was impacted in the shift from paternalism, because patients wanted more involvement and an equal footing in the decision-making process.[42] However, that shift has continued and has generally increased the emphasis of autonomy in the doctor-patient relationship.[43] At this time, since autonomy is held in high regard,

---

[35] Robert M. Arnold and Charles W. Lidz, "Informed Consent: Clinical Aspects of Consent in Health Care," 5.

[36] Stephen Wear, *Informed Consent,* 62, 66; Berdik, Chris, "Genetic Tests Give Consumers Hints About Disease Risk; Critics Have Misgivings," 3; Thomas Goetz, *The Decision Tree,* 122.

[37] Stephen Wear, *Informed Consent,* 62.

[38] Robert M. Arnold and Charles W. Lidz, "Informed Consent: Clinical Aspects of Consent in Health Care," 4–5; Tom Beauchamp, "Informed Consent," 191.

[39] John O. Beahrs and Thomas G. Gutheil, "Informed Consent in Psychotherapy," 8.

[40] Tom Beauchamp, "Informed Consent," 191.

[41] Jay Katz, "Physicians and Patients: A History of Silence," 136.

[42] Tom L. Beauchamp, "Informed Consent: Its History, Meaning, and Present Challenges," 516.

[43] Roberta M. Berry, "Informed Consent Law, Ethics, and Practice: From Infancy to Reflective Adolescence," 72.

generally the physician merely sees his role as informing the individual of the risks and benefits of a procedure or study. Howard Brody explains that typically doctors are responsible for the medical information and patients are responsible for that information within the context of their values. Usually, the physician or researcher imparts information and then allows the patient or subject to either sign the consent form or not. However, often there is little education and communication for the patient and/or subject to make an adequate informed decision. The current interaction with doctor-patient and researcher-subject is typically seen as more of an "informative," rather than an "interpretive" or "deliberative" role.[44]

However, even when there is a discussion about that information, sometimes the amount of doctor or researcher interference can be difficult to balance.[45] One example, the emergence of the so-called Nocebo Effect needs to be considered here. This Effect argues that providing patients or subjects with too much information can result in harm when the patients or subjects are not able to handle the amount of information properly.[46] The Nocebo Effect is also related to the placebo effect. The Nocebo Effect relates to PGT, because often there can be insufficient or overwhelming detail that can cause an increased risk to the patient and/or subject.[47] Doctor-patient and researcher-subject interaction in the current model is typically limited to presenting certain information while not allowing for adequate communication or education.

2). Communication and Education

At this time, more doctors are going into genetics and genomic medicine, and those doctors will have to educate patients appropriately about PGT. Francis Collins and Victor McKusick explain that this will necessitate more physicians understanding genetics.[48] Because patients generally do not understand PGT adequately by themselves, doctors play a crucial role in helping patients to make informed decisions about testing. However, some confusion can exist in the doctor-patient relationship about the appropriate level of communication and education.

The current model generally shows a lack of doctor-patient and researcher-subject education and communication. One study showed that if a doctor offered a test, generally patients assumed the test would be valuable. As a result, the patients agreed to testing and did not even consider the risks. While doctors would not recommend procedures that cause intentional harm, PGT is a little different in that

---

[44] Howard Brody, "The Physician-Patient Relationship," 78–79, 82.

[45] Wear, Stephen, *Informed Consent,* 172.

[46] Rebecca Erwin Wells and Ted J. Kaptchuk, "To Tell the Truth, the Whole Truth, May Do Patients Harm: The Problem of the Nocebo Effect for Informed Consent," 22–29.

[47] Chris Berdik, "Genetic Tests Give Consumers Hints About Disease Risk; Critics Have Misgivings," 1–2; Stephen Wear, *Informed Consent,* 61–62, 77, 82; Thomas Goetz, *The Decision Tree,* 215.

[48] Francis Collins and Victor McKusick, "Implications of the Human Genome Project for Medical Science," 477.

this testing almost always has potential benefits and harms. This study demonstrates that the physicians did not communicate adequately to the patients concerning the goals of testing. The patients were not educated enough to make an informed decision.[49] This area also applies to researchers and subjects. One study by Fitzgerald, Marotte, Verdier, et al. looked at the research consent procedures of Europe and the USA. This study demonstrated that the current guidelines requiring one discussion session with the researcher and subject was not necessarily enough, and the authors suggested creating better regulations.[50] With the amount of information that is becoming available with PGT, both physicians and researchers should encourage additional communication and education to promote informed decisions.[51]

2. Revised Model

Typically gene-related diseases involve probabilities that are difficult to calculate, such as environmental interactions. Since risk assessments are the foundation of PGT and are often very complex, it is essential that patients understand these related risk probabilities. This model enhances the link between risk and comprehension by looking at autonomy, understanding, and the doctor-patient relationship. The development of the relationship between autonomy and understanding is important when analyzing risk assessments for determining the likelihood of developing a disease.

a. Autonomy

Often respecting patients' rights and obtaining consent are the basic goals and guidelines for promoting autonomy.[52] James Childress explains that when people "acquiesce in another person's wishes, choices, and actions for that person's own benefit," autonomy is promoted.[53] The revised model adopts a personalized approach to consent that emphasizes extensive discussion with the patient as an autonomous agent. This section looks at personalization and competence first, and then it will discuss the impact of paternalism on autonomy.

---

[49] Robert Klitzman, "Misunderstandings Concerning Genetics Among Patients Confronting Genetic Disease," 443, 445.

[50] Daniel W. Fitzgerald, Cecile Marotte, Rose Irene Verdier, et al., "Comprehension during Informed Consent in a Less-Developed Country," 1301–1302.

[51] Robert Klitzman, "Misunderstandings Concerning Genetics Among Patients Confronting Genetic Disease," 444–445; Douglas Martin and Heather Greenwood, "Public Perceptions of Ethical Issues Regarding Adult Predictive Genetic Testing," 106.

[52] Onora O'Neill, "Gaining Autonomy and Losing Trust?" 16.

[53] James Childress, *Who Should Decide? Paternalism in Health Care*, 13.

1). Personalization and Competence

The revised model, rather than merely accepting or rejecting a physician's recommendation, enhances patient involvement by adopting a more personalized, extensive approach, described as a process rather than as an event.[54] Personalization of consent can be promoted in a couple of ways. First, the revised model takes into consideration the fact that PGT has risks and values at stake that can only be evaluated by the specific patient. The doctor has technical knowledge and experience; the patient has life circumstances.[55] As a result, the revised model assumes each person can contribute to the consent and decision-making process.[56] Utility of a genetic test cannot be presumed on the basis of availability as a medical test, but rather the individual patients and participants have to weigh the available information against their personal goals, values, and sometimes culture. Since expectations can be distorted at times, it is important to identify the benefits and risks such as psychological and social risks. Some risks can be more harmful than others, and as a result, having the individual evaluate the benefits even with future uncertainty can increase the individual's sense of autonomy.[57] Having a better sense of control and personal responsibility over an individual's health can assist in decision-making.[58]

Second, the revised model emphasizes heterogeneous decisions and informational needs of each patient. This model is against unrealistic demands of specific and explicit uniform processes of informed consent, because each person has different values and requests. Third, the revised model strives to turn abstract statistics and risks into more personalized medical information, which is an added measure for enhancing autonomy.[59] Hence, the patient's values and goals guide the outcome more clearly. Another way of noting this point is made by Lewis Vaughn when he points out that bioethicists promote informed consent and autonomy because "knowledgeable, autonomous patients who choose for themselves will advance their own best interests as they themselves conceive them."[60] Personalization of risk assessments is important for comprehension. An individual cannot make an

---

[54] Robert M. Arnold and Charles W. Lidz, "Informed Consent: Clinical Aspects of Consent in Health Care," 8–9.

[55] Stephen Wear, *Informed Consent*, 37–38.

[56] Robert M. Arnold and Charles W. Lidz, "Informed Consent: Clinical Aspects of Consent in Health Care," 5, 10.

[57] Michael Burgess, "Beyond Consent: Ethical and Social Issues in Genetic Testing," 508–509, 511; Hana Osman, "History and Development of the Doctrine of Informed Consent," 45–46; Constance MacIntosh, "Indigenous Self-Determination and Research on Human Genetic Material: A Consideration of the Relevance of Debates on Patents and Informed Consent, and the Political Demands on Researchers," 237–238.

[58] Terrence Ackerman, "Why Doctors Should Intervene," 76.

[59] Stephen Wear, *Informed Consent*. 67, 73, 95, 176; Thomas Goetz, *The Decision Tree*, xix, 141, 215; Neil C. Manson and Onora O'Neill, *Rethinking Informed Consent in Bioethics*, 80, 188–189; Edward Spencer, Ann Mills, Mary Rorty, and Patricia Werhane, *Organization Ethics in Health Care*, 36.

[60] Lewis Vaughn, *Bioethics: Principles, Issues, and Cases*, 144.

informed decision accurately, unless he or she recognizes the impact PGT can have on his or her life.[61] An individual's informed consent needs to be based on personal analysis rather than abstract, generic information.

Adapting consent to an individual's aptitude level can also help encourage understanding.[62] However, Joseph Goldstein argued against an emphasis on comprehension on the basis that sometimes people make choices for those with limited capacities which would limit autonomy.[63] Just because a person might have limited competence, does not necessarily mean he or she cannot make an informed decision with enough time and communication.[64] Sometimes situations that can limit capacity can be resolved or addressed, for example when a person is in pain, on strong medication, or in depression. As clarified by the Belmont Report, generally it is necessary to ensure a higher level of competency and decision-making capacity if the risks are greater than normal.[65] Sara Rosenthal states that capacity "operates on a sliding scale that permits lesser standards of capacity for less consequential medical decisions (such as getting a flu shot) and requires higher standards of capacity for decisions of greater consequence (such as consenting to high-dose radioactive iodine therapy)."[66] In many studies, the MacArthur Competency Assessment Tool-Clinical Research (MacCAT-CR) proved to be helpful in assessing an individual's level of capacity to make informed decisions.[67] If autonomy is based on the exercise of an individual to make a voluntary decision, often the number of potential choices will expand.[68] With PGT, because there is a wide range of possible decisions, ensuring comprehension before a decision is crucial.

2). Impact of Paternalism on Autonomy

The practices put in place as a result of the history of consent can guard against paternalism.[69] By respecting a person's choice, medical paternalism can be mini-

---

[61] Terrence Ackerman, "Why Doctors Should Intervene," 74.

[62] The National Commission for the Protection of Human Subjects of Biomedical and Behavioral Research, "The Belmont Report: Ethical Principles and Guidelines for the Protection of Human Subjects of Research," 768.

[63] Joseph Goldstein, "For Harold Lasswell: Some Reflections on Human Dignity, Entrapment, Informed Consent, and the Plea Bargain," 691–692, 701–702; Jessica Berg, Paul Appelbaum, Charles Lidz, and Lisa Parker, *Informed Consent Legal Theory and Clinical Practice,* 152.

[64] James Childress, *Who Should Decide? Paternalism in Health Care,* 136.

[65] The National Commission for the Protection of Human Subjects of Biomedical and Behavioral Research, "The Belmont Report: Ethical Principles and Guidelines for the Protection of Human Subjects of Research," 768; Terrence Ackerman, "Why Doctors Should Intervene," 74–75.

[66] M. Sara Rosenthal, "Informed Consent in the Nuclear Medicine Setting," 2.

[67] Debra Pinals and Paul Applebaum, "The History and Current Status of Competence and Informed Consent in Psychiatric Research," 88.

[68] H. Tristram Engelhardt Jr., *The Foundations of Bioethics,* 304.

[69] Jeffrey Carlisle and Ann T. Neulicht, "The Necessity of Professional Disclosure and Informed Consent for Rehabilitation Counselors," 28.

mized.[70] However, because of past abuses, the focus on paternalism was replaced with a strong focus on autonomy. While autonomy is typically beneficial, Berg, Applebaum, Lidz, and Parker argue that if there is too much of an emphasis on autonomy, physicians could be taken to court more often and patients might make increasingly inappropriate choices.[71]

Autonomy, justice, and beneficence need to be balanced. If not, opportunities can arise that might take advantage of other people and situations.[72] To illustrate the problems that can arise when those principles are not balanced, two models are analyzed briefly. First, the public health model of the past led to an increase in the eugenics movement. This model, more paternalistic in nature, focused primarily on the beneficence of the public, while often ignoring the rights of the individual. The second model, a newer model, is the personal service model which is based primarily on autonomy of the individual. This model argues that genetic tests are just medical services for people to take advantage of if desired. In this model, participating in PGT is based on an individual's decision, because how people use genetic information and services is up to them and not the public. Unfettered choice and an exaggerated emphasis on autonomy can lead to a different type of eugenics based on individual choice rather than the government coercion of the past. Having an improper view of autonomy can promote the freedom of choice of one person while infringing upon the autonomy of another. Even though autonomy can result in individual liberty to choose, unlimited autonomy should be regulated in PGT to prevent harm and promote justice.[73] Since both models have the opportunity for a level of discrimination and/or eugenics, a proper balance of autonomy and beneficence is necessary in order to promote comprehension.

b. Understanding Genetic Risks

The revised model focuses on a process that provides time for communication to foster an understanding of the complex meaning of PGT risk. The revised model seeks to encourage understanding and address the current model's misunderstandings of risk assessments. Stephen Wear suggests that understanding can be promoted through increased education and communication of related risk probabilities.[74]Clear communication of risk assessment and understanding of probabilities can often lead

---

[70] Lewis Vaughn, *Bioethics: Principles, Issues, and Cases,* 144.

[71] Jessica Berg, Paul Appelbaum, Charles Lidz, and Lisa Parker, *Informed Consent Legal Theory and Clinical Practice,* 152.

[72] Michael Brannigan and Judith Boss, *Healthcare Ethics in a Diverse Society,* 41.

[73] Allen Buchanan, Dan Brock, Norman Daniels, and Daniel Wikler, "From Chance to Choice: Genetics and Justice," 491–492.

[74] Stephen Wear, *Informed Consent,* 94–7; Robert Klitzman, "Misunderstandings Concerning Genetics Among Patients Confronting Genetic Disease," 445; Lori B. Andrews, *Future Perfect: Confronting Decisions about Genetics,* 166.

to increased patient satisfaction, better clinical outcomes, and adaptation to needs.[75] This section will describe the process approach and then look at methods to encourage understanding in the revised model.

1). Process Approach

Klitzman suggests that the current model views understanding as more static, but the revised model recognizes that understanding is continually developed through a process over time.[76] One study looking at procedures in Europe and the USA concluded that people can understand consent information if given adequate attention, and that the current procedures could be inadequate for understanding.[77] As a result, the revised model dedicates a significant amount of time to understanding and comprehending risk assessment probabilities through a process. The Institute of Medicine's Committee on Assessing Genetic Risks, consisting of Andrews, Fullarton, Holtzman, eds., et al., says that "An informed public is the best societal protection from possible abuses of genetic technology and information in the future."[78] An informed public implies that the "public" has been educated, but patient education is not adequate in itself. Neil Sharpe and Ronald Carter note that there is more to testing than just interpretation. Having appropriate communication, understanding, and genetic counseling can encourage a greater perspective.[79] In addition many times emotions and experiences have a higher impact on understanding than pure information or reasoning.[80] As a result, the process approach focuses on the "communicative, emotional, psychological needs to assist [the] patient to understand, adjust, and cope with implications posed by genetic test and information."[81] By analyzing each aspect over time, understanding can be achieved.[82]

2). Methods to Encourage Understanding

If a person does not understand the information appropriately, that misperception can lead to faulty consent. Even once the misunderstanding is corrected, patients

---

[75] Bill Runciman, Alan Merry, and Merrilyn Walton, *Safety and Ethics in Healthcare,* 94; Stephen Wear, *Informed Consent,* 54–55.

[76] Robert Klitzman, "Misunderstandings Concerning Genetics Among Patients Confronting Genetic Disease," 443.

[77] Daniel W. Fitzgerald, Cecile Marotte, Rose Irene Verdier, et al., "Comprehension during Informed Consent in a Less-Developed Country," 1301–1302.

[78] Lori Andrews, Jane Fullarton, Neil Holtzman, eds., et al., Committee on Assessing Genetic Risks, Institute of Medicine, *Assessing Genetic Risks: Implications for Health and Social Policy,* 195.

[79] Neil Sharpe and Ronald Carter, *Genetic Testing: Care, Consent, and Liability,* 364.

[80] Ian Young, *Introduction to Risk Calculation in Genetic Counseling,* 5.

[81] Neil F. Sharpe and Ronald Carter, *Genetic Testing,* 131.

[82] Tom Beauchamp and James Childress, *Principles of Biomedical Ethics,* 128.

can still choose to hold onto their incorrect views. As long as a person has a misconception about a certain aspect of the test or genetics that is important to decision-making, that individual's consent or refusal is suspect.[83]

The revised model promotes different ways to ensure patient understanding of risk assessment probabilities. First, many times understanding is impacted by the way risk is presented.[84] Often consent forms can be vague with inadequate information or with confusing information.[85] Breaking up large amounts of information into more manageable segments over a period of time can encourage appropriate communication.[86] If less information is presented at a time, then people might understand that information better before moving on to other information about risks. Thus, Pinals and Applebaum suggest making consent forms shorter to encourage increased understanding.[87] Second, statistical information can be simplified. Making comparisons of statistical information with typical risks the patient knows, like statistics for car accidents can help to increase understanding and make it practical.[88] Studies have shown people understand and apply risk better when actual risk is given than relative risk. Sometimes if relative risk is given, people can misinterpret the benefits of the treatment as being better than the actual risk.[89] Also when discussing risk, many times people like risks in terms of odds. One family wanted their risk information in gambling terms. So instead of saying.25, a physician could say there is a 1 in 4 chance of developing the disease or a 25 % chance. On the opposite side, a physician could say there is a 3 out of 4 chance the individual will not develop a disease. Third, patients should understand the meaning behind the results and be given more details about the risk.[90] Childress points out that risk could be in relation to developing a disease or complication in the future. While the severity of the disease cannot be predicted, the revised model can encourage understanding of the meaning of risk assessment for PGT so that people can make decisions based off of accurate views.[91]

---

[83] Tom Beauchamp and James Childress, *Principles of Biomedical Ethics*, 130–131.

[84] National Bioethics Advisory Commission, "Protecting Research Participants— A Time for Change," 374.

[85] David Wright, "Redesigning Informed Consent Tools for Specific Research," 151.

[86] Terrence Ackerman, "Why Doctors Should Intervene," 75–77; Allen Buchanan, "From Chance to Choice: Genetics and Justice," 491; Chris Berdik, "Genetic Tests Give Consumers Hints About Disease Risk; Critics Have Misgivings," 1–2; Stephen Wear, *Informed Consent,* 61–62, 77, 82; Thomas Goetz, *The Decision Tree,* 215; James Childress, *Who Should Decide? Paternalism in Health Care,* 135–136.

[87] Debra Pinals and Paul Applebaum, "The History and Current Status of Competence and Informed Consent in Psychiatric Research," 90.

[88] Tom Beauchamp and James Childress, *Principles of Biomedical Ethics*, 128.

[89] Patricia Kelly, "Cancer Risks in Perspective: Information and Approaches for Clinicians," 397.

[90] Ian Young, *Introduction to Risk Calculation in Genetic Counseling,* 4–5; Neil Sharpe and Ronald Carter, *Genetic Testing: Care, Consent, and Liability,* 2.

[91] James Childress, *Who Should Decide? Paternalism in Health Care,* 135–136.

c. Doctor-Patient Relationship

The revised model emphasizes the doctor-patient relationship as an interactive process to ensure sufficient education of the patient about the meaning of PGT. The additional time and complexity involved in comprehending the connection between risk and probability has significant implications for patient education by the doctor, thereby developing the meaning of the doctor-patient relationship.

1). Interactive Process

Wear explains that the revised model tries to eliminate the idea of "strangers taking care of strangers" by having an ongoing, interactive doctor-patient relationship that strives for comprehension.[92] In the revised model, doctor-patient and/or researcher-subject interaction and education are important aspects. The providers should educate and interact with patients and subjects about risk assessments and predictions to encourage understanding.[93] Often additional education can promote learning and understanding for testing.[94] Francis Collins and Victor McKusick suggest that public education should start now and be realistic about the risks and benefits of PGT in general.[95] By having increased public education of PGT and genetics, some of the misunderstandings of the current model might be eliminated. Research has suggested that education in science could encourage more understanding about risk assessments rather than just education in general, but no studies have looked specifically at different areas of education, just the quantity of education.[96] Education and interaction can prove beneficial in eliminating misunderstandings and encouraging comprehension. One study looked at the potential impact mental illness had on decision making capacity, and concluded that even those with limitations could improve their competency scores after having additional education and communication.[97] Thus Felt, Bister, Strassnig, and Wagner argue that if the goal is to develop patient understanding about the risks, benefits, and limits of genetics and science in general, then engaging patients at the beginning would be best. If not, then patients might not comply if trust is restricted.[98] Strengthening the doctor-

---

[92] Stephen Wear, *Informed Consent*, 95, 97.

[93] Thomas Goetz, *The Decision Tree*, xvii, 4; Stephen Wear, *Informed Consent*, 72–74; Robert M. Arnold and Charles W. Lidz, "Informed Consent: Clinical Aspects of Consent in Health Care," 4.

[94] Debra Pinals and Paul Applebaum, "The History and Current Status of Competence and Informed Consent in Psychiatric Research," 90.

[95] Francis Collins and Victor McKusick, "Implications of the Human Genome Project for Medical Science," 478.

[96] Robert Klitzman, "Misunderstandings Concerning Genetics Among Patients Confronting Genetic Disease," 442.

[97] Debra Pinals and Paul Applebaum, "The History and Current Status of Competence and Informed Consent in Psychiatric Research," 88.

[98] Ulrike Felt, Milena D. Bister, Michael Strassnig, and Ursula Wagner, "Refusing the Information Paradigm: Informed Consent, Medical Research, and Patient Participation," 103–104.

patient and researcher-subject relationship can encourage additional comprehension of risks involved with PGT.[99]

A study by Fitzgerald, Marotte, Verdier, et al., illustrates that having a couple of meetings to focus on education helped to increase patient comprehension. When presenting information to uneducated people, research has suggested that smaller amounts of information should be given at a time to increase understanding.[100] This process helps to ensure comprehension, and the interaction between doctor-patient and researcher-subject strengthens the relationship. One area which can be strengthened by this interactive process is the Nocebo Effect.[101] At times presenting too much information with PGT and risk assessments can be difficult for patients to comprehend and can cause additional stress in thinking about the potential options. Having too much information or too little information can be challenging for consent. Thus, the revised model encourages physicians to cut down on overloading patients with information and instead try to help patients organize and prioritize the information.[102] Pinals and Applebaum point out that since the current model does not emphasize a process, a large amount of information is typically given at one time. Asking the patient questions can help physicians identify which areas the patient understands and which areas need more discussion.[103] This process can also help to balance the doctor-patient and researcher-subject relationship.

2). Balancing the Doctor-Patient Relationship

Terrence Ackerman notes that respect for persons involves a more comprehensive view of the doctor-patient relationship. Ackerman argues that the current view of autonomy is based on the legalistic view of the doctor-patient relationship. This view falls short of the ideal, because it does not take into consideration how sickness affects independent decision-making. Sickness can hamper a patient's ability to have appropriate decision-making skills and relationships with the healthcare staff. The doctor's aim should be helping patients achieve their goals, and in order to do that, the physician has to have a personal interest in the patient. As a result, physicians should not have to be detached and uninvolved in order for autonomy to be emphasized. Instead of being inactive, physicians could encourage communication that fosters autonomy and freedom without needless limitations. If emotional

---

[99] Cynthia James, Gail Geller, Barbara Bernhardt, et al., "Are Practicing and Future Physicians Prepared to Obtain Informed Consent? The Case of Genetic Testing for Susceptibility to Breast Cancer," 203; Robert Klitzman, "Misunderstandings Concerning Genetics Among Patients Confronting Genetic Disease," 444–445.

[100] Daniel W. Fitzgerald, Cecile Marotte, Rose Irene Verdier, et al., "Comprehension during Informed Consent in a Less-Developed Country," 1302.

[101] Rebecca Erwin Wells and Ted J. Kaptchuk, "To Tell the Truth, the Whole Truth, May Do Patients Harm: The Problem of the Nocebo Effect for Informed Consent," 22–29.

[102] Tom Beauchamp and James Childress, *Principles of Biomedical Ethics*, 129–130.

[103] Debra Pinals and Paul Applebaum, "The History and Current Status of Competence and Informed Consent in Psychiatric Research," 90.

and societal aspects can influence autonomy, then doctors should evaluate the patients in regards to those issues.[104] This is the balance that exists between interference and noninterference in relation to autonomous actions.

The interactive process encouraged in the revised model inherently promotes a balance in the relationship. The revised model encourages doctors and researchers to take more of a guiding approach with patients and subjects. The physicians and researchers should educate the individual while helping to sort through the person's opinions about the decision. Having this supportive relationship with a doctor and/or researcher can help balance out the affiliation.[105] Physicians and researchers should communicate regularly and inquire openly as to what the patient and subjects wants to know. Howard Brody suggests that assuming certain information will not encourage a balanced relationship. Brody explains this further when he states, it "will not do to reduce communication to a cold and legalistic catalogue of medical facts, options, risks, and benefits. Real dialogue lies between these two extremes, but exactly where, for each relationship, is a tricky question."[106] Balancing these extremes can be problematic, but adhering to an interactive process can help to eliminate some of the difficulties within the relationship.

B. Disclosure to Select an Appropriate Treatment Option

In looking at the risks of research in the past, Jonsen and Dr. Katz realized that physicians had to change their way of thinking for disclosing information. It was no longer solely up to the physicians' views and the professional guidelines.[107] Instead throughout history, patients were progressively given more and more information in order to be able to make an appropriate decision. As a result, today there are clear guidelines on what to present to the patient and how to present that information in order to have an informed consent. This section will look at the standards for disclosure and genetic counseling in both the current and revised models for informed consent of PGT.

1. Current Model

In PGT, there are complex treatment options, including no treatment for some diseases, which require genetic counseling to select an appropriate option. This point develops the importance of disclosure in the current model. The first part will look

---

[104] Terrence Ackerman, "Why Doctors Should Intervene," 75–77; Allen Buchanan, "From Chance to Choice: Genetics and Justice," 491.

[105] Howard Brody, "The Physician-Patient Relationship," 82–83.

[106] Howard Brody, "The Physician-Patient Relationship," 85.

[107] Albert Jonsen, *The Birth of Bioethics*, 144–146.

at what information and options are typically disclosed in the current model. The second part will evaluate the current guidelines for genetic counseling.

a. Disclosure

The current model focuses on medical information in a standardized approach of consent. While patients can be educated about the procedure, selecting an appropriate treatment option can be more difficult.[108] There are studies that suggest disclosure of potential risks can sometimes cause patients to twist information or have unfounded worries.[109] Robert Arnold and Charles Lidz state that "using technical jargon, trying to give all of the available information in one visit, and not asking what the patient wants to know is a recipe for confusing even the most intelligent patient."[110] This section will discuss what to disclose and the guidelines that go along with disclosure.

1). Information to Disclose

If information material to a person's decision is left out of the disclosure, then informed consent will not be present. James, Geller, Bernhardt, et al. performed a study that looked at essential information for physicians to disclose to patients thinking about PGT. In comparing the levels of education, this study concluded that many of the levels had similar conclusions about what should be disclosed before making a decision about treatment. In the case study, the majority of physicians said if a test was positive, the likelihood of getting the cancer, the possible treatments to reduce the cancer, issues of the actual value and beneficence of the treatments, and insurance aspects should be discussed. The only difference in the results of the study was that medical students thought the more practical side of the disease or test should be discussed like the processes and painfulness of testing. James, Geller, Bernhardt, et al. argue that sometimes doctors can get caught up with more of the medical aspects and overlook the more practical side of PGT, which patients can be more interested in at times. Since those with a lower income and education can have a greater interest in the practical aspects, a more pronounced disparity among those groups can emerge if physicians do not discuss both the medical and practical factors involved in PGT.[111] However, the current model typically places more emphasis on disclosing the medical issues rather than the practical or non-medical issues.

---

[108] Stephen Wear, *Informed Consent,* 95–96; Neil C. Manson and Onora O'Neill, *Rethinking Informed Consent in Bioethics*, 70, 80; Robert M. Arnold and Charles W. Lidz, "Informed Consent: Clinical Aspects of Consent in Health Care," 11.

[109] Tom Beauchamp and James Childress, *Principles of Biomedical Ethics*, 130.

[110] Robert M. Arnold and Charles W. Lidz, "Informed Consent: Clinical Aspects of Consent in Health Care," 6.

[111] Cynthia James, Gail Geller, Barbara Bernhardt, et al., "Are Practicing and Future Physicians Prepared to Obtain Informed Consent? The Case of Genetic Testing for Susceptibility to Breast

2). Disclosure Guidelines

Disclosure for informed consent is more of a formal ritual, because often people can disregard disclosure guidelines and consent forms. In the current model, these guidelines focus on the standardized approach for disseminating information, which generally involves a physician or researcher giving information. Childress explains that simply presenting information, which people might or might not understand, does not fulfill the duty to disclose. Merely disclosing information without any support falls short of the ethical ideal. However, in certain instances, there are exceptions to disclosure. One exception that can apply to PGT is waiving a person's rights. If a patient waives his or her rights, then the doctor does not have a responsibility to inform the patient or to ensure the material is understood.[112] However, even if a person's rights are waived, the person still might want support with his or her decision. While physicians cannot force patients to reflect on disclosed information, the providers should support patients in order to be able to make an appropriate decision.

In the current model, many times the sole purpose of disclosure is to find out treatment options. Since PGT has numerous variables and uncertainty, the disclosure guidelines for PGT are often a little different. With PGT, there is often a lack of specific treatment options for many diagnosed genetic traits involved with PGT. However, some general possibilities include preventing the disease, lessening the severity, and monitoring the disease. Though with most diseases PGT tests for, Harris, Winship, and Spriggs explain that completely preventing the disease is typically rare. Since many of these diseases have no acceptable treatments, lessening the severity can be difficult. Thus, sometimes surveillance is the only option with PGT.[113] However, not all patients understand the problem of treatment options with PGT. The current disclosure guidelines for PGT do little to emphasize this potential lack of treatment options for PGT. By focusing mainly on medical information for treatment purposes, the current model can overlook some of the more relevant information which would be material to an informed decision. As a result, patients and subjects need more sophisticated consent approaches to disclose antecedently the treatment options, including the possibility of no treatment.

b. Genetic Counseling

Genetic counseling often includes information about a disease while looking at the emotional aspects of the at-risk diagnosis or the test.[114] These personal issues are

---

Cancer," 204, 207–210; Lewis Vaughn, *Bioethics: Principles, Issues, and Cases*, 146; Janet Dolgin and Lois Shepherd, *Bioethics and the Law*, 59.

[112] James Childress, *Who Should Decide? Paternalism in Health Care*, 135–136.

[113] Marion Harris, Ingrid Winship, Merle Spriggs, "Controversies and Ethical Issues in Cancer-Genetics Clinics," 301; Anita Silvers and Michael Ashley Stein, "An Equality Paradigm for Preventing Genetic Discrimination," 1348.

[114] Barbara Bowles Biesecker, "Privacy in Genetic Counseling," 108–109; Michael Arribas-Ayllon, Srikant Sarangi, and Angus Clarke, *Genetic Testing: Accounts of Autonomy, Responsibility and Blame*, 122.

crucial to the decision-making process. Angus Clarke suggests that genetic counseling emphasizes more of a listening and communication "process" rather than the "conclusion."[115] Genetic counseling can include looking into the family history, assessing a patient's understanding, discussing possible options, and making treatment decisions based on the person's values and opinions.[116]

The current model recommends non-directive counseling, and does not require counseling. While the current model emphasizes disclosure and signifies a decision is coming, mere disclosure is not enough.[117] In response, Stephen Wear argues that genetic counseling can supplement disclosure and help to enhance selection of an appropriate option.[118] However, even when counseling does occur, the process can be more difficult, since there are limited mechanisms in place to assess the patient. This section will look at the current counseling guidelines and counseling methods and then discuss disclosure to family.

1). Current Counseling Guidelines and Non-Directiveness

One potential problem with the current model in relation to PGT is the fact that often the people at increased risk for a particular disease are not having genetic counseling before or after PGT. Arribas-Ayllon, Sarangi, and Clarke note that the people who participate in genetic counseling often think like a consumer. Some people think if there is a test, then he or she should have it to know more about their future. One counselor said that he thought people should focus on being at risk first, and then after the implications of that settled in, the person can participate in PGT. Many times people are still in denial when participating in PGT. A person who assumes the test is going to be negative does not demonstrate an accurate understanding of the risks involved and is most likely rejecting the idea that he or she is at risk. Unless a person is prepared for the risks, benefits, and implications of PGT, this type of testing can cause more fear and uncertainty than is necessary.[119]

Typically when genetic counseling occurs, the counselor emphasizes non-directiveness. Since patients come in with different values than the counselor, the principle of non-directivess emphasizes "value neutrality" in counseling and requires the counselors not to judge other people's values.[120] This idea was made popular

---

[115] Angus Clarke, "Genetic Counseling," 132; Michael Arribas-Ayllon, Srikant Sarangi, and Angus Clarke, *Genetic Testing: Accounts of Autonomy, Responsibility and Blame,* 122.

[116] Jeffrey Carlisle and Ann T. Neulicht, "The Necessity of Professional Disclosure and Informed Consent for Rehabilitation Counselors," 29; Robin Bennett, *The Practical Guide to The Genetic Family History,* 253; Michael Arribas-Ayllon, Srikant Sarangi, and Angus Clarke, *Genetic Testing: Accounts of Autonomy, Responsibility and Blame,* 122.

[117] Lewis Vaughn, *Bioethics: Principles, Issues, and Cases,* 148.

[118] Stephen Wear, *Informed Consent,* 62, 66.

[119] Michael Arribas-Ayllon, Srikant Sarangi, and Angus Clarke, *Genetic Testing: Accounts of Autonomy, Responsibility and Blame,* 125–127.

[120] Barbara Bowles Biesecker, "Privacy in Genetic Counseling," 110–112.

after the harms of the past. This idea has both positive and negatives. The patient can benefit from this type of counseling since the counselor is not influencing the patient either way. As a result, Ensenauer, Michels, and Reinke explain that the patient can choose options that are based on their values and not another individual's values.[121] Also because the counselors do not have to be as involved personally, this type of counseling can protect against coercion and eugenics that were evident in the last chapter. However this view of counseling can also encourage information-oriented disclosure which can impact autonomy and reduce meaningful consent. As was seen before, the current model can emphasize a narrow, restricted form of autonomy as simple consent either accepting or rejecting a treatment.[122] As a result, the non-directiveness of typical genetic counseling can impede a more extensive, meaningful consent.

2). Disclosure to Family

Often people assume results need to be disclosed to family members, but disclosure is not always possible or emphasized for PGT.[123] Because information resulting from PGT often impacts family members, disclosure to family should be an important aspect, but the current model does not always emphasize the need to disclose to family members. One study suggests that while intentional nondisclosure was typically low, there were some people who were not informed about a relative's PGT results. Many factors can contribute to not disclosing information such as family dynamics, location, and communication problems. While counseling might help some people with disclosure efforts, counseling by itself does not always solve the problem. If part of the family has not talked in years, then disclosing information will be difficult. However, counseling and disclosure has the possibility to help some families work together to tell other members about an increased risk as a result of PGT results.[124]

2. Revised Model

This next section will look at both disclosure and genetic counseling in the revised model. The first section will look at the standards of disclosure and discuss the link

---

[121] Regina E. Ensenauer, Virginia V. Michels, and Shanda S. Reinke, "Genetic Testing: Practical, Ethical, and Counseling Considerations," 70.

[122] Michael Arribas-Ayllon, Srikant Sarangi, and Angus Clarke, *Genetic Testing: Accounts of Autonomy, Responsibility and Blame,* 122; Angus Clarke, "Genetic Counseling," 141–142; Barbara Bowles Biesecker, "Privacy in Genetic Counseling," 111–112.

[123] Kathryn Holt, "What Do We Tell the Children? Contrasting the Disclosure Choices of Two HD Families Regarding Risk Status and Predictive Genetic Testing," 262.

[124] Clara L. Gaff, Veronica Collins, Tiffany Symes, et al., "Facilitating Family Communication about Predictive Genetic Testing: Probands' Perceptions," 138.

between disclosure and decision-making. The second section will include an analysis of the purposes and goals of genetic counseling for the revised model.

a. Disclosure

The revised model addresses not only medical information but all other relevant information for the patient to consider for consent, including the fact that some PGT diseases might not have any available treatment. Manson and O'Neill suggest that if consent focuses mainly on standardized disclosure processes, then there is limited flexibility for personalized information which is often needed for decision-making.[125] This section will look at the information to disclose and the revised disclosure guidelines for PGT.

1). Information to Disclose

Since some genetic diseases have no cure or appropriate treatments, some of the important aspects of decision-making for consent can be nonmedical and family factors.[126] The revised model discloses both medical and non-medical information to patients before PGT in order to have a better grasp of possible future consequences. Many times the limitations of testing are not emphasized enough.[127] Trepanier, Ahrens, McKinnon, et al. suggest that one of the important areas with PGT is disclosing and understanding the severity of risk or the positive predictive value of the test.[128] Even if a person is at-risk for a particular disease, that does not mean the person will develop the disease.[129] If a patient assumes PGT is a diagnostic test, then he or she will have a faulty view of the potential treatment options and will most likely not chose appropriately.[130] A group at Johns Hopkins University concluded that after understanding the limits and predictive value of BRCA, women were less likely to get tested. The group cited the uncertainties of BRCA inheritance and treatment and the potential adverse consequences on employment and insurance as the main reasons for rejecting PGT.[131] Often the uncertainties continue even after testing. Young explains that the actual aspects of the disease are important as well. A

---

[125] Neil C. Manson and Onora O'Neill, *Rethinking Informed Consent in Bioethics*, 70, 80.

[126] Neil Sharpe and Ronald Carter, *Genetic Testing: Care, Consent, and Liability*. 131.

[127] Lori B. Andrews, *Future Perfect: Confronting Decisions about Genetics*, 83, 165.

[128] Angela Trepanier, Mary Ahrens, Wendy McKinnon, et al., "Genetic Cancer Risk Assessment and Counseling: Recommendations of the National Society of Genetic Counselors," 103, 105; Lori B. Andrews, *Future Perfect: Confronting Decisions about Genetics*, 125; Robert Klitzman, "Misunderstandings Concerning Genetics Among Patients Confronting Genetic Disease," 433–434.

[129] Leon Eisenberg, "Why has the Relationship Between Psychiatry and Genetics Been so Contentious?" 380.

[130] Jeffrey R. Botkin, Steven M. Teutsch, Celia I. Kaye, et al., "Outcomes of Interest in Evidence-Based Evaluations of Genetic Tests," 230–231.

[131] Lori B. Andrews, *Future Perfect: Confronting Decisions about Genetics*, 167.

study of genetic counseling concluded that actual risk was not necessarily as important as some of the practical aspects of the disease.[132] The treatment options need to be discussed even if there are no options other than surveillance.[133] Sometimes even surveillance can have risks associated with it like the radiation for mammograms.[134]

Some nonmedical factors are important as well such as the patient's objectives, concerns, and beliefs about genetic testing, the possibility of discrimination, privacy protections, and personal and family values.[135] One study concluded that less than half of the consent forms discussed anything about discrimination or privacy concerns.[136] David Orentlicher argues that because genetic information has implications for family members, if a person's privacy is violated, then family information could be violated as well.[137] Lori Andrews points out that sometimes because of a person's position in a company, that individual might be more likely to suffer adverse consequences of PGT.[138] Financial and psychological implications should also be considered and discussed with the counselor. Another important aspect is addressing the policies on what groups can see the test results after PGT.[139] Discussing a couple of future implications of having either a positive or negative test can help patients to understand their current and future options.[140] Anticipating some of the important factors and decisions that will need to be addressed after testing can help patients deepen their appreciation of the possible consequences.[141] Klitzman, Thorne, Williamson, et al., suggest that often PGT can have consequences on

---

[132] Ian Young, *Introduction to Risk Calculation in Genetic Counseling,* 5.

[133] Regina E. Ensenauer, Virginia V. Michels, and Shanda S. Reinke, "Genetic Testing: Practical, Ethical, and Counseling Considerations," 71.

[134] Lori B. Andrews, *Future Perfect: Confronting Decisions about Genetics,* 83.

[135] Neil Sharpe and Ronald Carter, *Genetic Testing: Care, Consent, and Liability,* 131; David Orentlicher, "Genetic Privacy in the Patient-Physician Relationship," 80; Bernard Lo, *Resolving Ethical Dilemmas,* 19; Angela Trepanier, Mary Ahrens, Wendy McKinnon, et al., "Genetic Cancer Risk Assessment and Counseling: Recommendations of the National Society of Genetic Counselors," 105–106; Jeffrey R. Botkin, Steven M. Teutsch, Celia I. Kaye, et al., "Outcomes of Interest in Evidence-Based Evaluations of Genetic Tests," 232.

[136] Lori B. Andrews, *Future Perfect: Confronting Decisions about Genetics,* 125.

[137] David Orentlicher, "Genetic Privacy in the Patient-Physician Relationship," 81.

[138] Lori B. Andrews, *Future Perfect: Confronting Decisions about Genetics,* 165.

[139] Regina E. Ensenauer, Virginia V. Michels, and Shanda S. Reinke, "Genetic Testing: Practical, Ethical, and Counseling Considerations," 71; Jeffrey R. Botkin, Steven M. Teutsch, Celia I. Kaye, et al., "Outcomes of Interest in Evidence-Based Evaluations of Genetic Tests," 234.

[140] Angus Clarke, "Genetic Counseling," 133–134; Lori B. Andrews, *Future Perfect: Confronting Decisions about Genetics,* 165, 167; Angela Trepanier, Mary Ahrens, Wendy McKinnon, et al., "Genetic Cancer Risk Assessment and Counseling: Recommendations of the National Society of Genetic Counselors," 103, 105; Katja Aktan-Collan, Jukka-Pekka Mecklin, Albert de la Chapelle, et al., "Evaluation of a Counselling Protocol for Predictive Genetic Testing for Hereditary Non-Polyposis Colorectal Cancer," 111.

[141] Regina E. Ensenauer, Virginia V. Michels, and Shanda S. Reinke, "Genetic Testing: Practical, Ethical, and Counseling Considerations," 70.

employment, insurance, and family aspects.[142] Disclosure for PGT should empha-size education and the rights of patients.[143]

2). Revised Disclosure Guidelines

The common belief demonstrated in the current model is that the exchange of infor-mation is enough for disclosure.[144] However, mere disclosure of information does not promote adequate decision-making. The revised model encourages additional communication between doctor and patient in order to promote appropriate deci-sion-making.[145] Open discussions and analysis of potential options can promote a patient's well-being. Doctors cannot predict how involved patients want to be unless asked. Arnold and Lidz point out that some patients do not always want to be involved in decision making, but many times the patients would like more infor-mation.[146] Often there is a discrepancy between what the physician discloses and what the patient would like to know.[147] The National Bioethics Advisory Commis-sion encourages disclosing information and understanding of that information over the formal consent documents. Disclosure of information and consent forms still need to take place, but the disclosure should be personalized more to the individual patient and flexible for different circumstances.[148]

Benjamin Freedman suggests that the amount of disclosure a patient wants to know should be established at the very beginning of the conversation. Giving the example of a cancer patient, he says that instead of focusing on competence and information at the outset, understanding how much information the patient really wants to know can help in the end. This method of disclosure can also help the fami-lies that might think disclosing every detail is not in the patient's best interest.[149] Instead of burdening the patient with unnecessary information, this approach can be more personalized and sensitive to different patient preferences for the amount of

---

[142] Robert Klitzman, Deborah Thorne, Jennifer Williamson, et al., "The Roles of Family Members, Health Care Workers, and Others in Decision-Making Processes about Genetic Testing among Individuals at Risk for Huntington Disease," 369; Lori B. Andrews, *Future Perfect: Confronting Decisions about Genetics*, 168.

[143] David Wright, "Redesigning Informed Consent Tools for Specific Research," 148.

[144] Jessica W. Berg, Paul S. Applebaum, Charles W. Lidz, and Lisa S. Parker, *Informed Consent: Legal Theory and Clinical Practice*, 66; Kathryn Holt, "What Do We Tell the Children? Contrast-ing the Disclosure Choices of Two HD Families Regarding Risk Status and Predictive Genetic Testing," 264.

[145] Lori B. Andrews, *Future Perfect: Confronting Decisions about Genetics*, 23.

[146] Robert M. Arnold and Charles W. Lidz, "Informed Consent: Clinical Aspects of Consent in Health Care," 5, 7.

[147] Lori B. Andrews, *Future Perfect: Confronting Decisions about Genetics*, 23.

[148] National Bioethics Advisory Commission, "Protecting Research Participants— A Time for Change," 374.

[149] Benjamin Freedman, "Offering Truth: Once Ethical Approach to the Uninformed Cancer Pa-tient," 113.

information desired.[150] Because of the large amount of information being presented, if there are no suitable options discussed, then coming to an appropriate course of action to take after PGT would be difficult. A study in *Genomics & Genetics Weekly,* looking into behavioral changes after PGT, suggested that actions were about the same before and after the test for breast cancer. It was also suggested that PGT for breast cancer could decrease people's need to alter their actions, because the people believed those risks were absolute.[151] Felt, Bister, Strassnig, et al. suggest that sometimes a person's lack of understanding about medicine and science can be deliberate, because the patient has no interest in the information that was disclosed. As a result, the revised model addresses the discrepancies between the current medical disclosure and the more personalized disclosure to ensure the information is understood and applied appropriately. The revised model emphasizes appropriate disclosure and counseling so that the medical aspects are merged with the patient's perspective in order to select a suitable option.[152]

b. Genetic Counseling

The revised model requires counseling both before and after testing. Michael Hayden suggests that counseling before testing should focus on reasons for participating in, emotions involved in consideration of, and an analysis of the possible risk with PGT.[153] Requiring genetic counseling can help understanding as well. Counseling programs have the opportunity to eliminate or reduce the psychological consequences that can come from PGT.[154] Having a better understanding of risk can also decrease emotional harms after testing.[155] While some patients might be nervous talking to a physician about certain issues, counselors can help patients relax

---

[150] Michael Brannigan and Judith Boss, *Healthcare Ethics in a Diverse Society,* 41.

[151] Genomics & Genetics Weekly staff, "Genetic Testing: Studies Point to Variable Prognostic Abilities and Question if Testing Results in Behavioral Change," 11–12.

[152] Ulrike Felt, Milena D. Bister, Michael Strassnig, et al., "Refusing the Information Paradigm: Informed Consent, Medical Research, and Patient Participation," 93; Marion Harris, Ingrid Winship, Merle Spriggs, "Controversies and Ethical Issues in Cancer-Genetics Clinics," 301; Anita Silvers and Michael Ashley Stein, "An Equality Paradigm for Preventing Genetic Discrimination," 1348.

[153] Michael Hayden, "Predictive Testing for Huntington's Disease: A Universal Model?" 141; Marita Broadstock, Susan Michie, Theresa Marteau, "Psychological Consequences of Predictive Genetic Testing: A Systematic Review," 734.

[154] Shoshana Shiloh and Shiri Ilan, "To Test or Not To Test? Moderators of the Relationship Between Risk Perceptions and Interest in Predictive Genetic Testing," 477; Michael Burgess, "Beyond Consent: Ethical and Social Issues in Genetic Testing," 508; Angela Trepanier, Mary Ahrens, Wendy McKinnon, et al., "Genetic Cancer Risk Assessment and Counseling: Recommendations of the National Society of Genetic Counselors," 88, 90, 103, 109.

[155] Marita Broadstock, Susan Michie, and Theresa Marteau, "Psychological Consequences of Predictive Genetic Testing: A Systematic Review," 736.

more and ask questions to evaluate the options and encourage open discussions.[156] Klitzman explains that since some misunderstandings can be very personal and hard to identify, doctors should look at the emotional issues behind misunderstandings such as control issues, feelings of vulnerability, confusion, and anxiety. Also patients might choose to believe they have the disease in order to eliminate feelings of vulnerability and helplessness. However, those assumptions can expose patients to increased risks, because the patients base their decisions off of inaccurate information.[157] Post-test counseling should focus on discussing the results, addressing the consequences of the results, and determining an acceptable treatment option.[158]

Since people often seek control of their lives, sometimes a lack of control over inheritance can cause problems when receiving the results. Depending on the results, people might try to take control of their health even if their decisions could have harmful consequences like agreeing to a prophylactic double mastectomy.[159] Ball, Tyler, and Harper note that counselors can help people examine their emotions so that the patients do not decide on something quickly in order to reduce the current amount of stress and anxiety.[160] When patients receive bad news or "toxic knowledge" in regards to PGT, genetic counselors can encourage enhanced decision-making skills by determining how people will react to the information.[161] Some people will be able to handle potentially bad news and some might become overwhelmingly distraught or permanently harmed. The medical staff should emphasize that communication is more important than disclosing information.[162] Having follow-up after PGT is important to discuss a person's reactions and encourage appropriate methods of coping with the results.[163] If the counselor feels that additional follow-

---

[156] Daniel W. Fitzgerald, Cecile Marotte, Rose Irene Verdier, et al., "Comprehension during Informed Consent in a Less-Developed Country," 1302; Robert M. Arnold and Charles W. Lidz, "Informed Consent: Clinical Aspects of Consent in Health Care," 5.

[157] Robert Klitzman, "Misunderstandings Concerning Genetics Among Patients Confronting Genetic Disease," 442, 444–445; Robin Bennett, *The Practical Guide to The Genetic Family History*, 253.

[158] Angela Trepanier, Mary Ahrens, Wendy McKinnon, et al., "Genetic Cancer Risk Assessment and Counseling: Recommendations of the National Society of Genetic Counselors," 107–108; Barbara Bowles Biesecker, "Privacy in Genetic Counseling," 108–109; Katja Aktan-Collan, Jukka-Pekka Mecklin, Albert de la Chapelle, et al., "Evaluation of a Counselling Protocol for Predictive Genetic Testing for Hereditary Non-Polyposis Colorectal Cancer," 111.

[159] Jeffrey R. Botkin, Steven M. Teutsch, Celia I. Kaye, et al., "Outcomes of Interest in Evidence-Based Evaluations of Genetic Tests," 232; Robert Klitzman, "Misunderstandings Concerning Genetics Among Patients Confronting Genetic Disease," 443.

[160] David Ball, Audrey Tyler, and Peter Harper, "Predictive Testing of Adults and Children," 70.

[161] Robert Wachbroit, "Disowning Knowledge: Issues in Genetic Testing," 497.

[162] Neil C. Manson and Onora O'Neill, *Rethinking Informed Consent in Bioethics*, 198.

[163] Katja Aktan-Collan, Jukka-Pekka Mecklin, Albert de la Chapelle, et al., "Evaluation of a Counselling Protocol for Predictive Genetic Testing for Hereditary Non-Polyposis Colorectal Cancer," 109; Regina E. Ensenauer, Virginia V. Michels, and Shanda S. Reinke, "Genetic Testing: Practical, Ethical, and Counseling Considerations," 71.

up might be needed, the counselor can monitor the consequences of the test at that time.[164]

In order to assist genetic counselors in their discussions with patients, Goetz argues that counselors should use patient assessment and feedback mechanisms like feedback loops, a decision tree, linear steps, and nomagrams. Through the use of a decision tree, patients can better internalize the risks, benefits, and future impact of their decision in order to facilitate appropriate decision making. Patient assessments in pre-test counseling can help to encourage additional questions about PGT. Also an IES questionnaire, another useful tool in both pre- and post-test counseling, can help to determine a patient's stress level and emotional status during this process of discussing new information.[165] This tool can help counselors predict the possibility of having severe emotional or psychological side effects after PGT. Feedback mechanisms and assessments are essential to the counseling process.

The revised model requires counseling and adopts value transparency and non-directive counseling. Leon Eisenberg suggests that counseling for PGT brings another level of difficulty, since the counselors are often discussing future risks that have not occurred yet.[166] PGT can be complex with implications for more than just the individual patient, and as a result the revised model requires genetic counseling both before and after testing.[167] One study in Canada concluded that risks were more tolerable when there was pre- and post-test counseling for PGT.[168] This model changes emphasis from simply information to a broader more in-depth focus on communication.[169] Thus the revised model requires genetic counseling in order to help clarify personal values, help establish patient views, and develop a treatment plan.[170] This section will look at non-directiveness and value transparency and disclosure to family.

1). Non-Directiveness and Value Transparency

While the current model often uses non-directive counseling to reduce the amount of external pressures or coercion put on patients, the amount of external pressures is not simply eliminated because the counselor did not give his or her own advice. Barbara Biesecker suggests that there are many social perspectives and influences

---

[164] David Ball, Audrey Tyler, and Peter Harper, "Predictive Testing of Adults and Children," 71.

[165] Thomas Goetz, *The Decision Tree*, xvii, 47–48, 67–68,141–142, 197, 215; Stephen Wear, *Informed Consent,* 122.

[166] Leon Eisenberg, "Why has the Relationship Between Psychiatry and Genetics Been so Contentious?" 380.

[167] Catherine Hayes, "Genetic Testing for Huntington's Disease—A Family Issue," 1451; Michael Hayden, "Predictive Testing for Huntington's Disease: A Universal Model?" 141–142.

[168] Michael Burgess, "Beyond Consent: Ethical and Social Issues in Genetic Testing," 508.

[169] Neil C. Manson and Onora O'Neill, *Rethinking Informed Consent in Bioethics,* 188–189.

[170] Regina E. Ensenaucr, Virginia V. Michels, and Shanda S. Reinke, "Genetic Testing: Practical, Ethical, and Counseling Considerations," 70; Stephen Wear, *Informed Consent,* 26, 45; Thomas Goetz, *The Decision Tree,* 138; Bernard Lo, *Resolving Ethical Dilemmas,* 276.

that are prevalent today. As a result, non-directiveness is not always practical even in counselor settings.[171] Even if this principle was realistic and could eliminate external pressures, non-directivess is not always a good method of counseling.[172] Sometimes non-directiveness promotes a distanced view between the patient and the counselor which can lead to patients feeling neglected or even more confused about potential options. Since most of the time patients do not know the important questions to ask, counselors are needed to give them additional information that might help. Arribas-Ayllon, Sarangi, and Clarke explain that there can be many sensible decisions, but often patients are helped more when counselors illustrate how to get to an intelligent decision. Thus counselors should give input on a patient's decision-making skills. Counselors should not exert pressure on a patient about PGT or the results, but counselors should be able to question and/or have the patients explain their decisions. Unless patients consider certain aspects of PGT, the patients will not be adequately informed about the decision and treatment option. Counselors can help patients evaluate and reflect on the possible consequences and future options of having a positive test.[173] If non-directiveness is emphasized solely, then counselors merely present the information so patients can make decisions which would be in line with the current model of consent.

Instead of value neutrality, which is really not achievable, there should be value transparency as argued by Diana Buccafurni. The revised model encourages value transparency, where the counselors make their values known before counseling.[174] Since all genetic counselors have certain views and biases, this idea promotes a more practical approach to addressing those opinions. The revised model encourages open communication and value clarification so patients and counselors can think through the entire process of PGT in order to arrive at a meaningful consent and appropriate course of action.

2). Disclosure to Family

The revised model encourages increased disclosure to family members. There can be increased disclosure by having genetic counselors help the patients in this aspect.[175] Counselors do not have to contact family members, but during the patient's counseling session, the patient can identify people who should know about the results. Then the patient and counselor can work together to encourage increased dis-

---

[171] Barbara Bowles Biesecker, "Privacy in Genetic Counseling," 111.

[172] Angus Clarke, "Genetic Counseling," 142.

[173] Michael Arribas-Ayllon, Srikant Sarangi, and Angus Clarke, *Genetic Testing: Accounts of Autonomy, Responsibility and Blame,* 123; David Ball, Audrey Tyler, and Peter Harper, "Predictive Testing of Adults and Children," 72.

[174] Diana Buccafurni, "Reconsidering the Facilitation of Autonomous Decision Making in Genetic Counseling," v, 3.

[175] Angus Clarke, "Genetic Counseling," 143.

closure to family members. Gaff, Collins, Symes, and Halliday studied the issue of family disclosure, and concluded that many people do not have a problem with medical centers telling family members about their increased risk for a certain disease. Another study suggested that counseling encouraged participants to disclose information and helped in knowing how to disclose certain information to family members.[176] There can be increased disclosure by having frequent discussions and establishing methods to help patients inform the family while in counseling both before and after testing.[177] Having more counseling has been shown to have improved family disclosure.[178] In the revised model, Catherine Hayes suggests that counselors can also encourage family members to come to the counseling sessions as well to consider the implications for both the patient and the family.[179] Then, after disclosure, the family members can have access to the same genetic services and resources to help them make an informed decision as well.[180] Another way to note this point is made by Angus Clarke when he argues that there is a moral responsibility to disclose information to family members so that those members will be able to participate in PGT as well if so desired.[181] In the revised model, proactively knowing when and how disclosure will take place is important to the counseling process.[182]

---

[176] Clara L. Gaff, Veronica Collins, Tiffany Symes, and Jane Halliday, "Facilitating Family Communication about Predictive Genetic Testing: Probans' Perceptions," 138–139; Kathryn Holt, "What Do We Tell the Children? Contrasting the Disclosure Choices of Two HD Families Regarding Risk Status and Predictive Genetic Testing," 263.

[177] Courtney Storm, Rinki Agarwal, and Kenneth Offit, "Ethical and Legal Implications of Cancer Genetic Testing: Do Physicians Have a Duty to Warn Patients' Relatives about Possible Genetic Risks?" 230.

[178] Laura E. Forrest, Jo Burke, Sonya Bacic, et al., "Increased Genetic Counseling Support Improves Communication of Genetic Information in Families," 171.

[179] Catherine Hayes, "Genetic Testing for Huntington's Disease—A Family Issue," 1451; Katja Aktan-Collan, Jukka-Pekka Mecklin, Albert de la Chapelle, et al., "Evaluation of a Counselling Protocol for Predictive Genetic Testing for Hereditary Non-Polyposis Colorectal Cancer," 111; Lori B. Andrews, "Gen-Etiquette: Genetic Information, Family Relationships, and Adoption," 271; Michael Arribas-Ayllon, Srikant Sarangi, and Angus Clarke, *Genetic Testing: Accounts of Autonomy, Responsibility and Blame,* 125.

[180] Courtney Storm, Rinki Agarwal, and Kenneth Offit, "Ethical and Legal Implications of Cancer Genetic Testing: Do Physicians Have a Duty to Warn Patients' Relatives about Possible Genetic Risks?" 230; Jeffrey R. Botkin, Steven M. Teutsch, Celia I. Kaye, et al., "Outcomes of Interest in Evidence-Based Evaluations of Genetic Tests," 233.

[181] Angus Clarke, "Genetic Counseling," 143; Lori B. Andrews, "Gen-Etiquette: Genetic Information, Family Relationships, and Adoption," 273; Michael Arribas-Ayllon, Srikant Sarangi, and Angus Clarke, *Genetic Testing: Accounts of Autonomy, Responsibility and Blame,* 123; Courtney Storm, Rinki Agarwal, and Kenneth Offit, "Ethical and Legal Implications of Cancer Genetic Testing: Do Physicians Have a Duty to Warn Patients' Relatives about Possible Genetic Risks?" 230; Laura E. Forrest, Jo Burke, Sonya Bacic, et al., "Increased Genetic Counseling Support Improves Communication of Genetic Information in Families," 171.

[182] Clara L. Gaff, Veronica Collins, Tiffany Symes, et al., "Facilitating Family Communication about Predictive Genetic Testing: Probans' Perceptions," 138–139.

Often counselors will look at a family history to help in knowing what relatives might be at-risk, recognizing some of the side effects their family had in the past, and assessing the risk of serious psychological factors in their family history.[183] While those practices are beneficial, the revised model promotes additional measures. Goetz and Wear suggest that individual patient concerns can be addressed by offering a more flexible and personalized consent process through ongoing counseling in order to recognize an individual's unique values and goals of testing.[184] Since a genetic counselor's training is different than what the revised model suggests, this model encourages changes to the curriculum and additional guidance with the updated goals of counseling and disclosure to facilitate better decision-making for PGT.[185]

C. Voluntariness

Consent is a deliberate action demonstrating understanding, and those actions should have limited controlling influences.[186] Roberta Berry notes that the views of autonomy as permission will have an impact on coercion and the voluntariness of consent.[187] Voluntariness requires autonomy and disclosure of appropriate information in order to be able to make a decision free from controlling interferences.[188] Coercion can be exhibited through many areas and based on varying justifications. Engelhardt suggests that medicine can be influenced by people voluntarily deciding on a course of treatment and by those wanting to do what is best for a patient even if those actions use intimidation or external pressures.[189]

This section will look at voluntariness in informed consent and apply it to PGT. The first part will look at the current model and discuss how coercion plays a part in informed consent and give some implications for family-related information on consent. The second part will develop the revised model of consent. The revised model will also look at coercion and family-related implications of this information. The principles of voluntariness will be applied to the revised model of consent for PGT.

---

[183] Robin Bennett, *The Practical Guide to The Genetic Family History,* 178, 181, 251–252; Angela Trepanier, Mary Ahrens, Wendy McKinnon, et al., "Genetic Cancer Risk Assessment and Counseling: Recommendations of the National Society of Genetic Counselors," 88.

[184] Stephen Wear, *Informed Consent,* 95; Thomas Goetz, *The Decision Tree,* 67–68; Neil C. Manson and Onora O'Neill, *Rethinking Informed Consent in Bioethics,* 85.

[185] Lori B. Andrews, *Future Perfect: Confronting Decisions about Genetics,* 165.

[186] Cynthia James, Gail Geller, Barbara Bernhardt, et al., "Are Practicing and Future Physicians Prepared to Obtain Informed Consent? The Case of Genetic Testing for Susceptibility to Breast Cancer," 203.

[187] Roberta M. Berry, "Informed Consent Law, Ethics, and Practice: From Infancy to Reflective Adolescence," 69.

[188] Lori B. Andrews, *Future Perfect: Confronting Decisions about Genetics,* 165.

[189] H. Tristram Engelhardt Jr., *The Foundations of Bioethics,* 358.

1. Current Model

Voluntariness is an important aspect of informed consent. Engelhardt suggests that both medicine and research has to emphasize consent without coercion.[190] In 1960 a study by Boston University's Law-Medicine Research Institute looked at issues of informed consent and research with children and prisoners. The study discussed the significance of coercion on consent and the issues of beneficence in research.[191]

The current model will look at coercion and family-related implication. Types and examples of coercion are discussed in relation to the current model of consent. Then family-related implications are discussed and analyzed further. Since genetic information affects more than the individual person, consent for PGT should emphasize some of those implications for families.

a. Coercion

Coercion exists if there is a threat so significant that a person has no other choice but to submit to the person's intimidation. Types of coercion and controlling influences include manipulation, not telling the truth, intimidation, and even kind actions for incentives. However, feeling vulnerable without an actual warning of intimidation is not enough to categorize that as credible coercion. Some controlling influences are more powerful than others, and some like persuasion are not controlling at all. Beauchamp and Childress explain that a persuasion to get treatment involves reasoning; on the other hand, controlling influences use emotions to intimidate.[192] A physician who says that medical treatment will stop if the patient does not follow instructions demonstrates coercion.[193] Tauber suggests that the differences of having influences that persuade and control are crucial for understanding the amount of coercion or voluntariness present in a person's consent.[194]

In the current model, there are no specific measures to address or avoid multiple sources of external pressures (such as pressures from relatives, the medical staff and community, and/or societal influences) which increase the possibility of coercion upon the individual. This section will discuss the importance of voluntariness on consent and analyze the external pressures in the current model.

---

[190] H. Tristram Engelhardt Jr., *The Foundations of Bioethics*, 331.

[191] Albert Jonsen, *The Birth of Bioethics*, 141–142.

[192] Lewis Vaughn, *Bioethics: Principles, Issues, and Cases*, 148; Tom Beauchamp, "Informed Consent," 201; Tom Beauchamp and James Childress, *Principles of Biomedical Ethics*, 94.

[193] Linda Farber Post, Jeffrey Blustein, Nancy Neveloff Dubler, *Handbook for Health Care Ethics Committees*, 42–43.

[194] Alfred Tauber, *Patient Autonomy and the Ethics of Responsibility*, 136.

1). Importance of Voluntariness on Consent

As history illustrates, voluntariness of consent was one of the most important aspects. Many of the medical and research failures seen in the past were because of coercion and a lack of voluntariness for consent. Generally voluntariness is linked with autonomy and decision-making that has limited controlling pressures. The problem with coercion is that it seeks to control another person's actions and behaviors and nullifies consent by eliminating voluntary choices.[195]

While autonomy and voluntariness have similar concepts, an autonomous patient can still disregard some options because of being uneducated or having influencing forces. Encouraging more than an autonomy-based justification for voluntariness, Beauchamp and Childress hold that a person should be able to choose an action free of controlling pressures. Voluntariness is a result of a patient making his or her own decisions based on individual goals, lifestyle, and available information without being pressured into an action. One example of voluntariness is illustrated by organ donation. Often questions arise as to the degree of voluntariness that can be present with living organ donors. Even a friendship can encourage coercive pressure and strain on a person to consent to donating an organ. While donating an organ does not in itself justify cause for coercion, often there are more emotions and hidden pressures at stake than is first evident.[196] Sometimes even liability can be a cause for coercion. Kilner, Pentz, and Young explain that the American College of Obstetricians and Gynecologists (ACOG) gave a statement in 1985 recommending physicians inform their patients about maternal serum alpha-fetoprotein screening. However, the group had previously taken the stance that the test had a high level of false results and uncertainty. Because there were some lawsuits against certain newborn diseases and defects, the group thought informing patients about the availability of that test would protect them from liability.[197] Both of these examples illustrate the importance of emphasizing voluntariness, while reducing external pressures like coercion.

2). External Pressures

All of the cases in the history of consent demonstrate the pressures of coercion on consent. One example in particular, the Nazis experiments, illustrates how dangerous presuppositions and thoughts affect consent. Glover explains that the attitudes of the Nazis, such as stigmatization, supremacy views, and eugenic thinking, can be just as harmful as the way in which many were killed during that time.[198] In order

---

[195] Bernard Lo, *Resolving Ethical Dilemmas,* 20.

[196] Tom Beauchamp and James Childress, *Principles of Biomedical Ethics,* 50, 58, 93; Linda Farber Post, Jeffrey Blustein, Nancy Neveloff Dubler, *Handbook for Health Care Ethics Committees,* 42.

[197] John Kilner, Rebecca Pentz, and Frank Young, eds., *Genetic Ethics,* 33.

[198] Jonathan Glover, "Eugenics: Some Lessons from the Nazi Experience," 472.

to fully understand voluntariness, it is important to point out the external pressures that might reduce voluntariness in the current model.

The current model illustrates some ways in which coercion can be common in consent. While not all pressures eliminate the freedom of choice, there should be extra measures in place to eliminate as many coercive influences as possible.[199] The current model of consent for PGT tries to promote voluntariness, but since there are multiple sources of external pressures for those undergoing PGT, the current model does not address each area adequately. As a result, people should try to eliminate coercion and deception by encouraging voluntariness.[200]

There are several different types of external pressures. Many times there can be emotional, social, institutional, and government pressures.[201] The first type of external pressure is emotional. As previously mentioned, living organ donation can cause pressures with friendships due to emotions.[202] Sometimes emotional reactions can lead to an individual pressuring or manipulating another individual. Second is social pressure. These social pressures are typically seen in areas of stigmatization and cultural norms. These cultural and social norms can often lead people to pressuring others in order to maintain the status quo.[203] Often decisions related to disabilities will have social and cultural pressures associated with them. Another example of social pressures can be the doctor-patient or researcher-subject relationship. Physicians can try to persuade an individual to make a decision, but sometimes that persuasion can lead to significant unwanted pressure.[204] The third type of pressure is institutional. Institutional pressures are illustrated by the ACOG case for liability concerns.[205] Liability concerns generally fall into pressures from professional and institutional guidelines and regulations. Professional guidelines such as the AMA can have some regulations that might put pressure upon individuals as well. Fourth, there can also be pressure from government regulations like the past group eugenics programs. These pressures are based on the views of the government or public policies of the top down approach.[206]

External pressures are often used to coerce and manipulate people into taking some action. Beauchamp and Walters suggest that PGT can lead to increased social and economic risks if coercion and external pressures are allowed in consent discussions.[207] However, Watson warns against having limits put on genetic testing and decision-making from societies' or the public's view, because often limitations like

---

[199] Tom Beauchamp, "Informed Consent," 201.

[200] H. Tristram Engelhardt Jr., *The Foundations of Bioethics*, 331.

[201] Torbjorn Tannsjo, *Coercive Care: The Ethics of Choice in Health and Medicine*, 9.

[202] Tom Beauchamp and James Childress, *Principles of Biomedical Ethics*, 50, 58, 93; Linda Farber Post, Jeffrey Blustein, Nancy Neveloff Dubler, *Handbook for Health Care Ethics Committees*, 42.

[203] Ruth Chadwick, "Genetic Screening," 197.

[204] Torbjorn Tannsjo, *Coercive Care: The Ethics of Choice in Health and Medicine*, 9.

[205] John Kilner, Rebecca Pentz, and Frank Young, eds., *Genetic Ethics*, 33.

[206] Jonathan Glover, "Eugenics: Some Lessons from the Nazi Experience," 472; Tom Beauchamp and LeRoy Walters eds., *Contemporary Issues in Bioethics*, 453.

[207] Tom Beauchamp and LeRoy Walters eds., *Contemporary Issues in Bioethics*, 452; Anita Silvers and Michael Ashley Stein, "An Equality Paradigm for Preventing Genetic Discrimination," 1347.

these will appear better than they actually are. The views can be based on positive principles, but the application and end results are often outward regulations that do little to promote genuine good.[208] Since there are not specific measures in place to address coercion and external pressures for PGT in the current model, the revised model will address those issues.

b. Family-Related Implications

PGT involves family-related information with accompanying implications that can compromise voluntariness. The current model does not take into consideration all family related implications which can lead to coercion of family members. This section looks at influencing pressures and discusses the concept of the right to know.

1). Influencing Pressures

Wear notes that PGT has the potential to cause discrimination, stress, fear, and coercion.[209] Since the results can impact the entire family, there is an opportunity for external pressures and coercion of the entire family which could result in negative feelings for the family as well. However, in the current model, the discussion of coercion typically emphasizes the specific patient, and not necessarily family pressures.

Typically when an individual consents to a particular treatment or test, the potential risk is specifically for that individual person. But with PGT, individual risks can be applied to the whole family if that individual is positive or at-risk for a genetic disease. As a result, family-related implications are not recognized as an influencing pressure in the current model. Often in the current model, family-related coercion is difficult to identify.[210] Thus, the revised model will address the problems with family-related implications in the current model.

2). Right to Know

The current model addresses this situation by recommending people tell their family about the possible results of PGT. Ideally, carriers should undergo PGT before the rest of the family in order to eliminate unnecessary testing. Michael Burgess expresses that a right not to know can make PGT more difficult. Typically PGT cannot be stopped by a family member who does not want to know certain information, but this example should raise additional concerns with consent for PGT and

---

[208] James Watson, "Genes and Politics," 483–484.

[209] Stephen Wear, *Informed Consent*, 62, 66; Thomas Goetz, *The Decision Tree*, 122.

[210] Lori B. Andrews, "Gen-Etiquette: Genetic Information, Family Relationships, and Adoption," 256.

family-related implications. Consent for groups with many different views is often complicated needing additional education and analysis.[211]

In America, the right to know discussion is often different than in cultures that emphasize community. Robert Wachbroit states, the "thought that someone ought to know seems to go against our cultural assumptions, interference in private relationship, [the] problem of solitary individuals contemplating whether or not to know is that it fits so few of us; decisions affect others as well."[212] In today's society, the people of America are thought of more as individuals rather than a community. As a result, individuals make decisions according to themselves and not family members or society as a whole. In the current model, physicians might recommend that patients inform family members, but the right of family members is typically not emphasized. As a result, sometimes family coercion can increase when family members are not included in a discussion of PGT results.

2. Revised Model

This third point of voluntariness develops the importance of avoiding coercion of both the patient and the patient's family when information is presented. The third distinctive characteristic of PGT is the relevance of genetic information for the patient's family. The revised model emphasizes the necessary inclusion of family implications to ensure the voluntary nature of consent.

The revised model analyzes coercion in the current model and addresses that coercion with an emphasis on voluntariness within the revised model of consent for PGT. Then the family-related implications of genetic information are discussed within the revised model of consent.

a. Coercion

As clarified by Arribas-Ayllon, Sarangi, and Clarke, many times people undergo PGT because of a feeling of responsibility towards their family.[213] PGT is personal, but this type of testing impacts both the individual and the family. Thus family coercion can be just as detrimental as or more than other sources of coercion.[214] Klitzman, Thorne, Williamson, et al. illustrate in their article that family pressure

---

[211] Michael Burgess, "Beyond Consent: Ethical and Social Issues in Genetic Testing," 510.

[212] Robert Wachbroit, "Disowning Knowledge: Issues in Genetic Testing," 499.

[213] Michael Arribas-Ayllon, Srikant Sarangi, and Angus Clarke, *Genetic Testing: Accounts of Autonomy, Responsibility and Blame,* 126; Kathryn Holt, "What Do We Tell the Children? Contrasting the Disclosure Choices of Two HD Families Regarding Risk Status and Predictive Genetic Testing," 262–263.

[214] Clara Gaff, Elly Lynch, and Lesley Spencer, "Predictive Testing of Eighteen Year Olds: Counseling Challenges," 249; Douglas Martin and Heather Greenwood, "Public Perceptions of Ethical Issues Regarding Adult Predictive Genetic Testing," 107.

has been used on many occasions.[215] The revised model shifts the focus from coercion of the patient alone to family-related coercion regarding PGT. However, this type of coercion is not the norm, because often the person making threats is the beneficiary of that decision as well.[216] Third party coercion is often more apparent in PGT, because of the nature of the family-related information with this testing.[217]

The revised model addresses external pressures on the patient and the family (such as pressures by the family for the patient to be tested and pressure upon the family regarding testing outcomes) to alleviate or resolve external coercion upon the patient. This section will analyze the external pressures and then discuss methods to reduce coercion in the revised model.

1). External Pressures

Often coercion and a lack of voluntary consent can come in many forms of subtle and obvious pressure.[218] There is the more dramatic type of coercion using a knife or weapon, but often there are lesser forms of coercion like being excluded. While everyone recognizes the coercive nature of bodily harm, Miller and Wertheimer express that the more emotional or social influences are more difficult to identify as coercion.[219] Even the subtle forms of negative influences like ostracism and peer pressure can arise among anyone applying enough pressure such as the patient's family. In PGT, coercion among family members can take on emotional intimidations or threaten to disrupt the family dynamics. A husband demonstrates coercion if he informs his wife that he will leave if she does not agree to have surgery for a condition.[220] The current model typically focuses on external pressures for the individual, but the revised model emphasizes the importance of both patient and family coercion.

2). Reducing Coercion

The revised model ensures voluntary consent by establishing procedures to avoid two forms of coercion: pressure by the family for the patient to be tested and pressure upon the family regarding the testing outcome. Coercion of the patient by the family is illustrated by the following example. If there is a family genetic trait al-

---

[215] Robert Klitzman, Deborah Thorne, Jennifer Williamson, et al., "The Roles of Family Members, Health Care Workers, and Others in Decision-Making Processes about Genetic Testing among Individuals at Risk for Huntington Disease," 367.

[216] Franklin Miller and Alan Wertheimer, *The Ethics of Consent*, 96.

[217] David Ball, Audrey Tyler, and Peter Harper, "Predictive Testing of Adults and Children," 73.

[218] John Kilner, Rebecca Pentz, Frank Young, eds., *Genetic Ethics*, 240.

[219] Franklin Miller and Alan Wertheimer, *The Ethics of Consent*, 15.

[220] Linda Farber Post, Jeffrey Blustein, Nancy Neveloff Dubler, *Handbook for Health Care Ethics Committees*, 42–43.

ready known, there can be pressure upon a child to be tested to ascertain if he or she is a carrier. If a trait emerges that affects other siblings, measures need to ascertain whether the sibling wants to know.[221] This example demonstrates the possible coercion of the family by the patient. Both examples can be addressed previously by discussions about the reasoning for participating in PGT and with the family beforehand in order to determine which family members want to know information and which if any do not want to know the results.

Often the level of voluntariness and coercion depends on a person's views and sensitivities to certain aspects.[222] Jehovah's Witnesses have certain religious views that result in the refusal of blood products. Ruth Macklin explains that when a person comes in with these views, before being allowed to refuse transfusions, the patients are encouraged to communicate their reasoning with a physician in order to ensure the voluntariness of their refusal.[223] In the revised model, the physician or counselor should also inquire into the possibility of family coercion if the entire family is Jehovah's Witnesses.[224] Laura Weiss Roberts proposes that discussing the patient's views without his or her family could sometimes help eliminate some of the family's pressure. Identifying and evaluating all the pressures involved can help to recognize and address some possible coercive situations or influences.[225]

Since physicians and researchers can help to identify where and when intimidating influences might arise, physicians and researchers have a role to play in encouraging the voluntariness of consent. If a doctor or researcher believes there is some sort of coercion being exerted on a patient, then it is the doctor's responsibility to inquire into the source of or reasoning behind the external influence. If the physician does not, then the consent is not adequately informed and the treatment options that were agreed upon would be subject to question.[226] Because those with limited autonomy and capacity to consent are often more affected by subtle pressures, those groups of people should be last in line to participate in research to protect against coercion. When those individuals are allowed to participate, then the justifications should be stronger and more persuasive, and the mechanisms to protect against coercion should be followed strictly.[227]

---

[221] Clara Gaff, Elly Lynch, and Lesley Spencer, "Predictive Testing of Eighteen Year Olds: Counseling Challenges," 249; Jeffrey R. Botkin, Steven M. Teutsch, Celia I. Kaye, et al., "Outcomes of Interest in Evidence-Based Evaluations of Genetic Tests," 233.

[222] Jessica W. Berg, Paul S. Applebaum, Charles W. Lidz, and Lisa S. Parker, *Informed Consent: Legal Theory and Clinical Practice*, 67.

[223] Ruth Macklin, "The Inner Workings of an Ethics Committee: Latest Battle over Jehovah's Witnesses," 233.

[224] Donna Dickenson, *Risk and Luck in Medical Ethics*, 173.

[225] Laura Weiss Roberts, "Informed Consent and the Capacity for Voluntarism," 709.

[226] Jessica W. Berg, Paul S. Applebaum, Charles W. Lidz, and Lisa S. Parker, *Informed Consent: Legal Theory and Clinical Practice*, 69–70; Robert Klitzman, Deborah Thorne, Jennifer Williamson, et al., "The Roles of Family Members, Health Care Workers, and Others in Decision-Making Processes about Genetic Testing among Individuals at Risk for Huntington Disease," 367.

[227] Albert Jonsen, *The Birth of Bioethics*, 151.

Ensuring voluntariness of consent involves paying attention to the patient and his or her situation, asking questions, and addressing certain family dynamics that might limit voluntariness.[228] PGT should not take place if there is any doubt as to the voluntariness of consent.[229] The revised model establishes more extensive processes to identify and address possible sources of external pressure. Unless policies or the ethical landscape changes, overt and subtle coercion will resume.[230]

b. Family-Related Implications

Since there is such an emphasis on patient autonomy in the United States, many times family members are not as involved with decision-making and participating in the treatment protocols.[231] Gaff, Lynch, and Spencer explain that the current model emphasizes and discloses information only to the specific patient, but the family has more at stake with PGT than other types of testing.[232] Since genetics is shared by family members, this model promotes more emphasis on the family for voluntariness.[233]

The revised model includes family-related concerns before testing and identifies ways to help the patient struggle with family-related PGT information. This section will analyze the right to know and discuss methods to identify family-related implications.

1). Right to Know

Because there are many implications that can affect other family members, some people have the view that genetics is family information and not just personal information.[234] Often the problem with focusing on the family as well as the individual patient is the inherent differences of the two arguments.

The right to know vs. the right not to know summarizes the potential conflicts.[235] Andrews suggests that many times the right not to know is harder to control. When

---

228 Laura Weiss Roberts, "Informed Consent and the Capacity for Voluntarism," 710.

229 David Ball, Audrey Tyler, and Peter Harper, "Predictive Testing of Adults and Children," 73.

230 John Kilner, Rebecca Pentz, Frank Young, eds., *Genetic Ethics,* 30.

231 Michael Brannigan and Judith Boss, *Healthcare Ethics in a Diverse Society,* 63.

232 Clara Gaff, Elly Lynch, and Lesley Spencer, "Predictive Testing of Eighteen Year Olds: Counseling Challenges," 250; Catherine Hayes, "Genetic Testing for Huntington's Disease—A Family Issue," 1450; Regina E. Ensenauer, Virginia V. Michels, and Shanda S. Reinke, "Genetic Testing: Practical, Ethical, and Counseling Considerations," 69.

233 Neil Sharpe and Ronald Carter, *Genetic Testing: Care, Consent, and Liability,* 364.

234 David Orentlicher, "Genetic Privacy in the Patient-Physician Relationship," 82–83; Lori B. Andrews, "Gen-Etiquette: Genetic Information, Family Relationships, and Adoption," 265–266; Catherine Hayes, "Genetic Testing for Huntington's Disease—A Family Issue," 1450.

235 Michael J. Green and Jeffrey R. Botkin, "'Genetic Exceptionalism' in Medicine: Clarifying the Differences between Genetic and Nongenetic Tests," 572; Michael Brannigan and Judith Boss, *Healthcare Ethics in a Diverse Society,* 264–265.

people undergo PGT, it is difficult to keep the results quietly contained to a couple of family members.[236] There is really not a right not to know, because often family members need to start thinking about the future consequences and options for themselves as well. A right not to know goes against autonomy, because if the person chooses not to know certain aspects, that person is not making a decision based off of accurate entire information. Since people often have less anxiety after finding out some results, the right not to know that information cannot be addressed by the principle of nonmaleficence. On the opposite side, some could argue that a family might be harmed because a person chooses not to know their risk-status for a disease like Huntington's. Sometimes people do not even participate, because the burdens of knowing can have harmful consequences for their relatives.[237]

The revised model emphasizes the importance of family-related information, and thus physicians and researchers should discuss those aspects before and after testing. If a patient or subject has a better idea of how the results will affect his or her family, then the individual will be able to communicate better with the family concerning the PGT results.

2). Identifying Family-Related Implications

While each family cannot consent separately, a discussion with the patient before testing should elucidate whether or not the patient has discussed testing options with his or her family. The first meeting with the counselor should address family implications, and if there has been no discussion with the family, then the physician or counselor should strongly recommend having the patient at least tell the family that he or she is considering PGT. Having a brief discussion will let the patient know the family's views and feelings on PGT for the future. Catherine Hayes suggests that sometimes when a patient chooses not to inform relatives, the patient demonstrates a lack of understanding or reflection about future implications of the results on either the family or him or herself personally.[238] The revised model encourages more attention on the family whether it is having additional family discussions or analysis of family dynamics for disclosure in counseling sessions.

Family members can have a significant impact on whether or not people participate in PGT. While families should know information that might affect them in the future and help them to make life choices, a family should not manipulate or threaten people into participating in PGT in order to identify future consequences.[239]

---

[236] Lori B. Andrews, "Gen-Etiquette: Genetic Information, Family Relationships, and Adoption," 265–266.

[237] Michael Brannigan and Judith Boss, *Healthcare Ethics in a Diverse Society,* 264–265.

[238] Catherine Hayes, "Genetic Testing for Huntington's Disease—A Family Issue," 1450; Michael Burgess, "Beyond Consent: Ethical and Social Issues in Genetic Testing," 510.

[239] Michael Brannigan and Judith Boss, *Healthcare Ethics in a Diverse Society,* 264–265.

D. Patient Safety

The revised model of consent requires an additional component to the traditionally recognized three components (comprehension, disclosure, voluntariness): the culture of patient safety. That is, the revised model of consent enhances the traditional components of consent within a medical culture that emphasizes patient safety. This emphasis has continued to grow in the area of medicine. Safety measures are related to systems and structure changes with an emphasis in organizational ethics.[240] By focusing on improving the system and processes of informed consent, Runciman, Merry, and Walter explain that risk factors can be decreased.[241] This culture of safety requires nationally established systems of accountability for PGT that implement the revised components of consent in a transparent manner to foster trust in the emerging system of genetic-related services. In order for this model to implement appropriate systems of accountability and transparency, Goetz argues that a shift from treatment and diagnosis to prevention and early detection needs to occur.[242] This shift will in turn emphasize a culture of patient safety in the area of PGT.

1. Current Model

This last section of patient safety is a new component for informed consent of PGT. Patient safety is not a component found in the current model of consent. Thomas Goetz expresses that without proper planning, genetic testing can result in "ambiguous probabilities and poorly calibrated risks."[243] In order to protect patients, the revised model adds a new component to informed consent, which is patient safety.

2. Revised Model

This section will look at accountability, transparency, trust, and patient safety systems in the revised model. All of these issues will focus on ways to promote the principles in the revised model, and in the end, those aspects will increase patient safety.

---

[240] William A. Nelson, Julia Neily, Peter Mills, et al., "Collaboration of Ethics and Patient Safety Programs: Opportunities to Promote Quality Care," 15, 17–18; Bill Runciman, Alan Merry, and Merrilyn Walton, *Safety and Ethics in Healthcare*, 6; Mary Ann Baily, Melissa Bottrel, Joanne Lynn, et al., "The Ethics of Using QI Methods to Improve Health Care Quality and Safety," S8.

[241] Bill Runciman, Alan Merry, and Merrilyn Walton, *Safety and Ethics in Healthcare*, 6.

[242] Thomas Goetz, *The Decision Tree*, xiv.

[243] Thomas Goetz, *The Decision Tree*, 122.

a. Accountability

The revised model encourages internal and external accountability by promoting communication among medical departments and institutional policies. David Shore suggests that the first part of increasing patient safety is the focus on accountability.[244] Accountability of the doctor and medical services arose during the history of consent, because sometimes there was limited accountability for doctors.[245] George Lundberg notes that without adequate regulations doctors have been known to do many unethical activities.[246] As a result, the revised model promotes accountability to increase patient safety. This section will focus on accountability and institutional policies.

1). Types of Accountability

Accountability is often broken up into two categories: internal and external accountability measures. Internal accountability measures are guidelines implemented by a specific hospital or medical practice, and external accountability measures are regulations that overarching groups or agencies establish like the AMA. Professional accountability typically falls into the external accountability measures, because those measures look at areas of physician licensing, specific medical qualifications and medical misconduct or litigation. In each of these categories, departments can hold other departments accountable for their actions.[247] Thus, by having greater communication among departments and professional groups, accountability of physicians and medical practices can be encouraged.

2). Consistent Institutional and Professional Policies

While there are general guidelines for physicians, the revised model also seeks to encourage accountability of PGT laboratories for informed consent. Since there is the possibility for patients to be harmed from misleading or faulty results, the revised model has more extensive system measures in place to ensure the accountability and quality of results and accuracy of information presented. The World Health Organization (WHO) suggests added communication with the labs and physicians about accountability measures.[248] The Clinical Laboratory Improvement Amendment (CLIA) Task Force proposes that laboratories should have some type of consent documentation before testing begins in order to promote accountability of the

---

[244] David Shore, *The Trust Prescription for Healthcare: Building Your Reputation with Consumers,* 110.

[245] Alfred Tauber, *Patient Autonomy and the Ethics of Responsibility,* 6–7.

[246] George Lundberg, *Severed Trust: Why American Medicine Hasn't Been Fixed,* 189–190.

[247] Mary Ann Baily, Melissa Bottrel, Joanne Lynn, et al., "The Ethics of Using QI Methods to Improve Health Care Quality and Safety," S21–22, S31.

[248] World Health Organization, "Quality & Safety in Genetic Testing: An Emerging Concern;" Thomas Goetz, *The Decision Tree,* xvi-xvii, 117; Bernard Lo, *Resolving Ethical Dilemmas,* 273.

labs and PGT in general.[249] Also in the revised model, the labs conducting PGT will be required to participate in a genetics quality assurance program. The American Society of Clinical Oncology (ASCO) explains that even though CLIA develops guidelines for quality, those regulations only recommend, not require, participation in specific genetics programs.[250] At this time CLIA is looking into establishing a genetics specialty, but clear guidelines have not yet been established.[251] However, WHO notes that genetic assessment evaluations can be done through the College of American Pathologists (CAP), the American College of Medical Genetics (ACMG), or American Society of Human Genetics (ASHG).[252] ASCO holds that programs to ensure accountability will look at measures within laboratories and testing clinics to confront regulatory challenges that can increase false accountability. Measures will also be in place to examine the accuracy of materials presented to both the patient and family.[253] As a result, the revised model will promote consistent, appropriate institutional and professional policies that ensure enhanced accountability measures.

There vised model promotes accountability measures to confront regulatory challenges that increase false accountability and decreased quality.[254] ASCO promotes the creation of nationally established measures to increase quality and accountability for PGT.[255] In order to adhere to appropriate accountability standards, the WHO is in the process of developing guidelines to assist with the quality and accountability of PGT.[256] When there are specific, consistent guidelines, an organization's accountability measures should be disclosed to patients in order to encourage understanding of the regulations and transparency of implementation.[257]

b. Transparency

The revised model requires transparency with physician discussions and consent requirements. Transparency along with accountability measures work to advance trust and patient safety of PGT. The revised model can have a stronger focus on

---

[249] Neil Holtzman and Michael Watson, eds., *Promoting Safe and Effective Genetic Testing in the United States*.

[250] American Society of Clinical Oncology, "American Society of Clinical Oncology Policy Statement Update: Genetic Testing for Cancer Susceptibility," 5–6; World Health Organization, "Case Study: United States of America;" Thomas Goetz, *The Decision Tree*, xvi-xvii, 117.

[251] Neil Holtzman and Michael Watson, eds., *Promoting Safe and Effective Genetic Testing in the United States*.

[252] World Health Organization, "Case Study: United States of America."

[253] American Society of Clinical Oncology, "American Society of Clinical Oncology Policy Statement Update: Genetic Testing for Cancer Susceptibility," 5–6, 9; Thomas Goetz, *The Decision Tree*, xvi-xvii, 117–118.

[254] Neil C. Manson and Onora O'Neill, *Rethinking Informed Consent in Bioethics*, 198.

[255] American Society of Clinical Oncology, "American Society of Clinical Oncology Policy Statement Update: Genetic Testing for Cancer Susceptibility," 5.

[256] World Health Organization, "Quality & Safety in Genetic Testing: An Emerging Concern."

[257] Mary Ann Baily, Melissa Bottrel, Joanne Lynn, et al., "The Ethics of Using QI Methods to Improve Health Care Quality and Safety," S16, S22.

accountability by having greater transparency in implementation.[258] This section will discuss medical transparency and methods to implement transparency.

1). Medical Transparency

Engelhardt points out that a medical practice can establish individual regulations, but transparency is needed to promote trust in that system.[259] Often with managed care, there is not enough time to clarify the aspects of informed consent such as the accountability or transparency measures.[260] However, the revised model recognizes that additional communication about the measures taken to ensure transparency is needed to promoting trust and patient safety.

Until recently, transparency measures were not emphasized much in regards to health care. Still, Goetz explains that at times encouraging public openness and evaluation is difficult for the medical community. However, if transparency is going to be emphasized, then the doctor needs to facilitate more openness concerning consent and decision-making, especially about PGT.[261] While decision-making for PGT is not as easy as a simple recommendation, the patient and physician could discuss possible suggestions and encourage added transparency within the revised model of consent.

2). Implementing Transparency

The revised model adheres to transparency measures that focus specifically on PGT. This model strives to improve the previous components by requiring transparency of implementation. Implementing the revised model in a transparent manner is crucial for patient safety and decision-making.If there is a lack of transparency, often communication with the doctors and counselors can suffer and lead to patient apprehension and a lack of trust. The revised model seeks to eliminate the idea of the "silent world" of doctors and patients so that communication and openness can flourish.[262] Howard Brody encouraged transparency for consent by suggesting that patients should be informed about the physicians reasoning for suggesting a course of action.[263] David Shore encourages medical practices and doctors to be open about the procedures and regulations that the organization and/or doctor is taking to produce trust or another goal like patient safety.[264]

---

[258] Kuala Lumpur, "Transparency, good governance also vital in healthcare," 24.

[259] H. Tristram Engelhardt Jr., *The Foundations of Bioethics*, 357.

[260] George Lundberg, *Severed Trust: Why American Medicine Hasn't Been Fixed*, 193.

[261] Thomas Goetz, *The Decision Tree*, xviii, 245.

[262] Kuala Lumpur, "Transparency, good governance also vital in healthcare," 24; Stephen Wear, *Informed Consent*, 72, 81, 95, 97.

[263] Howard Brody, *Transparency: Informed Consent in Primary Care*, 8–9.

[264] David Shore, *The Trust Prescription for Healthcare: Building Your Reputation with Consumers*, 155.

The revised model seeks to eliminate institutional barriers and establish a system of accountability and transparency in order to foster trust.[265] Whether it is due to fear of incomplete or inaccurate consent forms or other ideas, generally hospitals keep consent forms private. However, sometimes making forms openly accessible can encourage additional transparency and trust. Having consent forms available to the public on sites like ClincalTrials.gov could help patients evaluate whether or not they will participate in the study. If the forms are public, then more people can scrutinize the forms for accuracy which can encourage both accountability and transparency.[266] Since there are no internationally accepted consistent guidelines for implementing consent principles, the revised model of consent can help to improve regulatory standards by promoting transparency in implementation.[267]

c. Trust

Trust is the ultimate measure for a hospital and physician. However, trust can be harder to maintain at times, because of the abuses in the history of consent. As a result, if patients trust an institution or doctor, that practice will be recognized for its dependability.[268] The revised model encourages trust in the organizations and physicians by having open discussions with patient participation in the revised consent process. This section will look at the history and roles of trust and discuss trust in the revised model.

1). History and Roles of Trust in Medicine

In the beginning, people assumed that an increase in patient rights and autonomy would increase public trust in the ways medicine, science, and biotech were practiced and regulated. However even after promoting those two ideas, public trust was still not encouraged. O'Neill points out that the doctor-patient relationship has the potential to exploit patient trust as evidenced by paternalism.[269] Roberta Berry explains that while autonomy and patient rights were highlighted, trust became an unpopular area of emphasis due to its connection with paternalism at the time. However, trust became more important when people saw the shortcomings of autonomy in the doctor-patient relationship, when relationships were encouraged more than

---

[265] Stephen Wear, *Informed Consent*, 61, 72–73, 96, 173; Albert Jonsen, Mark Siegler, William Winslade, *Clinical Ethics: A Practical Approach to Ethical Decisions in Clinical Medicine*, 59.

[266] Jerry Menikoff, "Making Research Consent Transparent," 1713–1714.

[267] Martha Macintyre, "Informed Consent and Mining Projects: A View from Papua New Guinea," 53.

[268] David Shore, *The Trust Prescription for Healthcare: Building Your Reputation with Consumers*, xv; George Lundberg, *Severed Trust: Why American Medicine Hasn't Been Fixed*, 179.

[269] Onora O'Neill, "Gaining Autonomy and Losing Trust?" 16, 18.

individual actions, and when those interactions were threatened by medical systems like managed care.[270]

Trust in medicine is not the same as it once was when a physician would care for generations of family members. In the beginning, there was more emphasis on the doctor-patient relationship rather than the distanced business model of medicine today. The new commercialization and changing values of medicine has fostered mistrust in many areas.[271] As a result, David Shore notes that trust today often requires faith in procedures and organizations.[272] Traditional trust has been replaced with trust in contracts, because of the commercial focus of medicine and genetics. However, contracts alone cannot guarantee trust in the physicians or institutions, and as a result, trust has decreased over the years in medicine.[273]

Trust is foundational to informed consent. Since the patient is dependent on the doctor for information and recommendations, the doctor-patient relationship is based on fiduciary responsibilities which imply trust in the physician to act in the patient's best interest. Informed consent therefore assists patients in balancing trust in the physician with personal decision making.[274] Medicine is different than other professions, because the product of good medicine should be a trusting doctor-patient relationship.[275] David Shore argues that patients who trust their medical team are more likely to be responsible for their health leading to better outcomes and to have a stronger doctor-patient relationship causing patients to follow the physician's suggestions more.[276]

2). Trust within the Revised Model

Trust can be built when physicians help patients to understand their full potential in medical decision making.[277] When there is no clear treatment, the counselor can discuss the possible choices with the patient which can encourage trust.[278] Shore holds that trust is advanced by having better communication and recognizing that the doctor-patient relationship needs reciprocal disclosure to encourage patient par-

---

[270] Roberta M. Berry, "Informed Consent Law, Ethics, and Practice: From Infancy to Reflective Adolescence," 73.

[271] Alfred Tauber, *Patient Autonomy and the Ethics of* Responsibility, 7, 159, 167–168.

[272] David Shore, *The Trust Prescription for Healthcare: Building Your Reputation with Consumers,* 8, 12.

[273] Alfred Tauber, *Patient Autonomy and the Ethics of Responsibility,* 59, 159; Janet L. Dolgin, "The Legal Development of the Informed Consent Doctrine: Past and Present," 102.

[274] Roberta M. Berry, "Informed Consent Law, Ethics, and Practice: From Infancy to Reflective Adolescence," 73; David Orentlicher, "Genetic Privacy in the Patient-Physician Relationship," 84.

[275] Steve Lee, "The Physician as an Evolving Moral Actor," 682.

[276] David Shore, *The Trust Prescription for Healthcare: Building Your Reputation with Consumers,* xiii, 5; Stephen Wear, *Informed Consent,* 33, 50, 81; Roberta M. Berry, "Informed Consent Law, Ethics, and Practice: From Infancy to Reflective Adolescence," 73.

[277] Meredith Celene Schwartz, "Trust and Responsibility in Health Policy," 116, 122–123.

[278] Barbara Bowles Biesecker, "Privacy in Genetic Counseling," 112.

ticipation.[279] Steve Lee explains that patients have to have faith that the doctor is looking out for their best interest, because "If trust is lost, all is lost."[280] If patients do not believe physicians are promoting their beneficence, an increased skepticism can occur towards the physician's recommendations. If trust erodes in the physician or healthcare system, sometimes patients will try to address the mistrust themselves by attempting to reduce feelings of helplessness and protecting their welfare.[281] Sometimes those actions might be acceptable, but many times those actions can produce increased harm. If there is mistrust of the physician or institution, the utilization of other medical tests can be reduced as well.[282]

Trust is developed in the revised model by measures ensuring accountability of PGT regulations and transparency in implementation.[283] Accountability within laboratories and medical practices can promote trust in organizations and processes. When the revised model implements the informed consent components transparently, patients will be able to put more trust in the contracts and consent forms involved in PGT. When trust in the informed consent process is fostered for the emerging system of genetic services, the culture of patient safety is enhanced further.

d. Patient Safety Systems

The last aspect for the revised model of informed consent for PGT is patient safety systems. Patient safety is fostered by having systems of accountability and transparency to establish preventive measures as systems that promote the safety of patients considering PGT. This section will look at the systems of patient safety and preventive and organizational measures.

1). Systems of Patient Safety

Accountability and transparency are the two main aspects of having a system for patient safety. Lundberg explains that systems of protection can emerge in the form of accountability measures, and truthfulness can take the form of transparency measures for procedures and results. Both of these measures are needed in the revised model.[284] If those two requirements are met, then patients will have more confi-

---

[279] David Shore, *The Trust Prescription for Healthcare: Building Your Reputation with Consumers,* 72–73; Alfred Tauber, *Patient Autonomy and the Ethics of Responsibility,* 167–168.

[280] Steve Lee, "The Physician as an Evolving Moral Actor," 682.

[281] David Shore, *The Trust Prescription for Healthcare: Building Your Reputation with Consumers,* 63; Alfred Tauber, *Patient Autonomy and the Ethics of Responsibility,* 159, 167–168.

[282] Lori B. Andrews, *Future Perfect: Confronting Decisions about Genetics,* 165.

[283] Neil C. Manson and Onora O'Neill, *Rethinking Informed Consent in Bioethics,* 157–158; Robert M. Arnold and Charles W. Lidz, "Informed Consent: Clinical Aspects of Consent in Health Care," 5, 10; George Lundberg, *Severed Trust: Why American Medicine Hasn't Been Fixed,* 179; Stephen Wear, *Informed Consent,* 72, 81.

[284] George Lundberg, *Severed Trust: Why American Medicine Hasn't Been Fixed,* 176.

dence and trust in the revised system for consent of PGT. As a result of patient trust and an emphasis on prevention and early detection, the revised model will promote the culture of patient safety that is often sought in medicine.[285]

2). Preventive and Organizational Measures

By focusing on systems change, the revised model can encourage a broad, organized method to patient safety.[286] Nelson, Neily, Mills, et al. suggest that this model also uses preventive measures to increase patient safety for PGT. Rather than focusing on treatment like the current model, the revised model chooses to emphasize the value of prevention.[287]

The medical system focuses on incorrect principles. The revised model should be able to identify and address institutional and personal barriers to consent before PGT takes place. One barrier might include faulty reimbursement policies that favor treatment and advance potentially unnecessary medical services. Another barrier can be foundations of consent that seemingly allow for choice but do not adequately promote understanding, disclosure, or voluntariness.[288] By focusing on prevention instead of treatment, the revised model can reduce the amount of harm done to patients and improve patient safety. Education can help to prevent any future misunderstandings and concerns, which can led to patient safety in the end.[289] George Lundberg points out that looking at the organization, procedures, and end products can help to assess patient care. While all three are important, typically the end result is emphasized more, and in the revised model of consent for PGT, patient safety should be the outcome.[290]

E. Conclusion

If all people in society had the same ethics and values, then there would be no reason to have numerous laws and guidelines to protect patient's rights. However, the history of consent has illustrated what happens when there are no regulations in medicine. Because of the abuses of the past, there is a strong requirement to have

---

[285] Thomas Goetz, *The Decision Tree*, xiv.

[286] Bill Runciman, Alan Merry, and Merrilyn Walton, *Safety and Ethics in Healthcare*, 241; George Lundberg, *Severed Trust: Why American Medicine Hasn't Been Fixed*, 255.

[287] William A. Nelson, Julia Neily, Peter Mills, et al., "Collaboration of Ethics and Patient Safety Programs: Opportunities to Promote Quality Care," 20.

[288] Thomas Goetz, *The Decision Tree*, 247–248.

[289] Bonne Lorenzen, Constance Melby, and Barb Earles, "Using Principles of Health Literacy to Enhance the Informed Consent Process," 28.

[290] George Lundberg, *Severed Trust: Why American Medicine Hasn't Been Fixed*, 255.

ethics and informed consent in medicine and research.[291] Pellegrino argues that ethics is about protecting individuals from information and tests that do not benefit the patient. If medicine puts aspects like financial or social categories above patient beneficence, then medicine runs the risk of encouraging persecution and abuse and infringing upon rights.[292] Because respecting persons and encouraging beneficence are key elements of medicine, an appropriate model of informed consent is needed to support those principles.[293] Thus, the revised model strives to establish appropriate regulations in order to ensure an appropriate consent for PGT.

Broadstock, Michie, and Marteau explain that in the beginning of genetic services, there were more protections in place with required counseling and follow-up. But as genetic testing became more common and available in many different settings, the protections and regulations were relaxed.[294] Since genetics is central to us, if people get genetic information without adequately thinking through the consequences, then that can lead to unnecessary and possibly harmful outcomes for a patient and his or her family.[295] Thus, the revised model recognizes the importance of meaningful informed consent and regulations in the field of PGT.

The revised model tries to establish the necessary protections while still promoting accessibility and practicality. Tom Beauchamp notes that a balance between overly complex and excessively simplistic regulations for informed consent needs to be established. If guidelines are too challenging to adhere to like requiring complete disclosure, then getting consent will be too difficult and impractical. However on the other side, if consent is too simple focusing mainly on obtaining a signed consent form, then consent will emphasize the wrong values and will lose meaning.[296]

Kahn argues that consent should emphasize a process to promote meaningful decision making instead of focusing mainly on forms which can support a more legalistic view of consent.[297] In conclusion, according to Engelhardt, informed consent is justified when it authorizes an action, respects human dignity, supports individual freedom, encourages personalized evaluation of risks, promotes autonomous and voluntary decision-making, and recognizes the responsibility of a proper doctor-patient relationship that discloses appropriate information.[298] Thus, the healthcare system should promote a model of consent that has substantive information and guidelines in regards to PGT.[299]

---

[291] George Lundberg, *Severed Trust: Why American Medicine Hasn't Been Fixed,* 198.

[292] Edmund Pellegrino, "Nazi Doctors and Nuremberg: Some Moral Lessons Revisited," 307–308.

[293] Robert M. Arnold and Charles W. Lidz, "Informed Consent: Clinical Aspects of Consent in Health Care," 8.

[294] Marita Broadstock, Susan Michie, Theresa Marteau, "Psychological Consequences of Predictive Genetic Testing: A Systematic Review," 736.

[295] Lori B. Andrews, "Gen-Etiquette: Genetic Information, Family Relationships, and Adoption," 255.

[296] Tom Beauchamp, "Informed Consent," 191.

[297] Jeffrey Kahn, "Informed Consent in the Context of Communities," 919.

[298] Tristram Engelhardt Jr., *The Foundations of Bioethics,* 300.

[299] George Lundberg, *Severed Trust: Why American Medicine Hasn't Been Fixed,* 186.

Comprehension of risk assessment includes autonomy, understanding genetic risks, and the doctor-patient relationship. The current model uses a standardized approach to consent that typically focuses on the autonomous patient signing a consent form without much discussion. Since this model emphasizes the consent form, there is insufficient time and communication for understanding the meaning of PGT risk. The current doctor-patient relationship focuses upon the patient freely signing the consent form without sufficient education of the patient about the meaning of PGT. On the other hand, the revised model adopts a personalized approach to consent that emphasizes extensive discussion with the patient as an autonomous agent. The revised model focuses on a process that provides time for communication to foster an understanding of the complex meaning of PGT risk. The revised model emphasizes the doctor-patient relationship as an interactive process to ensure sufficient education of the patient about the meaning of PGT.

Disclosure to select an appropriate treatment option involves disclosure and genetic counseling. The current model focuses on medical information in a standardized approach of consent. The current model recommends non-directive counseling, and does not require counseling. Whereas, the revised model addresses not only medical information but all other relevant information for the patient to consider for consent, including the fact that some PGT diseases might not have any available treatment. The revised model requires counseling and adopts value transparency and non-directive counseling.

Voluntariness of consent discusses coercion and family-related implications. In the current model, there are no specific measures to address or avoid multiple sources of external pressures (such as pressures from relatives, the medical staff and community, and/or societal influences) which increase the possibility of coercion upon the individual. The current model does not take into consideration all family related implications which can lead to coercion of family members. Conversely, the revised model addresses external pressures on the patient and the family (such as pressures by the family for the patient to be tested and pressure upon the family regarding testing outcomes) to alleviate or resolve external coercion upon the patient. Because genetic information impacts the family, the revised model includes family-related concerns before testing and identifies ways to help the patient struggle with family-related PGT information.

Patient safety consists of accountability, transparency, trust, and patient safety. This is a new component that is not in the current model. The revised model encourages internal and external accountability by promoting communication among medical departments and institutional policies. The revised model requires transparency with physician discussions and consent requirements. The revised model encourages trust in the organizations and physicians by having open discussions with patient participation in the revised consent process. In the revised model, patient safety is fostered by having systems of accountability and transparency to establish preventive measures that promote the safety of patients considering PGT.

References

Ackerman, Terrence. "Why Doctors Should Intervene." In *Ethical Issues in Modern Medicine*, edited by Bonnie Steinbock, John Arras, and Alex John London, 73–77. Boston: McGraw Hill Publishing, 2009.

Aktan-Collan, Katja, Jukka-Pekka Mecklin, Albert de la Chapelle, et al. "Evaluation of a Counselling Protocol for Predictive Genetic Testing for Hereditary Non-Polyposis Colorectal Cancer." *Journal of Medical Genetics* 37:2 (February 2000): 108–113.

American Medical Association. "Direct-to-Consumer Genetic Testing." Accessed May 3, 2010. http://www.ama-assn.org/ama1/pub/upload/mm/464/dtc-genetic-test.pdf.

American Society of Clinical Oncology. "American Society of Clinical Oncology Policy Statement Update: Genetic Testing for Cancer Susceptibility." *Journal of Clinical Oncology* 21:12 (June 15, 2003): 1–10.

Andrews, Lori B. "Gen-Etiquette: Genetic Information, Family Relationships, and Adoption." In *Genetic Secrets: Protecting Privacy and Confidentiality in the Genetic Era*, edited by Mark Rothstein, 255–280. New Haven, CT: Yale University Press, 1997.

Andrews, Lori B. *Future Perfect: Confronting Decisions about Genetics*. New York: Columbia University Press, 2001.

Andrews, Lori, Jane Fullarton, Neil Holtzman, eds., et al., Committee on Assessing Genetic Risks, Institute of Medicine. *Assessing Genetic Risks: Implications for Health and Social Policy*. Washington, D.C.: National Academy Press, 1994.

Arnold, Robert M. and Charles W. Lidz. "Informed Consent: Clinical Aspects of Consent in Health Care." In *Taking Sides: Clashing Views on Bioethical Issues*, edited by Carol Levine, 4–14. Boston: McGraw Hill Higher Education, 2010.

Arribas-Ayllon, Michael, Srikant Sarangi, and Angus Clarke. *Genetic Testing: Accounts of Autonomy, Responsibility and Blame*. Abingdon, Oxon Oxford: Routledge Taylor and Francis Group, 2011.

Baily, Mary Ann, Melissa Bottrel, Joanne Lynn, et al. "The Ethics of Using QI Methods to Improve Health Care Quality and Safety." *The Hastings Center Report* 36:4 (July/August 2006): S1–S39.

Ball, David, Audrey Tyler, and Peter Harper. "Predictive Testing of Adults and Children." In *Genetic Counselling*, edited by Angus Clarke, 63–94. New York: Routledge, 1994.

Beahrs, John O. and Thomas G. Gutheil. "Informed Consent in Psychotherapy." *The American Journal of Psychiatry* 158:1 (January 2001): 4–10.

Beauchamp, Tom L. "Informed Consent." In *Medical Ethics*, edited by Robert Veatch, 185–208. Sudbury, MA: Jones and Bartlett Publishers, 1997.

Beauchamp, Tom L. "Informed Consent: Its History, Meaning, and Present Challenges." *Cambridge Quarterly of Healthcare Ethics* 20 (2011): 515–523.

Beauchamp, Tom and James Childress. *Principles of Biomedical Ethics*. New York: Oxford University Press, 2001.

Beauchamp, Tom and LeRoy Walters, eds. *Contemporary Issues in Bioethics*. Belmont, CA: Wadsworth Publishing Company, 2002.

Bennett, Robin. *The Practical Guide to The Genetic Family History*. Hoboken, NJ: John Wiley & Sons, Inc., 2010.

Berdik, Chris. "Genetic Tests Give Consumers Hints About Disease Risk; Critics Have Misgivings." *Washington Post*. (January 26, 2010): Special, 1–2.

Berg, Jessica W., Paul S. Applebaum, Charles W. Lidz, and Lisa S. Parker. *Informed Consent: Legal Theory and Clinical Practice*. New York: Oxford University Press, 2001.

Berry, Roberta M. "Informed Consent Law, Ethics, and Practice: From Infancy to Reflective Adolescence." *HealthCare Ethics Committee Forum* 17:1 (2005): 64–81.

Biesecker, Barbara Bowles. "Privacy in Genetic Counseling." In *Genetic Secrets: Protecting Privacy and Confidentiality in the Genetic Era*, edited by Mark Rothstein, 108–125. New Haven, CT: Yale University Press, 1997.

Botkin, Jeffrey R., Steven M. Teutsch, Celia I. Kaye, et al. from the EGAPP Working Group. "Outcomes of Interest in Evidence-Based Evaluations of Genetic Tests." *Genetics in Medicine* 12:4 (April 2010): 228–235.

Brannigan, Michael and Judith Boss. *Healthcare Ethics in a Diverse Society*. Mountain View, California: Mayfield Publishing Company, 2001.

Broadstock, Marita, Susan Michie, Theresa Marteau. "Psychological Consequences of Predictive Genetic Testing: A Systematic Review." *European Journal of Human Genetics* 8 (2000): 731–738.

Brock, Dan. "Patient Competence and Surrogate Decision-Making." In *The Blackwell Guide to Medical Ethics*, edited by Rosamond Rhodes, Leslie Francis, and Anita Silvers, 128–141. Malden, MA: Wiley-Blackwell Publishing, 2007).

Brody, Howard. "The Physician-Patient Relationship." In *Medical Ethics*, edited by Robert Veatch, 75–101. Sudbury, MA: Jones and Bartlett Publishers, 1997.

Brody, Howard. "Transparency: Informed Consent in Primary Care." *The Hastings Center Report* 19:5 (September- October 1989): 5–9.

Buccafurni, Diana. "Reconsidering the Facilitation of Autonomous Decision Making in Genetic Counseling." PhD diss., University of Utah, August, 2008.

Buchanan, Allen. "From Chance to Choice: Genetics and Justice." In *Contemporary Issues in Bioethics*, edited by Tom Beauchamp and LeRoy Walters, 485–495. Belmont, CA: Wadsworth Publishing Company, 1999.

Burgess, Michael. "Beyond Consent: Ethical and Social Issues in Genetic Testing." In *Contemporary Issues in Bioethics*, edited by Tom Beauchamp and LeRoy Walters, 507–512. Belmont, CA: Wadsworth Publishing Company, 1999.

Carlisle, Jeffrey and Ann T. Neulicht. "The Necessity of Professional Disclosure and Informed Consent for Rehabilitation Counselors." *Journal of Applied Rehabilitation Counseling* 41:2 (Summer 2010): 25–31.

Chadwick, Ruth. "Genetic Screening." In *The Concise Encyclopedia of the Ethics of New Technologies*, edited by Ruth Chadwick, 193–197. San Diego, CA: Academic Press, 2001.

Childress, James. *Who Should Decide? Paternalism in Health Care*. New York: Oxford University Press, 1982.

Clarke, Angus. "Genetic Counseling." In *The Concise Encyclopedia of the Ethics of New Technologies*, edited by Ruth Chadwick, 131–146. San Diego, CA: Academic Press, 2001.

Collins, Francis and Victor McKusick. "Implications of the Human Genome Project for Medical Science." In *Contemporary Issues in Bioethics*, edited by Tom Beauchamp and LeRoy Walters, 473–478. Belmont, CA: Wadsworth Publishing Company, 1999.

Dickenson, Donna. *Risk and Luck in Medical Ethics*. Cambridge, United Kingdom: Polity Press, 2003.

Dolgin, Janet L. "The Legal Development of the Informed Consent Doctrine: Past and Present." Special Section: Open Forum. *Cambridge Quarterly of Healthcare Ethics* 19 (2010): 97–109.

Dolgin, Janet and Lois Shepherd. *Bioethics and the Law*. New York: Aspen Publishers, 2005.

Eisenberg, Leon. "Why has the Relationship Between Psychiatry and Genetics Been so Contentious?" *Genetics in Medicine* 3:5 (September/October 2001): 377–381.

Engelhardt, H. Tristram, Jr. *The Foundations of Bioethics*. New York: Oxford University Press, 1996.

Ensenauer, Regina E., Virginia V. Michels, and Shanda S. Reinke. "Genetic Testing: Practical, Ethical, and Counseling Considerations." *Mayo Clinic Proceedings* 80:1 (January 2005): 63–73.

Felt, Ulrike, Milena D. Bister, Michael Strassnig, and Ursula Wagner. "Refusing the Information Paradigm: Informed Consent, Medical Research, and Patient Participation." *Health: An Interdisciplinary Journal for the Social Study of Health, Illness and Medicine* 13:1 (October 2009): 87–106.

Fitzgerald, Daniel W., Cecile Marotte, Rose Irene Verdier, Warren D. Johnson, et al. "Comprehension during Informed Consent in a Less-Developed Country." *The Lancet* 360:9342 (October 26, 2002): 1301–1302.

Forrest, Laura E., Jo Burke, Sonya Bacic, et al. "Increased Genetic Counseling Support Improves Communication of Genetic Information in Families." *Genetics in Medicine* 10:3 (March 2008): 167–172.

Freedman, Benjamin. "Offering Truth: Once Ethical Approach to the Uninformed Cancer Patient." In *Ethical Issues in Modern Medicine*, edited by Bonnie Steinbock, John Arras, and Alex John London, 110–116. Boston: McGraw Hill Publishing, 2009.

Gaff, Clara L., Veronica Collins, Tiffany Symes, and Jane Halliday. "Facilitating Family Communication about Predictive Genetic Testing: Probans' Perceptions." *Journal of Genetic Counseling* 14:2 (April 2005): 133–140.

Gaff, Clara, Elly Lynch, and Lesley Spencer. "Predictive Testing of Eighteen Year Olds: Counseling Challenges." *Journal of Genetic Counseling* 15:4 (August 2006): 245–251.

Genomics & Genetics Weekly staff. "Genetic Testing: Studies Point to Variable Prognostic Abilities and Question if Testing Results in Behavioral Change." *Genomics & Genetics Weekly* (June 1, 2001): 11–12.

Glover, Jonathan. "Eugenics: Some Lessons from the Nazi Experience." In *Contemporary Issues in Bioethics*, edited by Tom Beauchamp and LeRoy Walters, 467–472. Belmont, CA: Wadsworth Publishing Company, 1999.

Goetz, Thomas. *The Decision Tree.* New York: Rodale Inc., 2010.

Goldman, Alan. "The Refutation of Medical Paternalism." In *Ethical Issues in Modern Medicine*, edited by Bonnie Steinbock, John Arras, and Alex John London, 62–70. Boston: McGraw Hill Publishing, 2009.

Goldstein, Joseph. "For Harold Lasswell: Some Reflections on Human Dignity, Entrapment, Informed Consent, and the Plea Bargain." *Yale Law Journal* 84 (1975): 683–703.

Green, Michael J. and Jeffrey R. Botkin. "'Genetic Exceptionalism' in Medicine: Clarifying the Differences between Genetic and Nongenetic Tests." *Annals of Internal Medicine* 138:7 (April 1, 2003): 571–575.

Harris, Marion, Ingrid Winship, Merle Spriggs. "Controversies and Ethical Issues in Cancer-Genetics Clinics." *Lancet Oncology* 6 (2005): 301–310.

Hayden, Michael. "Predictive Testing for Huntington's Disease: A Universal Model?" *The Lancet Neurology* 2 (March 2003): 141–142.

Hayes, Catherine. "Genetic Testing for Huntington's Disease—A Family Issue." *The New England Journal of Medicine* 327:20 (November 12, 1992): 1449–1451.

Holt, Kathryn. "What Do We Tell the Children? Contrasting the Disclosure Choices of Two HD Families Regarding Risk Status and Predictive Genetic Testing." *Journal of Genetic Counseling* 15:4 (August 2006): 253–265.

Holtzman, Neil and Michael Watson, eds. *Promoting Safe and Effective Genetic Testing in the United States*. Washington, D.C.: National Institutes of Health- Department of Energy Working Group on Ethical, Legal and Social Implications of Human Genome Research, 1997. Accessed December 27, 2012. http://www.genome.gov/10002403.

James, Cynthia, Gail Geller, Barbara Bernhardt, et al. "Are Practicing and Future Physicians Prepared to Obtain Informed Consent? The Case of Genetic Testing for Susceptibility to Breast Cancer." *Community Genetics* 1 (1998): 203–212.

Jonsen, Albert. *The Birth of Bioethics*. New York: Oxford University Press, 1998.

Jonsen, Albert, Mark Siegler, and William Winslade. *Clinical Ethics: A Practical Approach to Ethical Decisions in Clinical Medicine*. New York: McGraw-Hill, 2006.

Kahn, Jeffrey. "Informed Consent in the Context of Communities." *The Journal of Nutrition* 135:4 (April 2005): 918–920.

Katz, Jay. "Physicians and Patients: A History of Silence." In *Contemporary Issues in Bioethics*, edited by Tom Beauchamp and LeRoy Walters, 135–138. Belmont, CA: Wadsworth Publishing Company, 1999.

Kelly, Patricia. "Cancer Risks in Perspective: Information and Approaches for Clinicians." In *Genetic Testing: Care, Consent, and Liability*, edited by Neil Sharpe and Ronald Carter, 382–397. Hoboken, New Jersey: John Wiley & Sons, Inc., 2006.

Kilner, John, Rebecca Pentz, Frank Young, eds. *Genetic Ethics*. Grand Rapids, MI: William B Eerdmans Publishing Company, 1997.

Klitzman, Robert. "Misunderstandings Concerning Genetics Among Patients Confronting Genetic Disease," *Journal of Genetic Counseling* 19:5 (October 2010): 430–446.

Klitzman, Robert, Deborah Thorne, Jennifer Williamson, et al. "The Roles of Family Members, Health Care Workers, and Others in Decision-Making Processes about Genetic Testing among Individuals at Risk for Huntington Disease." *Genetics in Medicine* 9:6 (June 2007): 358–371.

Lee, Steve. "The Physician as an Evolving Moral Actor." *Virtual Mentor: American Medical Association Journal of Ethics* 13:10 (October 2011): 681–683.

Levine, Robert J. "Informed Consent: Some Challenges to the Universal Validity of the Western Model." In *Contemporary Issues in Bioethics*, edited by Tom Beauchamp and LeRoy Walters, 143–148. Belmont, CA: Wadsworth Publishing Company, 1999.

Lo, Bernard. *Resolving Ethical Dilemmas*. Philadelphia, PA: Lippincott Williams and Wilkins, 2005.

Lorenzen, Bonne, Constance Melby, and Barb Earles. "Using Principles of Health Literacy to Enhance the Informed Consent Process." *AORN Journal*, 88:1 (July 2008): 23–29.

Lumpur, Kuala. "Transparency, good governance also vital in healthcare." *New Straits Times* (March 2, 2008): 24.

Lundberg, George. *Severed Trust: Why American Medicine Hasn't Been Fixed*. New York: Basic Books, 2000.

MacIntosh, Constance. "Indigenous Self-Determination and Research on Human Genetic Material: A Consideration of the Relevance of Debates on Patents and Informed Consent, and the Political Demands on Researchers." *Health Law Journal* 13 (2005): 213–251.

Macintyre, Martha. "Informed Consent and Mining Projects: A View from Papua New Guinea." *Pacific Affairs* 80:1 (Spring 2007): 49–65.

Macklin, Ruth. "The Inner Workings of an Ethics Committee: Latest Battle over Jehovah's Witnesses." In *Bioethics: An Introduction to the History, Methods, and Practice*, edited by Nancy Jecker, Albert Jonsen, and Robert Pearlman, 232–235. Sudbury, MA: Jones and Bartlett Publishers, 2007.

Manson, Neil C. and Onora O'Neill. *Rethinking Informed Consent in Bioethics*. New York: Cambridge University Press, 2007.

Marietta, Cynthia and Amy McGuire. "Direct-to-Consumer Genetic Testing: Is It the Practice of Medicine?" *Journal of Law, Medicine & Ethics* 37:2 (Summer 2009): 369–374.

Martin, Douglas and Heather Greenwood. "Public Perceptions of Ethical Issues Regarding Adult Predictive Genetic Testing." *Health Care Analysis* 18:2 (2010): 103–112.

Menikoff, Jerry. "Making Research Consent Transparent." *Journal of the American Medical Association* 304:15 (October 20, 1010): 1713–1714.

Miller, Franklin and Alan Wertheimer. *The Ethics of Consent*. New York: Oxford University Press, 2010.

National Bioethics Advisory Commission. "Protecting Research Participants—A Time for Change." In *Contemporary Issues in Bioethics*, edited by Tom Beauchamp and LeRoy Walters, 371–379. Belmont, CA: Wadsworth Publishing Company, 2003.

Nelson, William A., Julia Neily, Peter Mills, et al. "Collaboration of Ethics and Patient Safety Programs: Opportunities to Promote Quality Care." *HEC Forum*, 20:1 (2008): 15–27.

O'Neill, Onora. "Gaining Autonomy and Losing Trust?" In *Taking Sides: Clashing Views on Bioethical Issues*, edited by Carol Levine, 15–22. Boston: McGraw Hill Higher Education, 2010.

Orentlicher, David. "Genetic Privacy in the Patient-Physician Relationship." In *Genetic Secrets: Protecting Privacy and Confidentiality in the Genetic Era*, edited by Mark Rothstein, 77–91. New Haven, CT: Yale University Press, 1997.

Osman, Hana. "History and Development of the Doctrine of Informed Consent." *The International Electronic Journal of Health Education* 4 (2001): 41–47.

Paabo, Svante. "The Human Genome and Our View of Ourselves." In *Contemporary Issues in Bioethics*, edited by Tom Beauchamp and LeRoy Walters, 496–499. Belmont, CA: Wadsworth Publishing Company, 1999.

Pellegrino, Edmund. "Nazi Doctors and Nuremberg: Some Moral Lessons Revisited." *Annals of Internal Medicine* 127:4 (1997): 307–308.

Pinals, Debra and Paul Appelbaum. "The History and Current Status of Competence and Informed Consent in Psychiatric Research." *The Israel Journal of Psychiatry and Related Sciences* 37:2 (2000): 82–94.

Post, Linda Farber, Jeffrey Blustein, and Nancy Neveloff Dubler. *Handbook for Health Care Ethics Committees*. Baltimore: The John Hopkins University Press, 2007.

Roberts, Laura Weiss. "Informed Consent and the Capacity for Voluntarism." *The American Journal of Psychiatry* 159:5 (May 2002): 705–712.

Rosenthal, M. Sara. "Informed Consent in the Nuclear Medicine Setting." *Journal of Nuclear Medicine Technology* 39:1 (March 2011): 1–4.

Runciman, Bill, Alan Merry, and Merrilyn Walton. *Safety and Ethics in Healthcare*. Burlington, VT: Ashgate Publishing Company, 2007.

Schwartz, Meredith Celene. "Trust and Responsibility in Health Policy." *International Journal of Feminist Approaches to Bioethics* 2:2 (Fall 2009): 116–133.

Sharpe, Neil F. and Ronald Carter. *Genetic Testing: Care, Consent, and Liability*. Hoboken, New Jersey: John Wiley & Sons, Inc., 2006.

Shiloh, Shoshana and Shiri Ilan. "To Test or Not To Test? Moderators of the Relationship Between Risk Perceptions and Interest in Predictive Genetic Testing." *Journal of Behavioral Medicine* 28:5 (October 2005): 467–479.

Shore, David. *The Trust Prescription for Healthcare: Building Your Reputation with Consumers*. Chicago: Health Administration Press, 2005.

Silvers, Anita and Michael Ashley Stein. "An Equality Paradigm for Preventing Genetic Discrimination." *Vanderbilt Law Review* 55:1341 (2002): 1340–1395.

Spencer, Edward, Ann Mills, Mary Rorty, and Patricia Werhane. *Organization Ethics in Health Care*. New York: Oxford University Press, 2000.

Storm, Courtney, Rinki Agarwal, and Kenneth Offit. "Ethical and Legal Implications of Cancer Genetic Testing: Do Physicians Have a Duty to Warn Patients' Relatives about Possible Genetic Risks?" *Journal of Oncology Practice* 4:5 (September 2008): 229–230.

Tannsjo, Torbjorn. *Coercive Care: The Ethics of Choice in Health and Medicine*. New York: Routledge Taylor and Francis Group, 1999.

Tauber, Alfred. *Patient Autonomy and the Ethics of Responsibility*. Cambridge, MA: The MIT Press, 2005.

The National Commission for the Protection of Human Subjects of Biomedical and Behavioral Research. "The Belmont Report: Ethical Principles and Guidelines for the Protection of Human Subjects of Research." In *Ethical Issues in Modern Medicine*, edited by Bonnie Steinbock, John Arras, and Alex John London, 764–770. Boston: McGraw Hill Publishing, 2009.

Trepanier, Angela, Mary Ahrens, Wendy McKinnon, et al. "Genetic Cancer Risk Assessment and Counseling: Recommendations of the National Society of Genetic Counselors." *Journal of Genetic Counseling* 13:2 (April 2004): 83–114.

Vaughn, Lewis. *Bioethics: Principles, Issues, and Cases*. New York: Oxford University Press, 2009.

Veatch, Robert. "Abandoning Informed Consent." *The Hastings Center Report* 25:2 (1995): 5–12.

Wachbroit, Robert. "Disowning Knowledge: Issues in Genetic Testing." In *Bioethics: Principles, Issues, and Cases*, edited by Lewis Vaughn, 495–498. New York: Oxford University Press, 2010.

Wachbroit, Robert. "The Question Not Asked: The Challenge of Pleiotropic Genetic Tests." *Kennedy Institute of Ethics Journal* 8:2 (June 1998): 131–144.

Watson, James. "Genes and Politics." In *Contemporary Issues in Bioethics*, edited by Tom Beauchamp and LeRoy Walters, 479–484. Belmont, CA: Wadsworth Publishing Company, 1999.

Wear, Stephen. *Informed Consent: Patient Autonomy and Clinician Beneficence within Health Care*. Washington, DC: Georgetown University Press, 1998.

Wells, Rebecca Erwin and Ted J. Kaptchuk. "To Tell the Truth, the Whole Truth, May Do Patients Harm: The Problem of the Nocebo Effect for Informed Consent." *American Journal of Bioethics* 12:3 (March 2012): 22–29.

World Health Organization. "Case Study: United States of America." World Health Organization Genomic Resource Centre. Accessed December 27, 2012. http://www.who.int/genomics/policy/usa/en/index.html.

World Health Organization. "Quality & Safety in Genetic Testing: An Emerging Concern." World Health Organization Genomic Resource Centre. Accessed December 27, 2012. http://www.who.int/genomics/policy/quality_safety/en/index1.html.

Wright, David. "Redesigning Informed Consent Tools for Specific Research." *Technical Communication Quarterly* 21:2 (April- June 2012): 145–167.

Young, Ian, *Introduction to Risk Calculation in Genetic Counseling.* Leicester, United Kingdom: Oxford University Press, 2007.

Chapter 5
Application of the Revised Model

Since the Human Genome Project, the world of health care and medical intervention has rapidly been transformed into the genomic era, where the number of genetic interventions and tests are increasing at an alarming rate. There are a plethora of genetic tests, but this chapter will focus on direct-to-consumer (DTC) genetic testing and pleiotropic genetic testing. The revised model of informed consent will be applied to both of these tests. Both types of testing approach the subject of informed consent from a different perspective. DTC genetic testing focuses more on the research model of consent, and pleiotropic genetic testing emphasizes more of the patient treatment model. Because DTC genetic testing does not require physician involvement, the discussion around this type of testing focuses more on the results and the testing companies. Pleiotropic genetic testing emphasizes the education and disclosure needs in order to understand what this testing involves. All of those differences will be evident through each analysis.

Each section will give an introduction to and a discussion of the specific genetic test, apply the four components of the revised model, and then present a case study. Then, the chapter will conclude with summarizing the differences between these two types of genetic tests and discussing the implications for those tests in relation to informed consent.

A. DTC Genetic Testing and Informed Consent

Genetic testing is seen everywhere in health care, but most of the time physicians have to order the tests for their patients. Today however, consumers can go online and buy genetic tests themselves with DTC genetic testing. This section will analyze the ideas involved with DTC genetic testing.

The revised model will first be applied to DTC genetic testing. This section looks at the background of DTC testing, applies the revised model of consent, and analyzes a case study. First, the background of DTC genetic testing gives an introduction to this technology and different types of tests, evaluates the test results and

© Springer International Publishing Switzerland 2015
J. Minor, *Informed Consent in Predictive Genetic Testing,*
DOI 10.1007/978-3-319-17416-7_5

testing companies, and then analyzes the risks and benefits of this type of testing. Second, the four components of the revised model (comprehension, disclosure, voluntariness, and patient safety) are applied to DTC genetic testing. Third, the case study discusses the issues that are involved with DTC genetic testing and informed consent.

1. Background of DTC Genetic Testing

The first part will give an introduction to DTC genetic testing. This section will explain the meaning of DTC genetic testing, give an overview of the test results, and then evaluate the risks and benefits. Analyzing the risks and benefits will help to identify the areas that the revised model of informed consent needs to address.

a. DTC Genetic Testing

DTC genetic testing refers to genetic tests that are marketed and sold directly to consumers through the internet, television, or mail. There are numerous DTC genetic testing companies, including the two most popular in the United States, 23andMe and Navigenics. DTC genetic testing companies send consumers a test kit for collecting a DNA sample by either spitting into a tube or swabbing the inside of the mouth.[1] Within weeks, the consumer is given their results.

In order to understand what DTC genetic testing is, this section will look at the science of the testing and the types of testing available.

1). Science of DTC Genetic Testing

The science behind DTC genetic testing is just like the science of PGT. DTC genetic testing looks at the other samples and compares an individual's sample to the general population risk for a particular disease.[2] DTC genetic testing also looks at genetic variants in order to determine a person's risk of disease.[3] However, as was described before, different variants have different functions and significance.[4] While Huntington's disease only looks at a single genetic variant, many other diseases like the mutation for breast cancer, BRCA, analyze many genetic variants. Because part of this science depends on the number of variants analyzed and identified, DTC genetic testing companies should have a broad range of samples in order

---

[1] 23andMe, "Personal Genome Service: How it Works."

[2] Chris Berdik, "Genetic Tests Give Consumers Hints About Disease Risk; Critics Have Misgivings," 2.

[3] Francis Collins, *The Language of Life*, xxi–xxii.

[4] Cynthia Marietta and Amy McGuire, "Direct-to-Consumer Genetic Testing: Is It the Practice of Medicine?" 370.

to establish appropriate predictions.[5] Having a stronger database of samples could increase statistical probabilities when predicting genetic risks.

2). Types of DTC Genetic Tests

Since there are so many different tests a consumer can get, it is important to understand the different types of DTC genetic testing available. There are the more recreational types of testing including ancestry information and information about individual characteristics and traits such as athletic performance, eye color, and bitter taste perception. Some companies have nutritional and metabolic assessment testing including tests for caffeine metabolism, oxidative stress levels, and skin health. Then there are the more common genetic tests such as prenatal testing, newborn screening, pharmacogenomic testing, and diagnostic testing. Carrier testing is done to see if a person can pass on a disease to their children like cystic fibrosis, hemochromotosis, or Tay-Sachs. Some companies also participate in predisposition testing and genome wide association studies (GWAS). Predisposition testing will give your predicted risk for developing diseases like hereditary cancers, cardiovascular disease, depression, age-related macular degeneration, Celiac disease, Crohn's disease, Parkinson's disease, diabetes, and others. This section will focus on the predictive or predisposition testing for certain diseases.[6]

b. Test Results

Often, DTC genetic test results are very complicated. The first section will look at how to interpret the results. The second section will look at the DTC genetic testing companies and the viewpoints the companies have in regards to those results.

1). Meaning of the Results

Often with DTC genetic testing, consumers do not know what the results of a positive or negative risk assessment means. A test with a positive result means that the individual has a higher chance of developing the disease. While a negative test result means that the individual has the same percentage of risk as people in the general population.[7] Determining the meaning of the results can be very difficult, and

---

[5] Peter Kraft Ph.D., and David Hunter, "Genetic Risk Prediction – Are We There Yet?" 1701.

[6] Cynthia Marietta and Amy McGuire, "Direct-to-Consumer Genetic Testing: Is It the Practice of Medicine?" 369; Francis Collins, *The Language of Life*, 84; AMA, "Direct-to-Consumer Genetic Testing;" Andrew Pollack, "Consumers Slow to Embrace the Age of Genomics," B1.

[7] Marion Harris, Ingrid Winship, and Merle Spriggs, "Controversies and Ethical Issues in Cancer-Genetics Clinics," 302; Cynthia Marietta and Amy McGuire, "Direct-to-Consumer Genetic Testing: Is It the Practice of Medicine?" 370; Neil Sharpe and Ronald Carter, *Genetic Testing: Care, Consent, and Liability,* 269; AMA, "Direct-to-Consumer Genetic Testing."

many times these concepts are rarely discussed by the DTC genetic testing companies. Although, most companies recommend talking to their personal physician after the test in order to discuss the results. While some companies offer genetic counselors to interpret the test results, most do not require them.[8] As a result, many times the individual is responsible for determining what to do with the information.

2). DTC Genetic Testing Companies and Result Perspectives

Within the DTC genetic testing companies, there are different perspectives about the testing results and testing interpretation process. The two most popular DTC genetic testing companies in the United States are 23andMe and Navigenics. 23andMe has its foundation in the principle of autonomy and a fundamental right to know one's genetic makeup.[9] According to a recent article in the *New York Times,* 23andMe is the market leader for DTC genetic testing companies.[10] 23andMe puts more emphasis on the database collection, because the company believes the database will be worth a lot in the future. Navigenics, one of 23andMe's top competitors, has a more traditional approach to DTC genetic testing. Navigenics changed their model, and now their DTC genetic testing is to be used under a physician's supervision.[11] Also Navigenics is one of the only DTC genetic testing companies to have 5 genetic counselors on staff to discuss results with their consumers.[12] Navigenics thinks the best way to market DTC genetic testing is through a physician, which goes against 23andMe's foundation. Vance Vanier, the company's chief medical officer, says that DTC genetic testing is a "very young market and there's a lot of missing information and even misinformation. We're better off having trusted intermediaries through whom a customer gets their information."[13]

While these companies differ in their approaches to DTC genetic testing, there testing methods and end results are similar. These two companies illustrate the two approaches to DTC genetic testing. One approach looks at this testing as more informational, and thus the company does not see the need to involve medical professionals. The other approach sees the information as medical information, and therefore it needs to go through a physician. This is probably one of the biggest debates within DTC genetic testing. Because there are companies that perform both recreational tests and more of the medical test, the solution to informing people about their results is more complex. This issue will be discussed further in the application of the revised model of informed consent.

---

[8] Navigenics, "How our Services Work."

[9] 23andMe, "About Us."

[10] Andrew Pollack, "Consumers Slow to Embrace the Age of Genomics," B1.

[11] Mark Henderson, "Cashing in on Your Genes," 2.

[12] Jane Kaye, "The Regulation of Direct-to-Consumer Genetic Tests," 180.

[13] Mark Henderson, "Cashing in on Your Genes," 2.

c. Risk/Benefit Analysis

There are risks and benefits to almost every technology today. As such, this section performs a risk/benefit analysis of DTC genetic testing. Risks include inappropriate test utilization, misinterpretation of results, and a lack of necessary follow-up. Benefits can include consumer empowerment, lower chance of genetic discrimination, and assist in future planning and preventive measures.[14] The first section will analyze the risks of DTC genetic testing. The second section will evaluate the benefits of testing.

1). Risks

There are three main areas of risk within DTC genetic testing. First, inappropriate test utilization is the idea that people should not be participating in some of these tests. Often doctors will prescribe a patient a specific drug for a specific purpose. By applying the pharmaceutical example to DTC genetic testing, in effect, consumers could be able to buy prescriptions for everything even if a specific medication was not medically indicated. In DTC genetic testing, the consumer can buy any test he or she wants. The main concern is the fact that there are people participating in the tests who should not be. An excessive emphasis upon participation can be encouraged by misleading advertisements or just from the emphasis of consumer autonomy.[15] As a result, people could suffer from inappropriate test utilization by hearing about results for late-onset diseases like Alzheimer's and not being prepared for that knowledge. With this type of testing, harm could arise, because there is no gatekeeper to prevent consumers from buying tests that are unsuitable or that could be misinterpreted.[16]

Second, misinterpretation of results can come from the patient and/or the actual test results.[17] Misinterpretation can come from a lack of education on the part of the consumer so that the consumer misinterprets the results. Many times people do not understand what their results mean, because there is not enough consumer education and results are easily misunderstood.[18] The other aspect of misinterpretation lies in the testing itself. DTC genetic testing companies just take into account the genes and chromosomes, but the results do not take into account other areas of

---

[14] Chris Berdik, "Genetic Tests Give Consumers Hints About Disease Risk; Critics Have Misgivings," 1; Cynthia Marietta and Amy McGuire, "Direct-to-Consumer Genetic Testing: Is It the Practice of Medicine?" 370–371; Emily Singer, "Off-the-Shelf Genetic Testing on Display," 1.

[15] Kathy Beal, "Statement on Direct-to-Consumer Genetic Testing," 1; Cynthia Marietta and Amy McGuire, "Direct-to-Consumer Genetic Testing: Is It the Practice of Medicine?" 371; Emily Singer, "Off-the-Shelf Genetic Testing on Display," 1.

[16] Leslie Pray, "DTC Genetic Testing: 23andMe, DNA Direct and Genelex," 5; Daniel Farkas and Carol Holland, "Direct-to-Consumer Genetic Testing: Two Sides of the Coin," 2.

[17] Cynthia Marietta and Amy McGuire, "Direct-to-Consumer Genetic Testing: Is It the Practice of Medicine?" 370.

[18] Chris Berdik, "Genetic Tests Give Consumers Hint About Disease Risk; Critics Have Misgivings," 1.

medical information or environmental aspects.When analyzing a complex disease, all information relating to the person should be discussed including a family history, environmental interactions, lifestyle, and the person's current medications and medical condition.[19] Robert Green, a neurologist at Boston University, says "At this point, nongenetic factors, such as family history, body mass index, and history of smoking, often provide a better predictor of disease risk than does genetics."'[20] Unless all parts of a person's health are analyzed, results for an individual can be misinterpreted easily. While the major DTC genetic testing companies have a 99% accuracy rate in locating the genetic variants, not all the variants have equal meaning.Some SNPs can increase a person's disease risk by a 100%, while others only increase risk by 1 to 2%. Because of the uncertainty involved in this testing, there is a high risk for misinterpretation.[21]

Third, a lack of necessary follow-up is a risk and concern for DTC genetic testing. Some companies have genetic counselors and doctors for the consumers to talk to, but overall there is a lack of physician involvement and follow-up.[22] After positive results, a person might get extremely depressed or anxious, since the test shows there is a higher risk for developing a specific disease. However, there is also the fact that a person might have gotten a false reassurance. The person might assume a negative result meant that the individual would not get the disease. Sometimes poor health decisions can arise from that thinking as well.[23] If the individual does not share the results with a physician or counseling, he or she could be making medical decisions on misinterpreted and incomplete testing results causing harm to the individual.[24]Dr. Robert Marion, a clinical geneticist, says the main part of the problem for DTC genetic testing is that "without careful explanation, without accompanying genetic counseling to explain their meaning, the results are not only meaningless, they can actually be harmful."[25] Ignoring the communication process can cause faulty decisions and harm.[26] Follow-up and counseling are major areas that will be discussed more in the revised model.

2). Benefits

There are three potential benefits to DTC genetic testing. First, the advocates say it can help consumers feel empowered by knowing their genetic makeup, can cut

---

[19] AMA, "Direct-to-Consumer Genetic Testing."

[20] Emily Singer, "Off-the-Shelf Genetic Testing on Display," 1.

[21] Chris Berdik, "Genetic Tests Give Consumers Hints About Disease Risk; Critics Have Misgivings," 2.

[22] Daniel Farkas and Carol Holland, "Direct-to-Consumer Genetic Testing: Two Sides of the Coin," 264.

[23] Chris Berdik, "Genetic Tests Give Consumers Hints About Disease Risk; Critics Have Misgivings," 3.

[24] Mary Shedden, "Genetic Screenings are no Replacement for Medical Advice,"1; U.S. National Library of Medicine, "What is Direct-to-Consumer Genetic Testing?"

[25] Dr. Hsien-Hsien Lei, "Dr. Robert Marion on Direct-to-Consumer Genetic Testing."

[26] Kathy Beal, "Statement on Direct-to-Consumer Genetic Testing," 1.

down on the amount of genetic discrimination, and can help with future treatment plans. Consumers say that this type of testing is based on autonomy and a right to know one's genetic makeup, like the company 23andMe. If a person wants to claim more empowerment over their body, there are several DTC genetic testing companies that will fulfill this desire and satisfy curiosity. However, completely understanding the process of DTC genetic testing is essential for true autonomy and empowerment. While consumer empowerment might be a benefit to DTC genetic testing, consumer autonomy could be taken advantage of in this type of testing and could potentially cause harm to individuals.[27]

Second, oddly enough, genetic privacy was cited as a potential benefit for DTC genetic testing.Consumers thought that if they received their genetic testing results outside of their physician's office, then their genetic report would never make it into their medical records. This idea can point out the lack of information concerning genetic testing. Most, if not all, DTC genetic testing companies recommend going to your doctor to review the results of your genetic testing. Once a consumer goes to their doctor and discusses specific results, that information makes it onto a person's medical record. However, since the passing of the Genetic Information Non-Discrimination Act of 2008 (GINA), patients do not have to worry as much anymore about genetic discrimination.[28] Because of GINA, protecting genetic privacy and genetic discrimination is no longer a true benefit of DTC genetic testing. In fact, when looking at the possibility of the company selling consumer's DNA databases to scientists, there might be a risk to genetic privacy with this testing.

Third, helping patients with future treatment plans and preventive measures is another commonly cited benefit. Advocates say that once a person knows that he or she is at an increased risk for a particular disease, then the person will take precautionary measures such as having more screening tests or changing lifestyle habits.[29] The consumer will be more motivated and aware of his increased risk of disease, and as a result, he or she will therefore make better decisions.[30] A study, conducted in 2008, sent online surveys to 1,880 physicians asking if they had patients that had used DTC genetic testing. Out of the small percentage of patients that had used those services, the physicians said, after seeing the results, that about 75% of the cases had some change in the patient's care.[31] Participating in DTC genetic testing can be a benefit for preventive medicine, but there are also concerns with this point. The first is that while people say having a more active role in their health is a positive benefit for DTC genetic testing, there is no proof that that is what people are

---

[27] Chris Berdik, "Genetic Tests Give Consumers Hints About Disease Risk; Critics Have Misgivings," 1; Cynthia Marietta and Amy McGuire, "Direct-to-Consumer Genetic Testing," 370; Francis Collins, *The Language of Life*, 87–88; Daniel Farkas and Carol Holland, "Direct-to-Consumer Genetic Testing: Two Sides of the Coin," 1, 3; 23andMe, "About Us."

[28] Cynthia Marietta and Amy McGuire, "Direct-to-Consumer Genetic Testing," 370; B. Prainsack and J. Reardon, "Misdirected precaution," 34–35.

[29] Chris Berdik, "Genetic Tests Give Consumers Hints About Disease Risk; Critics Have Misgivings," 1–2; Leslie Pray, "DTC Genetic Testing: 23andMe, DNA Direct and Genelex," 4.

[30] Leslie Pray, "DTC Genetic Testing: 23andMe, DNA Direct and Genelex," 4.

[31] Jeff Evans, "DTC Genetic Tests Seen as Problematic," 4.

using these tests for.[32] In actuality, these tests could have the opposite effect either by instilling more anxiety or by creating an attitude of apathy. Another concern with this point is the fact that these treatment decisions could be based on inaccurate results, because there is no positive way of predicting a person's actual risk of developing a disease.

2. Application of the Revised Model

This section will apply the revised model of informed consent to DTC genetic testing. The four components of the revised model, comprehension, disclosure, voluntariness, and patient safety, will be applied to DTC genetic testing.

a. Comprehension

First, comprehension of DTC genetic testing will be analyzed. In this section, autonomy, genetic risks, and the doctor-patient relationship is discussed in regards to comprehension.

The current model uses a standardized approach to consent that typically focuses on the autonomous patient signing a consent form without much discussion. Since this model emphasizes the consent form, there is insufficient time and communication for understanding the meaning of PGT risk. The current doctor-patient relationship focuses upon the patient freely signing the consent form without sufficient education of the patient about the meaning of PGT. On the other hand, the revised model adopts a personalized approach to consent that emphasizes extensive discussion with the patient as an autonomous agent. The revised model focuses on a process that provides time for communication to foster an understanding of the complex meaning of PGT risk. The revised model emphasizes the doctor-patient relationship as an interactive process to ensure sufficient education of the patient about the meaning of PGT.

1). Autonomy

DTC genetic testing recognizes the importance of autonomy and self- determination. One company, 23andMe, has its foundation in the principle of autonomy and a fundamental right to know one's genetic makeup.[33] Since DTC genetic testing is different than some of the other types of testing in that it focuses on a patient and research subject model of consent, the application of autonomy can be a little different in this approach. Unlike the current model which uses a standardized approach

---

[32] Leslie Pray, "DTC Genetic Testing: 23andMe, DNA Direct and Genelex," 4.

[33] Cynthia Marietta, Amy McGuire, "Direct-to-Consumer Genetic Testing: Is It the Practice of Medicine?" 370; 23andMe, "About Us."

to consent, the revised model emphasizes more patient involvement through a process of increased education and discussion with the patient. In order to encourage enhanced autonomy and also understanding, the revised model encourages turning abstract statistics and risks into more personalized information.[34] Adopting a more personalized approach to consent with DTC genetic testing encourages the patient to act as an autonomous agent.

2). Understanding Genetic Risks

Risk assessments are often very complex to understand, but it is crucial that patients understand these assessments before making a decision based off of misunderstood information.[35] Having a positive result on a specific cancer test like prostate cancer does not mean that a person has prostate cancer right now, nor is it certain that he will ever get prostate cancer in the future.[36] The positive result just means that the individual has a higher risk of developing prostate cancer sometime in his life.

In order to enhance understanding of DTC genetic testing, the revised model focuses on a process that promotes increased time for patient education and communication with physicians or genetic counselors. Beauchamp and Childress point out one way understanding can be encouraged in the revised model. The authors explain that having an evaluation of other individuals after DTC genetic testing could help in the future. By having a post-test evaluation, individuals working for these companies can identify and address areas that other people did not understanding concerning genetic risks. One difficulty with understanding risk assessments for DTC genetic testing is the application of risk to the research realm. Because research seeks to gain knowledge, often the results of research do not benefit the individual subject at the time of the study. With DTC genetic testing, many times the individual functions as both a research subject and patient. As a result, the individual needs to understand both aspects of testing. In order to do that, the revised model encourages more time for communication. Research indicates that understanding can be increased with research subjects when there are one-on-one discussions with the individual and a "neutral educator."[37]

3). Doctor-Patient Relationship

The doctor-patient relationship is a little different with DTC genetic testing, because often there is no direct contact with a physician. Companies encourage discussing the results with a physician, but often discussions are limited with DTC genetic testing.

---

[34] Thomas Goetz, *The Decision Tree*, 215.

[35] Chris Berdik, "Genetic Tests Give Consumers Hint About Disease Risk; Critics Have Misgivings," 1.

[36] AMA, "Direct-to-Consumer Genetic Testing."

[37] Tom Beauchamp and James Childress, *Principles of Biomedical Ethics*, 129.

The current doctor-patient relationship focuses upon the patient freely signing the consent form without sufficient education of the patient about the meaning of PGT. The revised model emphasizes an interactive doctor-patient relationship to ensure sufficient education of the people participating in DTC genetic testing. In order to do that, physicians need to be able to educate patients adequately. However, an article in the *American Journal of Bioethics*, entitled "Direct to Confusion: Lessons Learned from Marketing BRCA Testing" illustrates that not all physicians are able to educate people participating in DTC genetic testing adequately. Matloff and Caplan point out that research "shows that physicians lack adequate knowledge of even basic genetic concepts, making them likely to mishandle, misinterpret, and misadvise these patients on what is one of the most important pieces of medical information they will ever receive."[38] As a result, the DTC genetic testing companies need to ensure that there are individuals, whether physicians or genetic counselors, that can explain the process and meaning of DTC genetic testing sufficiently.[39] Even though this testing is sent directly to the consumer, there still needs to be appropriate communication with a physician or counselor to ensure adequate understanding. The revised model ensures the doctor-patient relationship is an interactive process for encouraging understanding of DTC genetic testing.

The revised model adopts a personalized approach to consent that emphasizes extensive discussion with the patient as an autonomous agent. The revised model focuses on a process that provides time for communication to foster an understanding of the complex meaning of PGT risk. The revised model emphasizes the doctor-patient relationship as an interactive process to ensure sufficient education of the patient about the meaning of PGT.

b. Disclosure

Second, disclosure to select an appropriate treatment option involves disclosure and genetic counseling. Each area will be analyzed further. The current model focuses on medical information in a standardized approach of consent. The current model recommends non-directive counseling, and does not require counseling. Whereas, the revised model addresses not only medical information but all other relevant information for the patient to consider for consent, including the fact that some PGT diseases might not have any available treatment. The revised model requires counseling and adopts value transparency and non-directive counseling.

1). Disclosure Guidelines

The current model focuses on medical information in a standardized approach of consent. However, the revised model includes both medical and non-medical infor-

---

[38] Ellen Matloff and Arthur Caplan, "Direct to Confusion: Lessons Learned from Marketing BRCA Testing," 7.
[39] Jane Kaye, "The Regulation of Direct-to-Consumer Genetic Tests," 180; Mark Henderson, "Cashing in on Your Genes," 2.

mation within the disclosure processes. Disclosure also includes the fact that some diseases might not have any available treatment such as Huntington's disease (HD).

Most, if not all, companies use the samples for participation in research, but not all consumers are aware of this fact. The company 23andMe plans to sell their databases of DNA in the future so that other research companies can benefit from the amount of information. 23andMe combines customers' DNA samples and completed surveys on health information, and the company plans to sell those databases so that scientist can make new discoveries by comparing the samples with the survey information.[40] Thus, disclosure for DTC genetic testing should include disclosure information for research purposes as well as all other typical information like the risks, benefits, and purpose.[41]

Since this type of testing relies on large number of samples, disclosure should address the storage policies of these samples including the privacy regulations.[42] Individuals should be aware of who has access to their samples and information, how their privacy will be protected, and what the uses of their samples will be in the future. Beauchamp suggests that the "content of the consent will be roughly dictated by current and anticipated future uses of the samples."[43] The future uses of genetic samples are increasingly important with this type of testing when determining what to disclosure to an individual. Also another important aspect of disclosure for DTC genetic testing is the level of research. In order to establish better predictions, DTC genetic testing companies need to have a broad range of samples.[44] If the company has done little research and/or their database is relatively small, the results might be extremely varied or simply incorrect. As a result, disclosure for DTC genetic testing should discuss the level of research the results are based on. The companies should disclose the amount of information the results are based on. In order to protect against unsubstantiated claims, the revised model encourages adopting a research confidence rating system to illustrate the difference between preliminary and confirmed research.[45] This type of increased assurance can help the individual to be able to make a better decision about DTC genetic testing.

2). Genetic Counseling

With many DTC genetic testing companies, genetic counseling is not required.[46] However, unlike the current model, the revised model requires counseling and adopts value transparency and non-directive counseling. As Dr. Robert Marion

---

[40] Mark Henderson, "Cashing in on Your Genes," 2.

[41] Linda Farber Post, Jeffrey Blustein, and Nancy Neveloff Dubler, *Handbook for Health Care Ethics Committees*, 38–39.

[42] Angela Trepanier, Mary Ahrens, Wendy McKinnon, et al., "Genetic Cancer Risk Assessment and Counseling: Recommendations of the National Society of Genetic Counselors," 107.

[43] Tom L. Beauchamp, "Informed Consent: Its History, Meaning, and Present Challenges," 519–520.

[44] Peter Kraft Ph.D., and David Hunter, "Genetic Risk Prediction – Are We There Yet?" 1701.

[45] Kristine Goodwin, "Information Overload? National Conference of State Legislatures."

[46] Navigenics, "How our Services Work."

suggested, without an individual explaining and/or discussing the results, the person undergoing DTC genetic testing can be negatively impacted by the testing.[47] Having results that are not adequately explained can cause people to make harmful and risky decisions.[48]

The revised model requires genetic counseling both before and after testing to enhance decision making about appropriate options. Genetic counseling is needed for knowing when to utilize a certain test and then after the testing in order to evaluate the results.[49] Pre-test counseling can help with psychological assessments in order to evaluate whether the individual is competent and whether the individual will be able to handle the amount of information appropriately.[50] Post-test counseling ensures the patient meets to assess the results with either the DTC testing company or the patient's personal physician. While most companies only have a genetic counselor, Navigenics uses their testing under a physician's supervision.[51] One study by Aktan-Collan, Mecklin, de la Chapelle, et al. illustrates the basic foundations of pre- and post-test assessments. After disclosing the basic information needed, the study began with a pre-test assessment. This assessment included a questionnaire to evaluate the individual, pre-test counseling, a required wait time in between counseling and testing, and then a telephone call in order to find out about the individual's decision. Once the pre-test assessment concluded, if the person decided to participate in the test, the test was then performed. After completing the test, the study concluded with a post-test assessment which included post-test counseling and follow-up questionnaires for 1 month and 1 year after the test.[52] This example shows the general principles that guide pre- and post-test assessments for counselors. In the revised model, the consent process for DTC genetic testing should require some type of pre- and post-test counseling.

In the revised model, genetic counseling also should include patient assessment and feedback mechanisms. Feedback mechanisms like an Impact of Event Scale (IES) survey and a decision tree can encourage appropriate decision making about potential options. An IES is a survey that assesses the individual's ability to handle a lot of information. This survey can evaluate the amount of stress a person is likely to have with new a lot of information. Counselors can use this assessment in order to identify the people that might not be able to handle the amount of information DTC genetic testing reveals. Another assessment tool is a decision tree. A decision

---

[47] Dr. Hsien-Hsien Lei, "Dr. Robert Marion on Direct-to-Consumer Genetic Testing."

[48] Mary Shedden, "Genetic Screenings are no Replacement for Medical Advice," 1.

[49] Kathy Beal, "Statement on Direct-to-Consumer Genetic Testing," 1–2; Dr. Hsien-Hsien Lei, "Dr. Robert Marion on Direct-to-Consumer Genetic Testing;"Jane Kaye, "The Regulation of Direct-to-Consumer Genetic Tests," R180.

[50] Angela Trepanier, Mary Ahrens, Wendy McKinnon, et al., "Genetic Cancer Risk Assessment and Counseling: Recommendations of the National Society of Genetic Counselors," 93.

[51] Mark Henderson, "Cashing in on Your Genes," 2.

[52] Katja Aktan-Collan, Jukka-Pekka Mecklin, Albert de la Chapelle, et al., "Evaluation of a Counselling Protocol for Predictive Genetic Testing for Hereditary Non-Polyposis Colorectal Cancer," 109.

tree can break up the amount of information that is presented into more manageable segments by outlining the options, factors, and decisions. The decision tree can help patients determine whether or not to undergo testing and/or start a certain treatment. A patient can participate more in decision making by drawing or outlining the concepts involved in his/his decision.[53]

The following is an example of a decision tree for an individual that has a family history of cervical cancer. First, the patient asks the question of whether or not he or she should get tested for a particular gene mutation, in this case the BRCA mutation. If the patient decides to undergo testing and finds out she is positive for this mutation, then she needs to review the possible treatment options. After reviewing the options, then she needs to make a decision about whether she is going to under screening only or whether she will have a prophylactic surgery. If surgery is decided, then she needs to look at the different types of surgery. Once she decides on a type, then she needs to choose a doctor to perform the surgery. After identifying a doctor, the woman will need to decide when to have the surgery. If she decides to have both her ovaries and uterus taken out as part of the treatment, she needs to analyze whether or not she would like to have another child or whether she needs to wait until after breastfeeding her current child. All of these aspects need to be included when determining when to schedule the procedure. Then finally, if she is undergoing a mastectomy, she will need to look into reconstructive surgery. These are all areas that can be analyzed in a decision tree.[54]

Also within patient assessment and feedback, there needs to be time to think before making a final decision about DTC testing.[55] In one study by Aktan-Collan, Mecklin, de la Chapelle, et al., the pre-test counseling session was done and then a 2-week period was required before the individual participated in the test.[56] This time was given in order to reflect on the counseling sessions and the individual's concerns and values. The revised model requires at least 2 weeks before a final decision can be made to participate in DTC genetic testing. During this time, the individual can have a discussion with family members in order to determine their feelings on the test. By requiring genetic counseling with feedback and patient assessment mechanisms, the patient will be able to make an appropriate decision about possible options.

The revised model addresses not only medical information but all other relevant information for the patient to consider for consent, including the fact that some PGT diseases might not have any available treatment. The revised model requires counseling and adopts value transparency and non-directive counseling.

---

[53] Thomas Goetz, *The Decision Tree*, xii–xiii, 47–48, 197, 210.

[54] Thomas Goetz, *The Decision Tree*, 31.

[55] Stephen Wear, *Informed Consent*, 95; Thomas Goetz, *The Decision Tree*, 67–68.

[56] Katja Aktan-Collan, Jukka-Pekka Mecklin, Albert de la Chapelle, et al., "Evaluation of a Counselling Protocol for Predictive Genetic Testing for Hereditary Non-Polyposis Colorectal Cancer," 109.

c. Voluntariness

This section will look at the voluntariness of consent for DTC genetic testing. Since DTC genetic testing is a little different than other types of testing in that it does not always require a physician to be involved, the voluntariness focuses almost solely on family-related implications. As a result, the voluntary nature of consent is crucial in order to ensure meaningful consent for DTC genetic testing.[57] This section will look at coercion and family-related implications of consent in regards to DTC genetic testing.

In the current model, there are no specific measures to address or avoid multiple sources of external pressures (such as pressures from relatives, the medical staff and community, and/or societal influences) which increase the possibility of coercion upon the individual. The current model does not take into consideration all family related implications which can lead to coercion of family members. Conversely, the revised model addresses external pressures on the patient and the family (such as pressures by the family for the patient to be tested and pressure upon the family regarding testing outcomes) to alleviate or resolve external coercion upon the patient. Because genetic information impacts the family, the revised model includes family-related concerns before testing and identifies ways to help the patient struggle with family-related PGT information.

1). Coercion

Often the differences in negative and positive influences are the motivations and methods the individual uses to control or persuade. Sometimes external influences can actually support and benefit a person's decision-making by giving additional information. However, other times external influences exhibit deception, weakened choices, and faulty reasoning.[58] The detrimental influences most often "subvert autonomous action by distorting individual choice through coercion or deception."[59] Beauchamp says that in research, individuals should be protected from discrimination, stigmatization, and other pressures.[60] Thus the revised model of consent for DTC genetic testing seeks to avoid these types of detrimental influences.

In the current model, there are no specific measures to address or avoid multiple sources of external pressures (such as pressures from relatives, the medical staff and community, and/or societal influences) which increase the possibility of coercion upon the individual. On the other hand, the revised model addresses the

---

[57] Tom Beauchamp and James Childress, *Principles of Biomedical Ethics,* 79.

[58] Linda Farber Post, Jeffrey Blustein, and Nancy Neveloff Dubler, *Handbook for Health Care Ethics Committees,* 42–43.

[59] Linda Farber Post, Jeffrey Blustein, and Nancy Neveloff Dubler, *Handbook for Health Care Ethics Committees,* 42.

[60] Tom L. Beauchamp, "Informed Consent: Its History, Meaning, and Present Challenges," 519–520.

external pressures on the patient and the family (such as pressures by the family for the patient to be tested and pressure upon the family regarding testing outcomes) to alleviate or resolve external coercion upon the patient. In the revised model, the pretest questionnaires and surveys can help counselors to identify some of the external pressures that people might have before participating in DTC genetic testing. Pretest counseling can also help to identify individuals that might have more emotional or social pressures.[61]

Since DTC genetic testing can influence both the individual and his or her family, the revised model looks at family coercion as well.[62] The revised model ensures voluntary consent by establishing procedures to avoid two forms of coercion: pressure by the family for the patient to be tested and pressure upon the family regarding the testing outcome. If there is a known family genetic trait, there can be pressure on individuals to get DTC genetic testing done before becoming pregnant or just for informational purposes. On the other hand, if one sibling discovers a higher disease risk from a specific trait that can affect other siblings, the revised model ensures a process is undertaken to ascertain whether the other sibling wants to know. In order to avoid both types of coercion, the revised model encourages individuals to discuss his or her reasoning for and concerns of DTC genetic testing with a counselor and/or physician.[63] By assessing a patient's motives for DTC genetic testing, physicians and/or counselors should be able to identify any coercive elements. Tom Beauchamp and James Childress say that professionals in the healthcare and medical research areas should "probe for and ensure understanding and voluntariness" of consent.[64]

2). Family-Related Implications

Because genetic information impacts the family, the revised model includes family-related concerns before testing and identifies ways to help the patient struggle with family-related PGT information. Unlike the current model, the revised model strives to take into consideration all family related implications which can lead to coercion of family members.

Since DTC genetic testing produces results for many different diseases, the implications for the entire family is significant. Often those results cannot be contained with that single individual; at some point, the family will find out at least some of

---

[61] Franklin Miller and Alan Wertheimer, *The Ethics of Consent*, 15; Katja Aktan-Collan, Jukka-Pekka Mecklin, Albert de la Chapelle, et al., "Evaluation of a Counselling Protocol for Predictive Genetic Testing for Hereditary Non-Polyposis Colorectal Cancer," 109.

[62] Clara Gaff, Elly Lynch, and Lesley Spencer, "Predictive Testing of Eighteen Year Olds: Counseling Challenges," 249; Douglas Martin and Heather Greenwood, "Public Perceptions of Ethical Issues Regarding Adult Predictive Genetic Testing," 107; David Ball, Audrey Tyler, and Peter Harper, "Predictive Testing of Adults and Children," 73.

[63] Ruth Macklin, "The Inner Workings of an Ethics Committee: Latest Battle over Jehovah's Witnesses," 233.

[64] Tom Beauchamp and James Childress, *Principles of Biomedical Ethics*, 64.

the results.[65] As a result, the revised model addresses family-related implications by having the counselor or physician communicate those areas to the individual.

By having a discussion with the individual before participating in DTC genetic testing about family-related implications, the individual will have a better idea of what to discuss with his or her family.[66] Then, the individual can make a decision to participate voluntarily in DTC genetic testing based on a better view of the family-related implications.

The revised model addresses external pressures on the patient and the family (such as pressures by the family for the patient to be tested and pressure upon the family regarding testing outcomes) to alleviate or resolve external coercion upon the patient. Because genetic information impacts the family, the revised model includes family-related concerns before testing and identifies ways to help the patient struggle with family-related PGT information.

d. Patient Safety

DTC genetic testing has many possibilities for risk to patients. Some potential problems with this testing are stress, confusion, false assurances, and unreliable results. False assurances can come because either a certain genetic variance has not been identified yet or the test failed to detect the genetic variance.[67] Risks from false assurances and unreliable results can be minimized by adhering to the patient safety component within the revised model for PGT.

The revised model of consent requires nationally established systems of accountability for PGT that implement the revised components of consent in a transparent manner to foster trust in the emerging system of genetic-related services. One article in the *Journal of Molecular Diagnostics* said "It is the consumer's responsibility to exercise caution to avoid becoming a victim of marketing ploys that prey on humanity's innate curiosity and fears."[68] While ultimately DTC genetic testing is up to the consumer, there should also be mechanisms in place to ensure accountability, transparency, and trust in order to promote patient safety. This section will discuss accountability, transparency, trust, and patient safety within the context of consent for DTC genetic testing.

This is a new component that is not in the current model. The revised model encourages internal and external accountability by promoting communication among medical departments and institutional policies. The revised model requires

---

[65] Lori B. Andrews, "Gen-Etiquette: Genetic Information, Family Relationships, and Adoption," 265–266.

[66] Catherine Hayes, "Genetic Testing for Huntington's Disease—A Family Issue," 1450; Michael Burgess, "Beyond Consent: Ethical and Social Issues in Genetic Testing," 510.

[67] Cynthia Marietta and Amy McGuire, "Direct-to-Consumer Genetic Testing: Is It the Practice of Medicine?" 370; AMA, "Direct-to-Consumer Genetic Testing."

[68] Daniel Farkas, and Carol Holland, "Direct-to-Consumer Genetic Testing: Two Sides of the Coin," 3.

transparency with physician discussions and consent requirements. The revised model encourages trust in the organizations and physicians by having open discussions with patient participation in the revised consent process. In the revised model, patient safety is fostered by having systems of accountability and transparency to establish preventive measures that promote the safety of patients considering PGT.

1). Accountability

The revised model encourages internal and external accountability by promoting communication among medical departments and consistent institutional policies. Since DTC genetic testing companies can also conduct research from the samples being sent in, this area focuses on both the research subject and patient treatment models of informed consent.[69] As a result, accountability measures focus on the labs performing the research, the DTC genetic testing company, and the physician or counselor involved. Because individuals can be harmed by misleading or unsubstantiated info, labs conducting testing will be required to participate in genetics quality assurance program to ensure accuracy and validity of materials and results. This can help to ensure accountability, accuracy, and validity of materials and results.[70] Genetics quality assurance programs encourage consistent institutional policies for analyzing testing samples.

While the companies are giving consumers their results, those companies are also keeping the results to establish a database of DNA. The co-founder of 23andMe, Anne Wojcicki says that the company never gives out identifiable information to scientists unless consent of the person is given. She says that she is "careful when I say we're going to have a revenue stream from the database. We will not sell individuals' data, but the database as a whole will have enormous value."[71] To encourage accountability, the DTC genetic testing companies need to communicate the consent and research policies to the individuals and counselors or physicians. Accountability for DTC genetic testing is encouraged by having consistent policies and increased communication among testing labs, DTC genetic testing companies, physicians, and consumers.

2). Transparency

Since this is a new component not found in the current model, the revised model of consent also recognizes and emphasizes the significance of transparency in implementation. It is crucial to implement this model in a transparent manner in order

---

[69] Linda Farber Post, Jeffrey Blustein, and Nancy Neveloff Dubler, *Handbook for Health Care Ethics Committees*, 38–39.

[70] Thomas Goetz, *The Decision Tree*, xvi–xvii, 117; Bernard Lo, *Resolving Ethical Dilemmas*, 273.

[71] Mark Henderson, "Cashing in on Your Genes," 2.

to promote patient safety. The revised model requires transparency with physician discussions and consent requirements.

One aspect of transparency that is a little different with DTC genetic testing is research. There needs to be greater transparency with the patients concerning the research being done with their samples. While 23andMe says that consumer samples will not be sold with identifiable information, many individuals are not even aware their samples are being stored.[72] Thus physician and counselor discussions can help to encourage transparency in regards to research participation with DTC genetic testing. Another aspect of transparency in research is the reliability of the risk assessments. One DTC genetic testing company recognizes the need for increased transparency with reliable risk assessments. Anne Wojcicki from 23andMe says the company realizes the possibility "that people may misunderstand their genetic data if they are given incorrect or incomplete information."[73] She recognizes the company's responsibility towards their customers, and as a result, the company has tried to encourage transparency with their consumers. As a result, the company started a star system, a research confidence rating, which explains the amount of research the results are based off of. One star means that the results are based off of introductory research, and the rating goes up to four stars which means the research is reputable and well-recognized. 23andMe is trying to increase their transparency with consent requirements and consumers.[74] When consumers see the accountability and transparency measures that 23 and Me is starting to take, the level of trust can start to increase as well.

3). Trust

By having increased accountability and transparency measures, trust will be encouraged as well. The revised model encourages trust in the organizations and physicians by having open discussions with patient participation in the revised consent process.

Because genetic testing leads to very personal information, if there is not complete trust, then the individual and their family can be harmed from a lack of privacy and/or mistrust in the system. If a person does not trust his or her physician or counselor, then often that mistrust will continue into other areas which will eventually lead to mistrust of the medical organization.[75] An example of mistrust in medicine can occur among physicians and pharmaceutical companies. If a physician sells some patient information to drug companies, then the physician is not acting on the patient's best interest. David Orentlicher says that once physicians "become dual agents, they can no longer provide assurances to patients that it is safe to place their

---

[72] Peter Kraft Ph.D. and David Hunter, "Genetic Risk Prediction – Are We There Yet?" 1701; Mark Henderson, "Cashing in on Your Genes," 2.

[73] Kristine Goodwin, "Information Overload? National Conference of State Legislatures."

[74] Kristine Goodwin, "Information Overload? National Conference of State Legislatures."

[75] David Orentlicher, "Genetic Privacy in the Patient-Physician Relationship," 85.

trust in their physicians."[76] As a result, once trust is compromised, it is often hard to regain that trust in the process of informed consent.

Since DTC genetic testing has the opportunity to merge research with medical care, trust is extremely important to informed consent in this area. As a result, there should be trust among all the organizations including the researchers, the laboratories, the DTC genetic testing companies, and the medical professionals. There should also be trust in the consent process of the revised model. Trust in the revised model encourages physicians and counselors to make sure the individuals are in agreement with and have consented to the process of DTC genetic testing.[77] Trust among all levels of the DTC genetic testing process can help individuals to feel safe in giving his or her consent for testing. This new component of trust is important to the revised model of consent.

4). Patient Safety Systems

Patient safety is fostered by having systems of accountability and transparency to establish preventive measures that promote the safety of patients considering DTC genetic testing. By having more accountability and transparency measures, the revised model can encourage better systems of patient safety.[78] One aspect of patient safety involved with research participation is the Common Rule. This Rule, focusing on compliance, IRB reviews, and informed consent, can help to create better systems of patient safety for DTC genetic testing.[79]

Another aspect of patient safety in DTC genetic testing is preventive and organizational measures. By focusing on prevention and communication, the revised model decreases some of the institutional barriers of patient safety.[80] One example of a preventive measure is illustrated by a DTC genetic testing company, Psynomics. Psynomics offers testing for psychological problems like depression, mania, and bipolar disorders. This company has a different process of returning results. While most, if not all, companies return the results directly to the consumer, Psynomics returns the results to a physician of the patient's choice. By allowing the patient's doctor or a geneticist to discuss the results with the individual, the model that Psynomics takes encourages patient safety by preventive measures.[81] Patient

---

[76] David Orentlicher, "Genetic Privacy in the Patient-Physician Relationship," 84.

[77] Jeffrey Kahn, "Informed Consent in the Context of Communities," 919–920.

[78] Thomas Goetz, *The Decision Tree*, xiv.

[79] Dorene S. Markel and Beverly M. Yashar, "The Interface Between the Practice of Medical Genetics and Human Genetic Research: What Every Genetic Counselor Needs to Know," 356–357.

[80] William A. Nelson, Julia Neily, Peter Mills, et al., "Collaboration of Ethics and Patient Safety Programs: Opportunities to Promote Quality Care," 20; Thomas Goetz, *The Decision Tree*, 247–248.

[81] Philip B. Mitchell, Bettina Meiser, Alex Wilde, et al., "Predictive and Diagnostic Genetic Testing in Psychiatry," 226.

risks can be decreased by having "trusted intermediaries" to discuss concerns and results with.[82]

Another example of patient safety is the idea of opting out of or opting in for certain diseases. Donna Messner suggests that opting in is "preferable." In this case, people select which diseases or traits he or she would like to be tested for. By doing this, Donna Messner says that the individual "actively sets the parameters for the information she will receive; she is forced to make a conscious choice and is less likely to be frivolous in selection since each test is priced separately."[83] Instead of having the typical consent form, the form can have a list of which diseases or traits the individual is consenting for. This type of opting in could promote patient safety, because the individual is not getting risk information that he or she does not wish to know.[84] The revised model encourages patient safety of DTC genetic tests by focusing on accountability, transparency, and prevention.

The revised model encourages internal and external accountability by promoting communication among medical departments and institutional policies. The revised model requires transparency with physician discussions and consent requirements. The revised model encourages trust in the organizations and physicians by having open discussions with patient participation in the revised consent process. In the revised model, patient safety is fostered by having systems of accountability and transparency to establish preventive measures that promote the safety of patients considering PGT.

3. Case Study

This last section will present a case study that discusses DTC genetic testing and informed consent. The first part will present and discuss a case study about Josh. The second section will contrast the two models of informed consent in relation to the case study on DTC genetic testing.

a. Josh

Donna Messner describes and analyzes some case studies pertaining to DTC genetic testing. One of the case studies involved a man in his forties, Josh. Josh was employed in a medical research company, which was looking into PGT. In order to encourage better statistics, his company encouraged all workers to take part in the research study. Since he thought he might have a predisposition to type II diabetes, Josh thought the research study might be beneficial. Also because Josh understood

---

[82] Mark Henderson, "Cashing in on Your Genes," 2.

[83] Donna Messner, "Informed Choice in Direct-to-Consumer Genetic Testing for Alzheimer and Other Diseases: Lessons from Two Cases," 70.

[84] Donna Messner, "Informed Choice in Direct-to-Consumer Genetic Testing for Alzheimer and Other Diseases: Lessons from Two Cases," 68–69.

many of the techniques involved in medical research and testing, he thought he would be better able to interpret and handle the results. Thus he decided to participate. However, while it was his company that was doing the study, the company had an agreement with a DTC genetic testing company. The DTC genetic testing company would perform the research, but Josh's company was interested in the lifestyle choices the individuals made along with the research. Genetic counseling was optional through the DTC genetic testing company after the results were given. After reading and signing the informed consent form online, Josh gave a sample to the DTC genetic testing company. When the results returned, Josh discovered that he did not have a higher than normal susceptibility to type II diabetes, but that he did have a higher susceptibility to Alzheimer's disease. While he was ready for results about diabetes, he was not ready for results about Alzheimer's disease. After thinking about the results, Josh did remember that his family had a history of Alzheimer's disease, but at the same time, he was not ready to deal with that type of information yet. After calling the DTC genetic testing company for a counselor, the counselor informed him to eat better and exercise more. Josh did not feel that the advice was helpful, because he assumed all people should have a healthy diet and exercise regularly. He wanted to know about measures to predict or slow the progression of Alzheimer's disease, but in all his research he did not find any concrete preventive measures.[85]

b. Application

This section will apply the revised model of informed consent to the case study. In doing so, the contrast between the two models of consent will be evident. Each of the four components, including comprehension, disclosure, voluntariness, and patient safety, will be discussed.

Comprehension is one of the most important aspects of DTC genetic testing. First in the current model of consent, the consent form is emphasized for the standardized approach without much discussion. In this case study, Josh read and signed the consent form online, and after that, consent for DTC genetic testing was assumed. It should not be assumed that reading and signing a consent form online is enough to satisfy the requirements for an autonomous decision. However the revised model adopts a personalized approach to consent that emphasizes extensive discussion with the patient as an autonomous agent. Before signing the consent form, Josh's company or the DTC genetic testing company should have discussed the procedure and consent form with him. Second, in the current model, there is insufficient time and communication for understanding the meaning of PGT risk. In the case study, Josh did not have enough time or communication for adequate understanding. Even though Josh was educated and familiar with research protocols, he did not fully understand the meaning and results of DTC genetic testing. In the case study, Josh

---

[85] Donna Messner, "Informed Choice in Direct-to-Consumer Genetic Testing for Alzheimer and Other Diseases: Lessons from Two Cases," 63–65.

said that the results were confusing, because the DTC genetic testing company had his Alzheimer's risk at 69%, but that a study from Duke had it at 91%. He did not understand that companies could have different results because of the different variants being analyzed. The revised model focuses on a process that provides time for communication to foster an understanding of the complex meaning of PGT risk. In the revised model, Josh would have had time to ask questions and communicate adequately in order to foster understanding. Third, the current doctor-patient relationship focuses upon the patient freely signing the consent form without sufficient education of the patient about the meaning of PGT. This was clearly evidenced in the case study, because Josh signed the form without having a clear understanding about what DTC genetic testing entailed. Josh said that even after giving the results to his primary physician, the physician did not understand how to interpret the results.[86] However, the revised model emphasizes the doctor-patient relationship as an interactive process to ensure sufficient education of the patient about the meaning of PGT. In this model, the doctor needs enough information to be able to help Josh understand and comprehend what he is consenting to.[87]

Disclosure is another aspect of the current and revised models. First, the current model focuses on medical information in a standardized approach of consent. However, the revised model addresses not only medical information but all other relevant information for the patient to consider for consent, including the fact that some PGT diseases might not have any available treatment. This was probably one of the most important aspects for Josh in this case study. The DTC genetic testing company might have disclosed some important medical information, but the company did not see the need to inform Josh that there could be disease results for which there is no treatment. Second, the current model recommends non-directive counseling, and does not require counseling. This was evidenced in the case study. However, the revised model requires both pre- and post-test counseling and adopts value transparency and non-directive counseling. Josh said that if there had been pre-test counseling, most likely the counselor would have asked about medical conditions that ran in the family. He said that had he understood the fact that there could be results about Alzheimer's disease, then he would not have sent his sample in.[88] Pre- and post- test counseling is important to the revised model of consent.[89]

Voluntariness is the third aspect of the current and revised models. First in the current model, there are no specific measures to address or avoid multiple sources of external pressures (such as pressures from relatives, the medical staff and com-

---

[86] Donna Messner, "Informed Choice in Direct-to-Consumer Genetic Testing for Alzheimer and Other Diseases: Lessons from Two Cases," 63–65.

[87] Jane Kaye, "The Regulation of Direct-to-Consumer Genetic Tests," 180; Mark Henderson, "Cashing in on Your Genes," 2.

[88] Donna Messner, "Informed Choice in Direct-to-Consumer Genetic Testing for Alzheimer and Other Diseases: Lessons from Two Cases," 64–65.

[89] Angela Trepanier, Mary Ahrens, Wendy McKinnon, et al., "Genetic Cancer Risk Assessment and Counseling: Recommendations of the National Society of Genetic Counselors," 93; Kathy Beal, "Statement on Direct-to-Consumer Genetic Testing," 1–2; Dr. Hsien-Hsien Lei, "Dr. Robert Marion on Direct-to-Consumer Genetic Testing."

munity, and/or societal influences) which increase the possibility of coercion upon the individual. In this case study, Josh's company could have been a possible source of coercion, because the company encouraged all employees to participate. However, the case study did not mention the possibility of coercion. The fact that this case study did not specifically mention coercion illustrates the need for the revised model, because the revised model recognizes the need to specifically address coercion. The revised model addresses external pressures on the patient and the family (such as pressures by the family for the patient to be tested and pressure upon the family regarding testing outcomes) to alleviate or resolve external coercion upon the patient. Somebody in either Josh's company or the DTC genetic testing company should have inquired into the likelihood of Josh being coerced into participating. Second, the current model does not take into consideration all family related implications which can lead to coercion of family members. The companies did not discuss family-related implications at all. However after having the results, Josh was very concerned about his family. He said that while his family said the results did not matter much, Josh understood the implications for his entire family. He informed his family that "*you're* going to be suffering from this if I get sick! It's going to affect *you* more than it's going to affect me at some point in time."[90] Eventually the results had a harmful effect on his family relationships. Because genetic information impacts the family, the revised model includes family-related concerns before testing and identifies ways to help the patient struggle with family-related PGT information. Josh would have benefited from having a discussion about how the results would impact his family antecedently, rather than having to try to control the damage already done.[91]

Patient safety is a new component that is not in the current model. First, the revised model encourages internal and external accountability by promoting communication among medical departments and institutional policies. In this case study, there was a clear lack of communication among Josh's company and the DTC genetic testing company. Second, the revised model requires transparency with physician discussions and consent requirements. Transparency among the companies was not clear in this case. Third, the revised model encourages trust in the organizations and physicians by having open discussions with patient participation in the revised consent process. Because there were not clear discussions, trust was not evident in this case. Josh said that he "feels let down by a system that allowed him to have this information" while there was insufficient information about the preventive measures and inadequate support after testing.[92] As a result, trust in the entire process was distorted. Fourth, in the revised model, patient safety is fostered by having systems of accountability and transparency to establish preventive measures that

---

[90] Donna Messner, "Informed Choice in Direct-to-Consumer Genetic Testing for Alzheimer and Other Diseases: Lessons from Two Cases," 65.

[91] Catherine Hayes, "Genetic Testing for Huntington's Disease—A Family Issue," 1450; Michael Burgess, "Beyond Consent: Ethical and Social Issues in Genetic Testing," 510.

[92] Donna Messner, "Informed Choice in Direct-to-Consumer Genetic Testing for Alzheimer and Other Diseases: Lessons from Two Cases," 64.

promote the safety of patients considering PGT. Even after trying to get help from a psychologist, Josh felt that he had been harmed from knowing his susceptibilities. He concluded with the following: it "boggles my mind… I can't go into a laboratory and say, 'I think I have an infection. Can you please draw CBC on me?' [They'd] say, 'No, we have to have a physician's order.' And yet *anybody* can submit a saliva sample and get their genetic testing, which clearly is medical information…. I question whether it's ethical or not to be done that way."[93] Donna Messner takes Josh's conclusion further when she says that since there are so many problems with consent for multiplex testing, "then in the DTC environment informed choice is virtually impossible to achieve."[94]

By applying the revised model of consent to the case study, Josh could have had a better outcome for his testing process. The revised model of informed consent can encourage appropriate decision making for DTC genetic testing.

B. Pleiotropic Genetic Testing and Informed Consent

This part applies the revised model of informed consent to pleiotropic genetic testing. Pleiotropic genetic testing is where a gene has many different roles, and as a result pleiotropic genes give rise to multiple findings for one test.[95] This section will discuss how to handle informed consent when there is additional, and possibly unexpected findings.[96]

The first section will discuss the background of pleiotropic genetic testing. This includes the science of testing, some specific examples, and a risk/benefit analysis. The second section will apply all four components of the revised model of informed consent to pleiotropic genetic testing. The revised model will seek to encourage ethical informed consent when there are multiple findings. The third section will present a case study. This case study will discuss pleiotropic genetic testing and informed consent.

1. Background of Pleiotropic Genetic Testing

This first section, which discusses the background of pleiotropic genetic testing, is broken up into three aspects. The first aspect is the science of pleiotropic genetic testing which includes a discussion on the meaning of the test and the interpretation

---

[93] Donna Messner, "Informed Choice in Direct-to-Consumer Genetic Testing for Alzheimer and Other Diseases: Lessons from Two Cases," 64–65.

[94] Donna Messner, "Informed Choice in Direct-to-Consumer Genetic Testing for Alzheimer and Other Diseases: Lessons from Two Cases," 67–68.

[95] Ellen Wright Clayton, "Incidental Findings in Genetics Research Using Archived DNA," 289.

[96] Zachary Cooper, Robert Nelson, and Lainie Ross, "Informed Consent for Genetic Research Involving Pleiotropic Genes: An Empirical Study of ApoE Research," 1.

of the test results. The second aspect discusses examples of pleiotropic genes including a discussion on Alzheimer's disease and coronary artery disease (CAD). The third aspect looks at a risk/benefit analysis of pleiotropic genetic testing.

a. Pleiotropic Genetic Testing

In order to understand pleiotropic genetic testing, the meaning of pleiotropic genetic testing needs to be discussed. The first part of this section looks at the basic science of pleiotropy. The second part discusses the interpretation of the test results.

1). Science of Pleiotropic Genes

Pleiotropic genes can be traced back to Mendel with genetics. Pleiotropy was evident then when there was a disease that had several separate symptoms with a family link. However it was not until 1910 that this characteristic of gene expression was named. Ludwig Plate first discussed this concept as pleiotropy.[97]

Pleiotropy is where multiple diseases and/or traits can be expressed from one gene.[98] With this, a single gene can express many different phenotypes or physical characteristics.[99] A pleiotropic gene is one in which the same gene can have an influence on several different characteristics.[100] Another type of pleiotropy is antagonistic pleiotropy. This type of pleiotropy results in the same gene having a positive effect on one disease or characteristic while having a negative effect on a different disease.[101] An illustration of this is a type of dwarfism called Laron Syndrome. When a person has Laron Syndrome, the individual is less likely to have cancer or diabetes that a person without this Syndrome. Ashley Carter and Andrew Nguyen say that sometimes antagonistic pleiotropy can be disregarded, because many times the negative results get more attention in regards to research than the positive effects of a certain gene and/or allele.[102]

---

[97] Frank Stearns, "One Hundred Years of Pleiotropy: A Retrospective," 767.

[98] Tony McGleenan, "Genetic Testing for Cancer Predisposition- An Ongoing Debate- Genetic Screening Forum," 122–123; Frank Stearns, "One Hundred Years of Pleiotropy: A Retrospective," 767.

[99] Shanya Sivakumaran, Felix Agakov, Evropi Theodoratou, et al., "Abundant Pleiotropy in Human Complex Diseases and Traits," 607.

[100] Frederic Guillaume and Sarah Otto, "Gene Functional Trade-Offs and the Evolution of Pleiotropy," 1389.

[101] Colleen McBride, Deborah Bowen, Lawrence Brody, et al., "Future Health Applications of Genomics: Priorities for Communication, Behavioral, and Social Sciences Research," 559; Ashley Carter and Andrew Nguyen, "Antagonistic Pleiotropy as a Widespread Mechanism for the Maintenance of Polymorphic Disease Alleles," 2–3.

[102] Ashley Carter and Andrew Nguyen, "Antagonistic Pleiotropy as a Widespread Mechanism for the Maintenance of Polymorphic Disease Alleles," 2–3, 9.

In the study by Sivakumaran, Shanya, Felix Agakov, Evropi Theodoratou, James G. Prendergast, et al., there were 233 genes that were found to have pleiotropic characteristics. Pleiotropy is involved in approximately 17 % of the disease-related genes and 5 % of the SNPs. However, there are still many disease-related genes and SNPs that are currently unknown, and continual research could cause the number of pleiotropic genes and SNPs to rise.[103]

Since the relationship between some genes can be negligible, sometimes pleiotropic genes can be difficult to identify when studying the association between the two.[104] Frederic Guillaume and Sarah Otto explain that the degree of pleiotropy can differ between certain genes, because while most pleiotropic genes affect many different characteristics and/or behaviors, some pleiotropic genes are responsible for numerous differences and behaviors. Just like many of the genetic diseases, pleiotropic genes are multifactorial. Pleiotropic differences can depend on the "biochemical properties of coding genes," assortment and deviation of different characteristics of the genes resulting from biological selection, and the degree of gene and allele expression.[105]

2). Pleiotropic Genetic Testing Results

When performing genetic testing on pleiotropic genes, the test will result in information about two diseases or characteristics. A common example of this is coronary artery disease (CAD) and Alzheimer's disease. One of the genes identified to have an effect on CAD can also have an effect on the development of Alzheimer's disease.[106] When performing a genetic test to identify a person's susceptibility to CAD, the individual will also receive results about their susceptibility to adult on-set Alzheimer's disease. Pleiotropic genetic testing will produce information about multiple diseases and/or health characteristics. Because many diseases are multifactorial and involve multiple genetic variations, pleiotropic genetic testing can result in even more complicated information since one gene can return information for several different traits.[107]

The main complication of the results for pleiotropic genetic testing is unexpected findings.[108] Unless an individual is told about the possibility of multiple results, pleiotropic genetic testing can have some complications. Often for pleiotropic ge-

---

[103] Shanya Sivakumaran, Felix Agakov, Evropi Theodoratou, et al., "Abundant Pleiotropy in Human Complex Diseases and Traits," 610, 614.

[104] Frank Stearns, "One Hundred Years of Pleiotropy: A Retrospective," 767.

[105] Frederic Guillaume and Sarah Otto, "Gene Functional Trade-Offs and the Evolution of Pleiotropy," 1389, 1404.

[106] Tony McGleenan, "Genetic Testing for Cancer Predisposition- An Ongoing Debate- Genetic Screening Forum," 122–123.

[107] Matt Chamberlain, Paul Baird, Mohamed Dirani, et al., "Unraveling a Complex Genetic Disease: Age-related Macular Degeneration," 579.

[108] Ellen Wright Clayton, "Incidental Findings in Genetics Research Using Archived DNA," 289.

netic testing, there are some controversial aspects involved in the results of testing. One of the controversial aspects of testing for CAD is that the test returns results for a late-onset disease for which there is currently no treatment.[109] Another controversial aspect is the fact that many professional groups do not recommend PGT for Alzheimer's disease unless there is a family history of the disease.[110] Thus pleiotropic genetic testing can return information about untreatable diseases that most physicians and/or researchers do not assess in a typical practice. The next section will discuss some more examples of pleiotropic genes and the resulting diseases.

b. Examples of Pleiotropic Genes

There are numerous pleiotropic genes which can result in different diseases and/or genetic traits. This section will discuss examples of pleiotropic genes and diseases. Then there will be an in-depth discussion about one of the most commonly used examples of pleiotropic genetic testing, which is the relationship between CAD and Alzheimer's disease.

In one study by Shanya Sivakumaran, Felix Agakov, Evropi Theodoratou, et al. identified several pleiotropic genes. This study demonstrated that there were many variants associated with Crohn's disease such as leprosy, intracranial aneurysms, breast cancer, prostate cancer, type 2 diabetes, and several others. Sometimes there is a strong link between these diseases, but other times the link is relatively small. Some other examples include the relationship between fetal hemoglobin and malaria risk, serum campesterol and gallstones risk, and possibly narcolepsy and osteroarthritis.[111] Then some common examples of antagonistic pleiotropy include people with Huntington's disease and sickle cell anemia. Those with Huntington's disease have a lower incidence of cancer. Those with sickle cell anemia have a higher protection against malaria, which can sometimes cause resistance to the disease. These examples are only some of the previously identified pleiotropic genes. However there are many other pleiotropic and antagonistic pleiotropic genes and alleles that have yet to be discovered.[112]

The next section will discuss the apolipoprotein E gene (APOE). This gene has several alleles or segments, and each of the alleles have one difference in their DNA nucleotide sequence. Chamberlain, Matt, Paul Baird, Mohamed Dirani, et al. say that that slight difference can be enough to change the risk predictions for age-

---

[109] Hyman Schipper, "Presymptomatic Apolipoprotein E Genotyping for Alzheimer's Disease Risk Assessment and Prevention," e118.

[110] J. Scott Roberts and Wendy Uhlmann, "Genetic Susceptibility Testing for Neurodegenerative Diseases: Ethical and Practice Issues," 90.

[111] Shanya Sivakumaran, Felix Agakov, Evropi Theodoratou, et al., "Abundant Pleiotropy in Human Complex Diseases and Traits," 613, 615.

[112] Ashley Carter and Andrew Nguyen, "Antagonistic Pleiotropy as a Widespread Mechanism for the Maintenance of Polymorphic Disease Alleles," 3, 5, 8.

related macular degeneration, Alzheimer's disease, and cardiovascular diseases.[113] The ε4 allele on the APOE gene can affect the disease risk for both Alzheimer's disease and CAD.[114] As a result, the first part will discuss Alzheimer's disease and analyze genetic testing for Alzheimer's disease. The second part will look at CAD and analyze genetic testing for CAD.

1). Alzheimer's Disease

Alzheimer's disease is a progressive neurological disease that is incurable. This disease typically occurs in the middle to late years of an adult. Alzheimer's affects the memory, standard living practices, motor skills, and reasoning.[115] The current treatments only slow the progression of the disease, but eventually the disease will lead to death. In the United States there are about 4.5 million cases of Alzheimer's disease. However, Hyman Schipper suggests that the cases of Alzheimer's disease will increase to more than 13 million by the year 2050. Alzheimer's disease involves several genes, which can be affected by genetics, environmental factors, and/or lifestyle choices.[116] However with this disease, probably one of the most important factors is age. Donna Messner says that the risk of Alzheimer's "doubles every 5 years after age 65."[117]

The most common form of Alzheimer's disease is late-onset which is affected by the APOE gene. This gene has 3 alleles, ε2, ε3, and ε4, on chromosome 19.[118] While all of the alleles can affect Alzheimer's disease, the ε4 allele has a higher predictive value for Alzheimer's.[119] If a person inherits this allele, the risk of developing Alzheimer's disease could increase by three times, from 9% to about 29%, with

---

[113] Matt Chamberlain, Paul Baird, Mohamed Dirani, et al., "Unraveling a Complex Genetic Disease: Age-related Macular Degeneration," 578.

[114] Tony McGleenan, "Genetic Testing for Cancer Predisposition- An Ongoing Debate- Genetic Screening Forum," 122–123; Robert Wachbroit, "The Question Not Asked: The Challenge of Pleiotropic Genetic Tests," 131; Zachary Cooper, Robert Nelson, and Lainie Ross, "Informed Consent for Genetic Research Involving Pleiotropic Genes: An Empirical Study of ApoE Research," 1.

[115] Donna Messner, "Informed Choice in Direct-to-Consumer Genetic Testing for Alzheimer and Other Diseases: Lessons from Two Cases," 60–61; Peter St. George-Hyslop and Agnes Petit, "Molecular Biology and Genetics of Alzheimer's Disease," 120.

[116] Hyman Schipper, "Presymptomatic Apolipoprotein E Genotyping for Alzheimer's Disease Risk Assessment and Prevention," e118; Donna Messner, "Informed Choice in Direct-to-Consumer Genetic Testing for Alzheimer and Other Diseases: Lessons from Two Cases," 60–61.

[117] Donna Messner, "Informed Choice in Direct-to-Consumer Genetic Testing for Alzheimer and Other Diseases: Lessons from Two Cases," 60–61.

[118] Peter St. George-Hyslop and Agnes Petit, "Molecular Biology and Genetics of Alzheimer's Disease," 122; Philip Mitchell, Bettina Meiser, Alex Wilde, et al., "Predictive and Diagnostic Genetic Testing in Psychiatry," 233; Theresa Marteau, Scott Roberts, Susan LaRusse, et al., "Predictive Genetic Testing for Alzheimer's Disease: Impact upon Risk Perception," 398.

[119] Sebastián Cervantes, Lluís Samarancha, José Manuel Vidal-Taboadaa, et al., "Genetic Variation in *APOE* Cluster Region and Alzheimer's Disease Risk," 2107.e13; Peter St. George-Hyslop and Agnes Petit, "Molecular Biology and Genetics of Alzheimer's Disease," 122.

just one copy of the ε4 allele.[120] Those with two copies of this allele can increase their risk of Alzheimer's disease by about fifteen-thirty times the standard risk.[121] However because of the polygenic nature of Alzheimer's disease, even with this increased risk, this allele is not required in order for a person to develop Alzheimer's. Having the ε4 allele is only one of the factors for predicting this disease. As a result, there are concerns about using this as a predictor for genetic testing.[122]

Due to the uncertainty of the predictive value of Alzheimer's, there are many professional groups that do not recommend using the APOE gene for PGT of Alzheimer's disease. Rather, many of those groups encourage clinical diagnosis over PGT for Alzheimer's, because a clinical diagnosis is more accurate.[123] This is illustrated by the study conducted by Mayeux, R., M. Saunders, S. Shea, et al. The study explains that when compared to a clinical diagnosis with a sensitivity of 93 % and a specificity of 55 %, genetic testing using the APOE gene for analysis only has 65 % sensitivity and 68 % specificity.[124] While a clinical diagnosis has more accurate and valid results, the APOE gene with the ε4 allele is still probably one of the best indicators to predict late-onset Alzheimer's disease.[125]

Even though the predictive value of the APOE gene is uncertain, genetic testing of this gene can help to identify the progression of the disease and to analyze the effectiveness of different treatments in research. As a result, many health centers today test for the APOE gene in the elderly when there are questions about cognition, and more neurological research tests for the presence of this gene in healthy participants.[126] However, unless there is a family history of the disease and there is an "identified gene mutation" in the family, PGT for Alzheimer's disease is not the recommended standard of care in those without symptoms.[127]

---

[120] Hyman Schipper, "Presymptomatic Apolipoprotein E Genotyping for Alzheimer's Disease Risk Assessment and Prevention," e119.

[121] Donna Messner, "Informed Choice in Direct-to-Consumer Genetic Testing for Alzheimer and Other Diseases: Lessons from Two Cases," 61; Theresa Marteau, Scott Roberts, Susan LaRusse, et al., "Predictive Genetic Testing for Alzheimer's Disease: Impact upon Risk Perception," 398.

[122] Theresa Marteau, Scott Roberts, Susan LaRusse, et al., "Predictive Genetic Testing for Alzheimer's Disease: Impact upon Risk Perception," 398; J. Scott Roberts and Wendy Uhlmann, "Genetic Susceptibility Testing for Neurodegenerative Diseases: Ethical and Practice Issues," 90.

[123] Peter St. George-Hyslop and Agnes Petit, "Molecular Biology and Genetics of Alzheimer's Disease," 125; Hyman Schipper, "Presymptomatic Apolipoprotein E Genotyping for Alzheimer's Disease Risk Assessment and Prevention," e119; J. Scott Roberts and Wendy Uhlmann, "Genetic Susceptibility Testing for Neurodegenerative Diseases: Ethical and Practice Issues," 90.

[124] R. Mayeux, M. Saunders, S. Shea, et al., "Utility of the Apolipoprotein E Genotype in the Diagnosis of Alzheimer's Disease," 506.

[125] Michael Cassidy, J. Scott Roberts, Thomas Bird, et al., "Comparing Test-specific Distress of Susceptibility versus Deterministic Genetic Testing for Alzheimer's Disease," 407; Ging-Yuek Robin Hsiung and A. Dessa Sadovnick, "Genetics and Dementia: Risk Factors, Diagnosis, and Management," 422; Hyman Schipper, "Presymptomatic Apolipoprotein E Genotyping for Alzheimer's Disease Risk Assessment and Prevention," e119.

[126] American College of Medical Genetics/American Society of Human Genetics Working Group on ApoE and Alzheimer disease, "Statement on Use of Apolipoprotein E Testing for Alzheimer Disease," 1628–1629; Hyman Schipper, "Presymptomatic Apolipoprotein E Genotyping for Alzheimer's Disease Risk Assessment and Prevention," e119.

[127] J. Scott Roberts and Wendy Uhlmann, "Genetic Susceptibility Testing for Neurodegenerative Diseases: Ethical and Practice Issues," 92.

2). Coronary Artery Disease

CAD is another polygenic disease.[128] The American Heart Association explains that CAD can lead to coronary heart disease (CHD). Sometimes people use these names to refer to the same disease. However in CAD, the plaque builds up in the arteries, and typically when it gets severe, the plaque continues to the arteries of the heart leading to CHD. When there is enough plaque build-up, the arteries will constrict, and this leads to decreased blood flow to the heart. As a result, CAD can lead to heart attacks and ischemia.[129] CHD is one of the leading causes of death in the United States. Approximately 13 million people have CHD, and this disease is responsible for about 1 million deaths per year.[130] However if CAD is caught early enough, there are several treatment measures that can prevent the disease from getting worse and developing plaque in the arteries of the heart.[131] Since CAD is preventable, there are reliable tests which can diagnose CAD and determine the risk of CAD.

The genetic test that analyzes an individual's risk of developing CAD looks at the APOE gene and the ε4 allele. The study by Bassam Nassar, Kenneth Rockwood, Susan Kirkland, et al. confirms that there is a higher frequency of the APOE gene with the ε4 allele and BChE-K in those with early-onset CAD than those with late-onset CAD.[132] As a result, looking at the ε4 allele can help to predict a person's risk of CAD. However, since the ε4 allele can also return results for predicting Alzheimer's disease, PGT for CAD will produce a person's risk of developing both CAD and Alzheimer's disease.[133] This illustrates the pleiotropic effects of the ε4 allele on the APOE gene.[134]

If the PGT for CAD comes back positive, then the individual has several treatment options and lifestyle changes that can eliminate plaque build-up and CAD. However, since the test was positive for the ε4 allele on the APOE gene, the test results mean that the individual also has a higher risk for developing late-onset Alzheimer's disease. As was discussed before, there are no treatment options for Alzheimer's disease. Knowing a person is at risk might make pleiotropic genetic testing more of a problem[135] Tony McGleenan says that a person "cannot enjoy

---

[128] Bassam Nassar, Kenneth Rockwood, Susan Kirkland, et al., "Improved Prediction of Early-onset Coronary Artery Disease using APOE ε4, BChE-K, PPARγ2 Pro12 and ENOS T-786C in a Polygenic Model," 109.

[129] The American Heart Association, "Coronary Artery Disease- Coronary Heart Disease."

[130] Diddahally Govindaraju, L. Adrienne Cupples, William B. Kannel, et al., "Genetics of the Framingham Heart Study Population," 35.

[131] The American Heart Association, "Coronary Artery Disease- Coronary Heart Disease."

[132] Bassam Nassar, Kenneth Rockwood, Susan Kirkland, et al., "Improved Prediction of Early-onset Coronary Artery Disease using APOE ε4, BChE-K, PPARγ2 Pro12 and ENOS T-786C in a Polygenic Model," 111.

[133] Ellen Wright Clayton, "Incidental Findings in Genetics Research Using Archived DNA," 289.

[134] Diddahally Govindaraju, L. Adrienne Cupples, William B. Kannel, et al., "Genetics of the Framingham Heart Study Population," 46.

[135] Robert Wachbroit, "The Question Not Asked: The Challenge of Pleiotropic Genetic Tests," 133; Ruth Hubbard and R.C. Lewontin, "Genetic Testing for Disease Predisposition, Pitfalls of

the therapeutic benefits of one without being burdened with predictive information about the other."[136] This is the crux of the controversy concerning pleiotropic genetic testing. This problem carries over into the discussion of informed consent, because normally the patient has only given consent to find out about their risk for CAD. But since there are additional risk predictions, now the doctor has to determine whether or not to present the patient with the risk predictions for Alzheimer's disease as well.[137]

c. Risk/Benefit Analysis

Since one gene could determine the predictive risks to many unrelated diseases, there are several ethical issues involved with this type of testing. Some ethical issues include the use of pleiotropic tests in general, the idea of screening for a disease with no treatments, the ethics of doctor/patient disclosure about pleiotropic results, informed consent, and an obligation to disclose or an obligation to know the results.[138]

In order to fully understand the implications of pleiotropic genetic testing, the risks and benefits need to be analyzed. The first part of this section will analyze and discuss the risks of pleiotropic genetic testing. Then the second part will look at some of the benefits of testing.

1). Risks

Since there are often many implications of pleiotropic genetic testing, the risks need to be identified before participating in the testing. One of the risks with pleiotropic genetic testing is the predictability of disease. Since pleiotropic genetic testing looks at susceptibility of certain diseases, sometimes people assume the test results are more predictive than they really are. However as was discussed with PGT, many times risk predictions are uncertain, and since many genetic diseases are multifactorial, disease prediction is based off of many different factors and not just genetic variants.[139] However with pleiotropic genes, sometimes the level of risk can be even more complicated to identify. When one gene has implications on multiple traits and diseases, the degree to which the gene affects both of the diseases or traits is not always well known. Sometimes a gene can simply add to the risk which would only

---

Genetic Testing," 360–362.

[136] Tony McGleenan, "Genetic Testing for Cancer Predisposition- An Ongoing Debate- Genetic Screening Forum," 122–123.

[137] Lewis Vaughn, *Bioethics: Principles, Issues, and Cases*, 465–66.

[138] Robert Wachbroit, "The Question Not Asked: The Challenge of Pleiotropic Genetic Tests," 131–136; Ruth Hubbard and R.C. Lewontin, "Genetic Testing for Disease Predisposition, Pitfalls of Genetic Testing," 360–362.

[139] Martin Richards, "How Distinctive is Genetic Information?" 678–679.

result in a minimal addition of risk; while other times the gene can compound the risk which would result in a much greater degree of risk. Since not all pleiotropic gene interactions are studied in great detail yet, the predictability of risk can be very complicated.[140]

Another risk is the misinterpretation of the results. There can be the concern that getting a negative result for a PGT like Alzheimer's disease could cause people to overlook some possible preventive measures or beneficial lifestyle changes. However the REVEAL study, which looked at Alzheimer's disease, showed that with appropriate education and communication, most people understood the test results. Although, some without the APOE gene ε4 allele thought he or she had a much lower chance of developing Alzheimer's than even the general population. Also since not all the variants of a particular disease are always known, classifying a gene or allele as pleiotropic can sometimes be misleading. If a gene is assumed to be pleiotropic, then that gene has implications on multiple diseases or traits. However, if the gene is not really pleiotropic, then the gene only has implications for one disease or trait. Thus, the results would be misunderstood and misrepresented.[141]

Sometimes there can be psychological problems, depression, and/or worry with pleiotropic genetic testing.[142] If the test returns results for multiple findings, then the individual could be depressed after finding out additional unexpected information, especially if the information is about an incurable disease like Alzheimer's.[143] However if the individuals are informed about having additional results and what those results could include, research has shown that depression is not as common as once thought.[144] The REVEAL study demonstrated that with pre- and post-test counseling, there were fewer psychological problems when looking at Alzheimer's disease risk results. However there can still be harmful psychological problems even with counseling and education. In regards to Huntington's disease, a study of approximately 5000 people showed that there were still some serious adverse events, like suicide or psychological traumas, in about 1 % of the individuals tested. Most of those serious events occurred in people with positive tests for Huntington's.[145] While many of the diseases involved in pleiotropic genetic testing are not as severe

---

[140] Matt Chamberlain, Paul Baird, Mohamed Dirani, et al., "Unraveling a Complex Genetic Disease: Age-related Macular Degeneration," 578.

[141] J. Scott Roberts and Wendy Uhlmann, "Genetic Susceptibility Testing for Neurodegenerative Diseases: Ethical and Practice Issues," 94; Shanya Sivakumaran, Felix Agakov, Evropi Theodoratou, James G. Prendergast, et al., "Abundant Pleiotropy in Human Complex Diseases and Traits," 616.

[142] Colleen McBride, Deborah Bowen, Lawrence Brody, et al., "Future Health Applications of Genomics: Priorities for Communication, Behavioral, and Social Sciences Research," 561.

[143] Shanya Sivakumaran, Felix Agakov, Evropi Theodoratou, et al., "Abundant Pleiotropy in Human Complex Diseases and Traits," 616.

[144] Philip Mitchell, Bettina Meiser, Alex Wilde, et al., "Predictive and Diagnostic Genetic Testing in Psychiatry," 236.

[145] J. Scott Roberts and Wendy Uhlmann, "Genetic Susceptibility Testing for Neurodegenerative Diseases: Ethical and Practice Issues," 94; Hyman Schipper, "Presymptomatic Apolipoprotein E Genotyping for Alzheimer's Disease Risk Assessment and Prevention," e119, e121..

and certain as Huntington's disease, the research still illustrates that there can be a possibility for some serious adverse psychological harms in those with positive test results, especially if people are not expecting some of the results.

Also discrimination can sometimes result after pleiotropic genetic testing.[146] Because this test has the potential for multiple disease results, discrimination can occur for certain disease predictions. In regards to testing the ε4 allele on the APOE gene, discrimination can occur with long-term care insurance, because of the risk for Alzheimer's disease. The REVEAL study showed that there were small differences with the long-term care insurance for those with the ε4 allele than without the allele.[147] Pleiotropic test results can also have an impact on life and disability insurance and job discrimination.[148]

2). Benefits

Sometimes pleiotropic genetic testing can result in information that would help in treatment guidelines and options. Genetic testing for presence of the ε4 allele with the APOE gene could prove beneficial for treating and/or preventing CAD and CHD.[149] Sometimes pleiotropic genetic testing can help to increase information on prevention and treatment options.[150] If a pleiotropic genetic test is performed, most of the time the test is needed to find out the risk of a treatable disease. Once the results come back, the individual can start on a treatment that will either cure or reduce the disease. Risks can come when information for the secondary disease is not handled properly.

Another benefit can be future planning.[151] Pleiotropic genetic testing can return information that can be helpful for long-term goals and personal decision making.[152] Planning benefits can range from helping to make life decisions, career options, and the possibility of children.[153]

---

[146] Colleen McBride, Deborah Bowen, Lawrence Brody, et al., "Future Health Applications of Genomics: Priorities for Communication, Behavioral, and Social Sciences Research," 561.

[147] Hyman Schipper, "Presymptomatic Apolipoprotein E Genotyping for Alzheimer's Disease Risk Assessment and Prevention," e121.

[148] J. Scott Roberts and Wendy Uhlmann, "Genetic Susceptibility Testing for Neurodegenerative Diseases: Ethical and Practice Issues," 95, 97; Hyman Schipper, "Presymptomatic Apolipoprotein E Genotyping for Alzheimer's Disease Risk Assessment and Prevention," e120.

[149] Martin Richards, "How Distinctive is Genetic Information?" 678.

[150] Matt Chamberlain, Paul Baird, Mohamed Dirani, et al., "Unraveling a Complex Genetic Disease: Age-related Macular Degeneration," 577.

[151] J. Scott Roberts and Wendy Uhlmann, "Genetic Susceptibility Testing for Neurodegenerative Diseases: Ethical and Practice Issues," 92.

[152] Hyman Schipper, "Presymptomatic Apolipoprotein E Genotyping for Alzheimer's Disease Risk Assessment and Prevention," e120.

[153] J. Scott Roberts and Wendy Uhlmann, "Genetic Susceptibility Testing for Neurodegenerative Diseases: Ethical and Practice Issues," 95.

Also while pleiotropic genetic testing can result in additional information, if that information is explained properly, the added information can promote healthy behaviors and choices.[154] Sometimes having additional information can help motivate people to make better lifestyle decisions that can prevent or slow down the progression of diseases. In the REVEAL study, those with an increased risk of Alzheimer's disease adopted lifestyle and behavior changes to encourage the prevention of the disease. Some of the changes included increased exercise, taking supplements, and altering their diet.[155] Even if information is only needed for one disease, if there is enough education and counseling, pleiotropic genetic testing can encourage healthy living.

One example of the complexity of screening for some diseases is the story of the Wexler sisters. Like Alzheimer's disease, there is no significant treatment for Huntington's disease. However, unlike Alzheimer's, the certainty of Huntington's disease is almost 100% if the test comes back positive. Because her whole family had suffered from Huntington's disease, Nancy Wexler was an advocate for finding the Huntington's gene. She was a supporter of creating a pre-symptomatic genetic test for this disease. But when the gene was actually found, and the pre-symptomatic test was developed, Nancy Wexler and her sister Alice changed their position. In fact, both of the sisters became an advocate for not getting the pre-symptomatic genetic test for Huntington's disease. In an article entitled "On Not Taking the Test," Alice Wexler said "I'd rather work at learning to live with a certain amount of insecurity than have to adjust to a grim future even before the symptoms begin."[156] The sisters understood the complexity of that decision, and as a result cautioned people against making a decision without adequately looking at the risks and benefits. Because of the complexity and predictive value of pleiotropic genetic testing, the same caution should be used before an individual decides to undergo testing. The risks and benefits of testing need to be analyzed.[157]

2. Application of the Revised Model

In the second part, each of the components of the revised model of consent will be applied to pleiotropic genetic testing. Comprehension, disclosure, voluntariness, and patient safety will be discussed in relation to pleiotropic genetic testing.

---

[154] Colleen McBride, Deborah Bowen, Lawrence Brody, et al., "Future Health Applications of Genomics: Priorities for Communication, Behavioral, and Social Sciences Research," 561; J. Scott Roberts and Wendy Uhlmann, "Genetic Susceptibility Testing for Neurodegenerative Diseases: Ethical and Practice Issues," 94.

[155] Hyman Schipper, "Presymptomatic Apolipoprotein E Genotyping for Alzheimer's Disease Risk Assessment and Prevention," e121-e122.

[156] Alice Wexler, "On Not Taking the Test."

[157] Martin Richards, "How Distinctive is Genetic Information?" 768; J. Scott Roberts and Wendy Uhlmann, "Genetic Susceptibility Testing for Neurodegenerative Diseases: Ethical and Practice Issues," 94.

a. Comprehension

The first component of the revised model of informed consent is comprehension. This section will look at autonomy, genetic risks, and the doctor-patient relationship. Each area will be discussed and analyzed further.

In the current model, a standardized approach to consent is used, this approach typically focuses on the autonomous patient signing a consent form without much discussion. Since this model emphasizes the consent form, there is insufficient time and communication for understanding the meaning of PGT risk. The current doctor-patient relationship focuses upon the patient freely signing the consent form without sufficient education of the patient about the meaning of PGT. On the other hand, the revised model adopts a personalized approach to consent that emphasizes extensive discussion with the patient as an autonomous agent. The revised model focuses on a process that provides time for communication to foster an understanding of the complex meaning of PGT risk. The revised model emphasizes the doctor-patient relationship as an interactive process to ensure sufficient education of the patient about the meaning of PGT.

1). Autonomy

Informed consent for pleiotropic genetic testing cites autonomy as one of the foundational principles of testing. The ideas behind autonomy and pleiotropic testing are that patients have the right to decide for themselves whether or not to be tested for the pleiotropic gene.[158] However, unless the individual understands the ideas behind and implications of pleiotropic genetic testing, the individual cannot truly make an autonomous decision.

Autonomy should be more than just a chance to accept or reject testing for the pleiotropic gene.[159] The revised model of consent encourages patient involvement through a more extensive process of consent. Patients undergoing pleiotropic genetic testing need to be able to process the information and be able to make a decision about testing. Personalization of that information can be helpful in encouraging autonomy for each patient. This model recognizes the differences among the patients and suggests having more flexible consent for each patient in identifying their particular needs.[160] The revised model adopts a personalized approach to consent that emphasizes extensive discussion with the patient as an autonomous agent.

2). Understanding Genetic Risks

It is important to understand the ideas of genetic risks associated with pleiotropic genetic testing. Genetic risks of pleiotropic genetic testing are generally the same

---

[158] Lewis Vaughn, *Bioethics: Principles, Issues, and Cases*, 465–66.

[159] Robert M. Arnold and Charles W. Lidz, "Informed Consent: Clinical Aspects of Consent in Health Care," 8–9.

[160] Tom Beauchamp and James Childress, *Principles of Biomedical Ethics*, 127.

as PGT. Since the current model of consent emphasizes the consent form, there is insufficient time and communication for understanding the meaning of PGT risk. However the revised model focuses on a process that provides time for communication to foster an understanding of the complex meaning of PGT risk.

Patients and research participants need to understand the genetics behind susceptibility testing, what the implications are of that testing, and how to interpret the results of testing.[161] It is important to help the individuals to understand that most of the pleiotropic diseases are multifactorial, meaning that the predictive value is based on genetics, environmental factors, social aspects, and lifestyle choices. In the REVEAL study, the participants were told the risks assessments included "the best available information," but were also told that other factors like social and environmental interactions were not included in the assessments.[162] In relation to pleiotropic genes, since one gene can affect multiple traits, it is also important that the individuals understand the complexity of the relationship among the genes and/ or alleles.

Ellen Wright Clayton illustrates the difference between pleiotropic genetic testing and some other types of testing that would identify a mutation. She says that people would typically recognize the distinction between "incidental detection of a mutation in the APC gene that will cause them to develop colon cancer if their colon is not removed and a mutation that mildly increases their risk of developing hypertension, a disorder that would ordinarily be detected in the course of routine care."[163] Participating in a test that can return unexpected genetic results can be difficult to handle and understand the genetic risks. However, the difference in testing needs to be understood in order to be able to make an appropriate decision about testing.

Research shows that the pubic needs more genetic literacy, because many do not understand the concepts of genetic risks. Colleen McBride, Deborah Bowen, Lawrence Brody, et al. suggests that people base their understanding of genetics and risks on several factors including the nature of the disease and inheritance, possible personal or family experience, treatment options, and communication and discussion of the risks. In order to increase the understanding of genetic risks, doctors or counselors should make the risk easier to understand by applying the risk information to normal everyday occurrences, adding visual aspects as well like charts or graphs, giving the individual information to take home, and encouraging additional communication for support.[164]

---

[161] Theresa Marteau, Scott Roberts, Susan LaRusse, et al., "Predictive Genetic Testing for Alzheimer's Disease: Impact upon Risk Perception," 398, 401.

[162] J. Scott Roberts and Wendy Uhlmann, "Genetic Susceptibility Testing for Neurodegenerative Diseases: Ethical and Practice Issues," 93.

[163] Ellen Wright Clayton, "Incidental Findings in Genetics Research Using Archived DNA," 290.

[164] Colleen McBride, Deborah Bowen, Lawrence Brody, et al., "Future Health Applications of Genomics: Priorities for Communication, Behavioral, and Social Sciences Research," 559; J. Scott Roberts and Wendy Uhlmann, "Genetic Susceptibility Testing for Neurodegenerative Diseases: Ethical and Practice Issues," 94.

The revised model promotes additional conversations and education of the patient in order to cultivate understanding when thinking about risk assessments. When discussing risk assessments and probabilities, it is important to turn conceptual risks into more personal and identifiable risks in order to encourage understanding and comprehension. The revised model focuses on a process that provides time for communication to foster an understanding of the complex meaning of pleiotropic genetic testing which can result in multiple findings.

3). Doctor-Patient Relationship

The doctor-patient relationship is important in promoting education and understanding of risk assessments for pleiotropic genetic testing. One study suggests that not many researchers communicate the ideas of pleiotropic genetic testing fully to their participants.[165] In the article "Informed Consent for Genetic Research Involving Pleiotropic Genes: An Empirical Study of ApoE Research," a study was done that looked at pleiotropic research and informed consent with the participants. Zachary Cooper, Robert Nelson, and Lainie Ross said that despite the fact that the study was on the ApoE gene and pleiotropy, "only four of 41 researchers (10%) indicated that they discussed the multiple associations of ApoE (pleiotropy) in their consent forms. Only one of the 15 consent forms (7%) that we analyzed mentioned that ApoE had pleiotropic implications."[166] The authors go on to say that even though the researchers might have thought the pleiotropic nature of the gene was not pertinent to their research, the omission could have serious impact on the informed consent process resulting in failed consent. Zachary Cooper, Robert Nelson, and Lainie Ross say that the participants should be informed of the pleiotropic nature of the gene being researched "because it could affect their perception of the risks and benefits of participating for themselves, and it could influence the impact their participation has on their families, and their communities."[167] Knowing there is a risk of finding out more information than the person would like might be enough to forgo testing. The Nocebo Effect can also have implications for comprehension of pleiotropic genetic testing, because sometimes having too much information can actually cause harm to the patient.[168] The revised model of consent looks at education and communication in order to ensure additional understanding and comprehension.

In the revised model, doctors should participate more in educating patients and encouraging discussions about risk in order to foster understanding. However in

---

[165] KG Fulda and Lykens K., "Ethical Issues in Predictive Genetic Testing: A Public Health Perspective," 143–7; Zachary Cooper, Robert Nelson, and Lainie Ross, "Informed Consent for Genetic Research Involving Pleiotropic Genes: An Empirical Study of ApoE Research," 6–9.

[166] Zachary Cooper, Robert Nelson, and Lainie Ross, "Informed Consent for Genetic Research Involving Pleiotropic Genes: An Empirical Study of ApoE Research," 6–9.

[167] Zachary Cooper, Robert Nelson, and Lainie Ross, "Informed Consent for Genetic Research Involving Pleiotropic Genes: An Empirical Study of ApoE Research," 6–9.

[168] Rebecca Erwin Wells and Ted J. Kaptchuk, "To Tell the Truth, the Whole Truth, May Do Patients Harm: The Problem of the Nocebo Effect for Informed Consent," 22–29.

order to do that, doctors and researchers need to be able to make more time available for their patients and research participants. Just like with PGT, doctors need to have enough knowledge in order to be able to help their patients understand genetic risk assessments for pleiotropic genetic testing. In the REVEAL study, the doctors discussed the limitations of risk assessments for Alzheimer's disease in order to help the participants understand better.[169] Also as was previously addressed, another important aspect of the doctor-patient relationship is the need for doctors to address the nature of pleiotropy.[170] For example, if testing for CAD, the doctors should make the patients aware of the complication of having risk information for Alzheimer's disease as well. The revised model emphasizes the doctor-patient relationship as an interactive process to ensure sufficient education of the patient about the meaning of PGT.

The revised model adopts a personalized approach to consent that emphasizes extensive discussion with the patient as an autonomous agent. The revised model focuses on a process that provides time for communication to foster an understanding of the complex meaning of PGT risk. The revised model emphasizes the doctor-patient relationship as an interactive process to ensure sufficient education of the patient about the meaning of PGT.

b. Disclosure

In order to have appropriate informed consent, disclosure of certain information is necessary.[171] Dorene S. Markel and Beverly M. Yashar say that informed consent should present all the needed information in a "factual, complete, and accurate manner."[172] Because pleiotropic genetic testing has many complex treatment options and can result in unexpected findings, the revised model requires disclosure and genetic counseling in order to select an appropriate option. This section will discuss each of those aspects in detail. The first section will look at the disclosure guidelines, and the second section will look at the genetic counseling for pleiotropic genetic testing.

The current model focuses on medical information in a standardized approach of consent. The current model recommends non-directive counseling, and does not require counseling. Whereas, the revised model addresses not only medical information but all other relevant information for the patient to consider for consent, including the fact that some PGT diseases might not have any available treatment. The revised model requires counseling and adopts value transparency and non-directive counseling.

---

[169] J. Scott Roberts and Wendy Uhlmann, "Genetic Susceptibility Testing for Neurodegenerative Diseases: Ethical and Practice Issues," 93–94.

[170] Hyman Schipper, "Presymptomatic Apolipoprotein E Genotyping for Alzheimer's Disease Risk Assessment and Prevention," e122.

[171] J. Scott Roberts and Wendy Uhlmann, "Genetic Susceptibility Testing for Neurodegenerative Diseases: Ethical and Practice Issues," 93.

[172] Dorene S. Markel and Beverly M. Yashar, "The Interface Between the Practice of Medical Genetics and Human Genetic Research: What Every Genetic Counselor Needs to Know," 360.

1). Disclosure Guidelines

Sometimes disclosure can be difficult with pleiotropic genetic testing, because not all of the risks and benefits might be known at the time.[173] However in order to encourage better disclosure, the revised model addresses not only medical information but all other relevant information for the patient to consider for consent, including the fact that some pleiotropic diseases might not have any available treatment.[174]

One of the most important areas to disclose is the basic nature of pleiotropic genes. If the nature of pleiotropic genes were not clearly communicated antecedently, disclosure of this type of information can be difficult to communicate.[175] For example when testing the APOE gene, patients might not be expecting to hear about the risks for developing Alzheimer's disease. Disclosure should focus on what testing means and discuss the nature of both diseases that the pleiotropic genetic test might find. If the APOE gene is being tested, information on both CAD and Alzheimer's disease needs to be disclosed, because of the effect of pleiotropic genes.[176] In regards to research participation, Ellen Wright Clayton says that there is still debate about what to disclose when participating in research with a pleiotropic gene.[177] However, even though research participation is a little different, in order to have adequate informed consent, the participant still needs to be aware of the fact that there can be unexpected results and information on multiple disease susceptibilities.

Another important area of disclosure should be the predictive values of the diseases. Risk assessment values need to be disclosed for both the general population and in relationship to the individual. In the REVEAL study, researchers told the participants about the standard risk for developing Alzheimer's disease, which was about 10–15 % for the general population. Also if the ε4 allele on the APOE gene is being tested, people should understand the risk for having either one or two copies of the ε4 allele. If an individual has two copies of the allele, then the individual's risk for CAD and Alzheimer's disease increases even more.[178]

Some other areas of disclosure include privacy and confidentiality measures that will be taken when the results come back. The doctor and patient can also discuss whether all of the information will go in the medical record. If the APOE test comes

---

[173] J. Scott Roberts and Wendy Uhlmann, "Genetic Susceptibility Testing for Neurodegenerative Diseases: Ethical and Practice Issues," 93.

[174] Dorene S. Markel and Beverly M. Yashar, "The Interface Between the Practice of Medical Genetics and Human Genetic Research: What Every Genetic Counselor Needs to Know," 362.

[175] KG Fulda and Lykens K., "Ethical Issues in Predictive Genetic Testing: A Public Health Perspective," 143–7; Ellen Wright Clayton, "Incidental Findings in Genetics Research Using Archived DNA," 290.

[176] Robert Wachbroit, "The Question Not Asked: The Challenge of Pleiotropic Genetic Tests," 133; Annelien L. Bredenoord, Hester Y. Kroes, Edwin Cuppen, et al., "Disclosure of Individual Genetic Data to Research Participants: The Debate Reconsidered," 41–42.

[177] Ellen Wright Clayton, "Incidental Findings in Genetics Research Using Archived DNA," 290.

[178] Theresa Marteau, Scott Roberts, Susan LaRusse, et al., "Predictive Genetic Testing for Alzheimer's Disease: Impact upon Risk Perception," 399.

back positive, the patient might not want the increased risk for Alzheimer's disease to be included in his or her record.[179]

In order to encourage adequate disclosure, the REVEAL study suggests that better decisions can be made when disclosure uses both written and verbal aspects. Also the revised model encourages better decision making by ensuring all of the important information is disclosed before testing occurs. If the physician or researcher does not ask the patient or participant antecedently which results he or she wants to know, there can be significant problems with the disclosure process.[180] Then if the physician discloses unexpected and unwanted information without explicit consent, the patient could be harmed, and the informed consent process will have been inadequate.

Thus significant harm can come if doctors or researchers do not address antecedently the nature of pleiotropy and the fact that there will be multiple result findings. As a result, more counseling is encouraged before testing in order to help the patients or research participants to grasp the information that might result.[181]

2). Genetic Counseling

Dorene S. Markel and Beverly M. Yashar say that a genetic counselor is "uniquely positioned to play an important role in understanding the nuances of the genetic research interface between basic/clinical science and genetic counseling."[182] The current model recommends non-directive counseling, and does not require counseling. However, in the revised model, genetic counseling is required both before and after testing to ensure the selection of an appropriate option.[183] Also, the counselor should ensure there is enough time between the pre-test counseling and the actual test procedure in order to make an appropriate, informed decision.[184]

The pre-test counseling should focus on what the information will mean to the patient, since the test returns results for two diseases.[185] Serious problems can occur if a doctor has already performed genetic testing without discussing the nature of pleiotropy with the patient. This is why pre-test counseling is so important. The

---

[179] Dorene S. Markel and Beverly M. Yashar, "The Interface Between the Practice of Medical Genetics and Human Genetic Research: What Every Genetic Counselor Needs to Know," 363–364.

[180] J. Scott Roberts and Wendy Uhlmann, "Genetic Susceptibility Testing for Neurodegenerative Diseases: Ethical and Practice Issues," 94, 97.

[181] Ellen Wright Clayton, "Incidental Findings in Genetics Research Using Archived DNA," 289.

[182] Dorene S. Markel and Beverly M. Yashar, "The Interface Between the Practice of Medical Genetics and Human Genetic Research: What Every Genetic Counselor Needs to Know," 366.

[183] Dorene S. Markel and Beverly M. Yashar, "The Interface Between the Practice of Medical Genetics and Human Genetic Research: What Every Genetic Counselor Needs to Know," 364.

[184] Katja Aktan-Collan, Jukka-Pekka Mecklin, Albert de la Chapelle, et al., "Evaluation of a Counselling Protocol for Predictive Genetic Testing for Hereditary Non-Polyposis Colorectal Cancer," 112.

[185] Robert Wachbroit, "The Question Not Asked: The Challenge of Pleiotropic Genetic Tests," 131–132; Lewis Vaughn, Bioethics: Principles, Issues, and Cases, 465–66.

counselor should also ask about disclosure of results. The counselor should inquire into whether or not the patient wants to know his or her Alzheimer's risk.[186] By planning ahead, the doctor and patient should be able to arrive at an acceptable course of action before the results are returned. Post-test counseling ensures a doctor has discussed the results with the patient. As suggested by the REVEAL study, sometimes bringing a support person like a spouse or friend to the post-test counseling session can help the patient or participant as an added resource. After post-test counseling there should also be appropriate follow-up after the test. The REVEAL study had follow-up at 6 weeks, 6 months, and a year after the test.[187]

Genetic counseling can help with the complex nature of pleiotropy and is essential to the decision making process for pleiotropic genetic testing.[188] Genetic counselors can help educate the patient further about pleiotropic genetic testing and can encourage the patients to make an appropriate decision about testing.[189] Also since the revised model adopts value transparency and non-directive counseling, the counselors and physicians can give their input and advice if there is a particular treatment or test that might be best for the patient. The revised model encourages physician and counselor participation and recommendations.[190]

The revised model also emphasizes the necessary inclusion of feedback and patient assessment mechanisms as a tool for genetic counseling. Feedback mechanisms and patient assessments like a decision tree will be applied to the patient in order to encourage appropriate selection of the options. One of the important assessment measures specifically for pleiotropic genetic testing is the IES survey. The REVEAL study that analyzed Alzheimer's risk sent out IES surveys. These surveys can help professionals to identify whether or not the individual is comfortable with the new information received. This survey analyzes a person's stress level with a particular incident. Since pleiotropic genetic testing produces results for two diseases, the IES survey can be helpful in predicting a person's reactions to testing. IES surveys can be great indicators of a person's possible stress after having pleiotropic genetic test results disclosed. The survey asks people to determine the frequency with which he or she thought the survey comments were true during the week. Some of the comments included "I thought about it when I didn't mean to"

---

[186] Ruth Hubbard and R.C. Lewontin, "Genetic Testing for Disease Predisposition, Pitfalls of Genetic Testing," 360–362; Lewis Vaughn, *Bioethics: Principles, Issues, and Cases*, 465–66; Robert Wachbroit, "The Question Not Asked: The Challenge of Pleiotropic Genetic Tests," 133–136.

[187] Michael Cassidy, J. Scott Roberts, Thomas Bird, et al., "Comparing Test-specific Distress of Susceptibility versus Deterministic Genetic Testing for Alzheimer's Disease," 407–408, 411; Angus Clarke, "Genetic Counseling," 133.

[188] Dorene S. Markel and Beverly M. Yashar, "The Interface Between the Practice of Medical Genetics and Human Genetic Research: What Every Genetic Counselor Needs to Know," 366.

[189] J. Scott Roberts and Wendy Uhlmann, "Genetic Susceptibility Testing for Neurodegenerative Diseases: Ethical and Practice Issues," 93.

[190] Angus Clarke, "Genetic Counseling," 142; Diana Buccafurni, "Reconsidering the Facilitation of Autonomous Decision Making in Genetic Counseling," v, 3; Tom Beauchamp and James Childress, *Principles of Biomedical Ethics*, 79; Angus Clarke, "Genetic Counseling," 142.

or "I tried to remove it from my memory."[191] Based off of the person's answers, the survey can tell if people will either avoid stressful information and not deal with it or handle the information.

The results of REVEAL study showed that there was not a significant difference in the IES ratings for people with the εe4 allele on the APOE gene and people without the ε4 allele. It also showed that there was really not a large difference in the "distress" ratings. However, the study required education sessions, counseling, and follow-up of participants.[192] Thus if there are studies with inadequate education, counseling, and follow-up, the distress levels after disclosing Alzheimer's disease risk might be a lot higher. By focusing on genetic counseling and patient feedback mechanisms, the revised model should ensure appropriate decision making.

The revised model addresses not only medical information but all other relevant information for the patient to consider for consent, including the fact that some PGT diseases might not have any available treatment. The revised model requires counseling and adopts value transparency and non-directive counseling.

c. Voluntariness

The third section is voluntariness. Voluntariness is extremely important when discussing informed consent. This section will look at coercion and family-related implications. Each area will be discussed in relation to pleiotropic genetic testing.

In the current model, there are no specific measures to address or avoid multiple sources of external pressures (such as pressures from relatives, the medical staff and community, and/or societal influences) which increase the possibility of coercion upon the individual. The current model does not take into consideration all family related implications which can lead to coercion of family members. Conversely, the revised model addresses external pressures on the patient and the family (such as pressures by the family for the patient to be tested and pressure upon the family regarding testing outcomes) to alleviate or resolve external coercion upon the patient. Because genetic information impacts the family, the revised model includes family-related concerns before testing and identifies ways to help the patient struggle with family-related PGT information.

1). Coercion

Coercion and voluntariness are key aspects of informed consent. If a physician or researcher presents an individual with unwanted information that is involved with the pleiotropic test results, the voluntariness of the individual can be questioned. Ellen Wright Clayton says that presenting "incidental findings to unsuspecting people

[191] Michael Cassidy, J. Scott Roberts, Thomas Bird, et al., "Comparing Test-specific Distress of Susceptibility versus Deterministic Genetic Testing for Alzheimer's Disease," 408.

[192] Michael Cassidy, J. Scott Roberts, Thomas Bird, et al., "Comparing Test-specific Distress of Susceptibility versus Deterministic Genetic Testing for Alzheimer's Disease," 408–411.

who had not previously thought about the issue just does not seem right."[193] It is up to the patient to voluntarily consent to testing and to reveal any information he or she wishes.[194] Tom Beauchamp and James Childress categorize voluntariness as a precondition of consent.[195]

External pressures and controlling influences are commonly seen in many different areas. Sometimes even genetic counselors, doctors, and researchers can demonstrate the underpinnings of coercion implicitly.[196] Since it is common to perceive external pressures in most decisions, this third point develops the importance of avoiding coercion of both the patient and the patient's family when information is presented. There can also be internal pressure as well. One question that illustrates the internal pressure of pleiotropic genetic testing is the following. Ellen Wright Clayton suggests one of the important questions of this testing is "How can I say I do not want to know when someone says they have important information about me?"[197] However the revised model strives to address the possible sources of coercion and external pressures.

Sometimes manipulation and coercion can emerge from the education process. Alfred Tauber in his book *Patient Autonomy and the Ethics of Responsibility* says, "At one end of the spectrum, patients require instruction, which embeds certain subjective points of view, values, and assumptions."[198] In pleiotropic genetic testing, manipulation can arise from the physicians misrepresenting the nature of pleiotropic genes.[199] Coercion can arise from family members with strong opinions on either wanting or not wanting to know additional at-risk information for possible Alzheimer's disease. Also voluntariness can be impacted by the way a doctor or relative explains the information or views of pleiotropic genetic testing.[200] In order to keep the integrity, the consent process needs "continual attention to the purpose, process, and impact of external influences."[201]

In contrast to the current model which has no specific measures in place to address or avoid multiples sources of external pressures, the revised model addresses external pressures on the patient and the family (such as pressures by the family for the patient to be tested and pressure upon the family regarding testing outcomes) to alleviate or resolve external coercion upon the patient.

---

[193] Ellen Wright Clayton, "Incidental Findings in Genetics Research Using Archived DNA," 290–291.

[194] Barbara Bowles Biesecker, "Privacy in Genetic Counseling," 111.

[195] Tom Beauchamp and James Childress, *Principles of Biomedical Ethics*, 79.

[196] John Kilner, Rebecca Pentz, and Frank Young, eds., *Genetic Ethics*, 33.

[197] Ellen Wright Clayton, "Incidental Findings in Genetics Research Using Archived DNA," 290.

[198] Alfred Tauber, *Patient Autonomy and the Ethics of Responsibility*, 136.

[199] Bernard Lo, *Resolving Ethical Dilemmas*, 20.

[200] Tom Beauchamp and James Childress, *Principles of Biomedical Ethics*, 95.

[201] Linda Farber Post, Jeffrey Blustein, and Nancy Neveloff Dubler, *Handbook for Health Care Ethics Committees*, 42–43.

2). Family-Related Implications

Pleiotropic genetic information has implications and consequences for the whole family. The implications can even carry over into family-planning decisions.[202] While the current model does not take into consideration all family related implications, the revised model ensures voluntary consent by establishing procedures to avoid two forms of coercion: pressure by the family for the patient to be tested (eg, if heart disease runs in the family, there can be pressure upon a younger individual to be tested in to see if s/he is at-risk etc); and pressure upon the family regarding the testing outcome (eg, if the patient finds out s/he is at an increased risk for Alzheimer's disease, there can be pressure on other individuals in the family to get tested for the disease as well). Avoiding coercion of the patient and the patient's family helps to ensure meaningful consent for pleiotropic genetic testing.

The revised model takes additional measures to protect family members. Only the necessary information should be given, and any additional information that could have implications for family members should be addressed and analyzed before the test to prevent harm to the family. In order to protect the individuals, family-related implications first need to be identified. Once the individual recognizes the family-related implications, the physician or counselor can encourage the patient or participant to discuss these implications with his or her family before participating in the test. While consent from all the family members is not required, the revised model encourages family discussions of the consequences of pleiotropic genetic testing. Also during the discussion sessions, privacy and confidentiality measures can be identified so that the family members can feel protected against unwanted discrimination or harm. While discussing the test with family members, the revised model encourages the individual to find out whether or not the family wants to know the results of the test. While some members might want to know this information, others might not want to know. Thus, having discussions with the family is extremely important when determining disclosure of results to family members. The revised model seeks to ensure the voluntariness of consent and to protect against possible coercion of family members.[203] Because genetic information impacts the family, the revised model includes family-related concerns before testing and identifies ways to help the patient struggle with family-related PGT information.

The revised model addresses external pressures on the patient and the family (such as pressures by the family for the patient to be tested and pressure upon the family regarding testing outcomes) to alleviate or resolve external coercion upon the patient. Because genetic information impacts the family, the revised model includes family-related concerns before testing and identifies ways to help the patient struggle with family-related PGT information.

---

[202] Martin Richards, "How Distinctive is Genetic Information?" 681.

[203] Dorene S. Markel and Beverly M. Yashar, "The Interface Between the Practice of Medical Genetics and Human Genetic Research: What Every Genetic Counselor Needs to Know," 363–364; Tony McGleenan, "Genetic Testing for Cancer Predisposition- An Ongoing Debate- Genetic Screening Forum," 122–123.

d. Patient Safety

The last component of the revised model of informed consent is patient safety. Patient safety consists of accountability, transparency, trust, and patient safety. Pleiotropic genetic testing needs to emphasize a culture of safety in the revised model. This culture of safety in the revised model needs nationally established systems of accountability that implements this model in a transparent manner in order to foster trust with pleiotropic genetic testing services. The revised model applies systems changes in order to increase patient safety and decrease risk for informed consent of pleiotropic genetic testing.

This is a new component that is not in the current model. The revised model encourages internal and external accountability by promoting communication among medical departments and institutional policies. The revised model requires transparency with physician discussions and consent requirements. The revised model encourages trust in the organizations and physicians by having open discussions with patient participation in the revised consent process. In the revised model, patient safety is fostered by having systems of accountability and transparency to establish preventive measures that promote the safety of patients considering PGT.

1). Accountability

While this is a new component not found in the current model, the revised model seeks to establish accountability measures for pleiotropic genetic testing procedures and results.[204] Accountability of results and practices is crucial to ensure patient safety of pleiotropic genetic testing.

The revised model of informed consent ensures accountability by adhering to nationally established systems for PGT. This model promotes accountability by encouraging additional communication between the doctors and laboratories performing the tests. Since there is a possibility of finding out too much information with pleiotropic genetic testing, the area of accountability of results is crucial to ensure patient safety. One of the most important aspects of accountability of pleiotropic genetic testing is communication among the different departments and professional groups.[205] Establishing consistent guidelines among the departments can help to encourage further accountability of pleiotropic genetic testing. One of the consistent policies among all departments for the testing should be to require physicians and researchers to discuss the nature of pleiotropy before participating in the test. Accountability measures also include the validity and accuracy of results and tests.[206]

---

[204] Thomas Goetz, *The Decision Tree,* xvi–xvii, 117; Bernard Lo, *Resolving Ethical Dilemmas,* 273.

[205] Linda Farber Post, Jeffrey Blustein, and Nancy Neveloff Dubler, *Handbook for Health Care Ethics Committees,* 38–39.

[206] Dorene S. Markel and Beverly M. Yashar, "The Interface Between the Practice of Medical Genetics and Human Genetic Research: What Every Genetic Counselor Needs to Know," 364.

When a person is participating in a research study, IRBs note the importance of having tests that are confirmed and results that are valid.[207] The revised model encourages internal and external accountability by promoting communication among medical departments and institutional policies.

2). Transparency

Transparency in implementing the revised model of consent will also help to ensure patient safety for pleiotropic genetic testing. Often specific accountability and transparency measures are hard to identify in informed consent, but the revised model seeks to enhance and clarify those measure for pleiotropic genetic testing.[208]

Transparency can be maintained by the doctors and counselors when educating and communicating with the patient about pleiotropic testing. A positive doctor-patient relationship is cultivated by an interactive process of communication in the revised model of informed consent. When discussing risks and options with patients, doctors and counselors should be especially attentive to bringing out the differences of pleiotropic genetic testing in order to promote transparency of information and procedures. Transparency is crucial for both accountability and trust in the revised model.

Because patients typically do not assess their physician's performance due to the complexity of the testing, transparency of the medical staff is extremely important.[209] The transparency of the revised model addresses conflicts of interests and third-party interests. For example, financial conflicts of interests often put "the interests of patients and doctors in direct conflict"[210] If a researcher is more focused on the financial backing of a trial involving the APOE gene, the researcher might not recognize some of the possible harms of the trial. In the revise model, physicians can eliminate conflicts of interests by encouraging transparency of the test procedures, test results, and interaction among the medical staff.[211] Physician transparency is also relevant when looking at what to disclose to third parties in relation to pleiotropic genetic testing.[212] The revised model requires transparency with physician discussions and consent requirements.

3). Trust

Trust in the medical system and staff is important to all aspects of genetic testing. Research has shown that if a patient trusts his or her physician, the individual

---

[207] Ellen Wright Clayton, "Incidental Findings in Genetics Research Using Archived DNA," 290.

[208] KG Fulda and Lykens K., "Ethical Issues in Predictive Genetic Testing: A Public Health Perspective," 143–7.

[209] David Orentlicher, "Genetic Privacy in the Patient-Physician Relationship," 84.

[210] Alfred Tauber, *Patient Autonomy and the Ethics of Responsibility,* 168.

[211] David Orentlicher, "Genetic Privacy in the Patient-Physician Relationship," 84.

[212] Hyman Schipper, "Presymptomatic Apolipoprotein E Genotyping for Alzheimer's Disease Risk Assessment and Prevention," e122.

is more likely to adhere to the doctor's recommended treatment plan or behavior changes that can help to prevent the disease.[213]

When the revised model promotes patient safety, accountability, and transparency in implementation, trust is encouraged in the system of pleiotropic genetic testing. After establishing additional measures, trust is easier to build and maintain in the revised model of informed consent. After implementing transparency measures, trust can be easier to establish. By promoting confidentiality and eliminating some conflicts of interest, trust in the medical staff can be promoted. If the physician is an instrument of any other person or entity, trust is much harder to create and sustain. If the patient or research participant feels their interests are not being promoted, trust will be almost impossible to maintain.[214]

The revised model seeks to eliminate the "organizational pressures" that are responsible for creating barriers to trust.[215] Organizational systems can be responsible for creating disproportionate power among patients and medical facilities and staff.[216] As a result, the revised model encourages trust in the organizations and physicians by having open discussions with patient participation in the revised consent process.

4). Patient Safety Systems

Unlike the current model, the revised model of informed consent will promote additional patient safety in the area of pleiotropic genetic testing. The revised model encourages system-thinking in order to promote patient safety. Because of the complexity of pleiotropic genetic testing, the typical individual approach cannot handle the amount of information, the multifactorial nature of many diseases, and the consequences of having multiple findings for one test.[217] The system of patient safety includes the accountability and transparency measures.[218]

Also the revised model adheres to a proactive, preventive approach to patient safety.[219] The revised model encourages adopting organizational measures in order to protect patients from harm and promote patient safety.[220] In pleiotropic genetic testing, the revised model of informed consent needs to emphasize preventive measures in order to help patients understand the idea of pleiotropic genes before seri-

---

[213] David Shore, *The Trust Prescription for Healthcare: Building Your Reputation with Consumers*, xiii.

[214] David Orentlicher, "Genetic Privacy in the Patient-Physician Relationship," 83–84.

[215] David Shore, *The Trust Prescription for Healthcare: Building Your Reputation with Consumers*, 40.

[216] Bill Runciman, Alan Merry, and Merrilyn Walton, *Safety and Ethics in Healthcare*, 96.

[217] Colleen McBride, Deborah Bowen, Lawrence Brody, et al., "Future Health Applications of Genomics: Priorities for Communication, Behavioral, and Social Sciences Research," 562.

[218] George Lundberg, *Severed Trust: Why American Medicine Hasn't Been Fixed,* 176.

[219] Colleen McBride, Deborah Bowen, Lawrence Brody, et al., "Future Health Applications of Genomics: Priorities for Communication, Behavioral, and Social Sciences Research," 563.

[220] Bill Runciman, Alan Merry, and Merrilyn Walton, *Safety and Ethics in Healthcare*, 241; George Lundberg, *Severed Trust: Why American Medicine Hasn't Been Fixed,* 255.

ous problems arise.[221] In the revised model, patient safety is fostered by having systems of accountability and transparency to establish preventive measures that promote the safety of patients considering PGT.

The revised model encourages internal and external accountability by promoting communication among medical departments and institutional policies. The revised model requires transparency with physician discussions and consent requirements. The revised model encourages trust in the organizations and physicians by having open discussions with patient participation in the revised consent process. In the revised model, patient safety is fostered by having systems of accountability and transparency to establish preventive measures as systems that promote the safety of patients considering PGT.

3. Case Study

The last section will look at a case study concerning pleiotropic genetic testing and informed consent. The case study will be presented. Then, the case study will apply the revised model of informed consent.

a. Morgan

This case study looks at Morgan, who is a 20 year old college student. Morgan started running track and field when he was a 19 year old freshman at his school. After winning several races, he wanted to broaden his running and start training for a triathlon. However, just recently his father died from a heart attack due to severe coronary heart disease (CHD). Morgan also remembers that another relative had CHD as well. Because of the level of endurance training and strenuous activity he has to do to prepare for the triathlon, Morgan is concerned about his risk of heart disease. While he has no symptoms of heart disease or CAD, he does not want to take an unnecessary risk. As a result, Morgan decides to go to his doctor and ask about PGT for CAD.

Morgan's doctor discusses his increased risk due to the family history of CAD and CHD and the recommendation of the American Heart Association (AHA) and the American College of Sports Medicine (ACSM) that there should be a doctor's approval before strenuous exercise if there is a heart condition.[222] As a result, the doctor informs Morgan that he might want to participate in PGT for the APOE gene which can determine an individual's risk of developing CAD. Even though he is asymptomatic at the moment, Morgan is concerned about the stress and excessive exercise involved in training for a triathlon.

---

[221] Robert Wachbroit, "The Question Not Asked: The Challenge of Pleiotropic Genetic Tests," 131–132; Lewis Vaughn, *Bioethics: Principles, Issues, and Cases*, 465–66.

[222] Michael Shipe, "Exercising with Coronary Heart Disease."

After asking about the risks and benefits of testing, his doctor informs him that the APOE gene also has implications for Alzheimer's disease. When testing the APOE gene for CAD, having a positive test for the ε4 allele means that the individual has a higher risk for developing hyperlipidemia and atherosclerosis which would result in a higher incidence of heart attacks. However, if the individual tested positive for the ε4 allele on the APOE gene, the individual also has a higher risk of developing Alzheimer's disease later in life.[223]

However, his doctor also informs him that if he does have a higher risk of CAD, then he could have increased heart problems while training for the triathlon. While exercise can help those with CAD, continual, strenuous activity, like training for a triathlon, can reduce arterial function which could increase the likelihood of having a heart attack.[224] While sudden cardiac death occurs more often in those with heart deformities, sometimes sudden death can occur in younger individuals involved in strenuous sports due to a heart attack in those with a family history of severe CAD.[225]

As a result of all of this information, Morgan is not quite sure whether or not he should participate in PGT for the APOE gene. Because of the complicated information presented, his doctor recommends participating in genetic counseling. At the end of the visit, Morgan decides to go home and discuss the information with his family.

b. Application

This section will apply the revised model of informed consent to the case study involving Morgan's decision. Contrasting the current and revised models of consent can help to establish the importance of the revised model. By applying the revised model of informed consent, Morgan can be better prepared to make the decision of whether or not to get tested for the APOE gene.

Comprehension is one of the first components of the revised model of informed consent. First, the current model uses a standardized approach to consent that typically focuses on the autonomous patient signing a consent form without much discussion. On the other hand, the revised model adopts a personalized approach to consent that emphasizes extensive discussion with the patient as an autonomous agent. In this case, Morgan's doctor has discussed many of the implications of pleiotropic testing. The revised model encourages additional personalization of

---

[223] Robert Wachbroit, "The Question Not Asked: The Challenge of Pleiotropic Genetic Tests," 133.

[224] Ellen A. Dawson, Greg P. Whyte, Mark A. Black, et al., "Changes in Vascular and Cardiac Function after Prolonged Strenuous Exercise in Humans," 1564–1565; Hope Gillette, "Strenuous Exercise Puts Heart Health at Risk, Study Says."

[225] Leonard Cobb and W. Douglas Weaver, "Exercise: A Risk for Sudden Death in Patients with Coronary Heart Disease," 215; Timothy Noakes, "Sudden Death and Exercise."

information such as the information that Morgan started training for a triathlon.[226] The information involved in an autonomous decision for PGT is different for almost all patients. Second, since the current model emphasizes the consent form, there is insufficient time and communication for understanding the meaning of PGT risk. However, in this case, the doctor took time to explain the meaning of pleiotropic genetic testing for the APOE gene. The revised model focuses on a process that provides time for communication to foster an understanding of the complex meaning of PGT risk. Third, the current doctor-patient relationship focuses upon the patient freely signing the consent form without sufficient education of the patient about the meaning of PGT. On the other hand, the revised model emphasizes the doctor-patient relationship as an interactive process to ensure sufficient education of the patient about the meaning of PGT. In this case, Morgan's doctor took the time and effort to explain the testing. Overall, the revised model encourages more education in order to be able to understand the implications of pleiotropic genetic testing.[227]

Disclosure is the second aspect of both the current and revised models of informed consent. First, the current model focuses on medical information in a standardized approach of consent. As previously described, the study by Cooper, Nelson, and Ross illustrated that not a lot of researchers discussed the idea of having multiple findings for APOE testing in the consent form.[228] However, in this study, Morgan's doctor informed Morgan about the risks and benefits of pleiotropic genetic testing including the fact that if Morgan tests positive for an increased risk of CAD, then he could also have a higher risk of developing Alzheimer's disease.[229] The revised model addresses not only medical information but all other relevant information for the patient to consider for consent, including the fact that some PGT diseases might not have any available treatment. Second, the current model recommends non-directive counseling, and does not require counseling. In this case study, Morgan's doctor recommends genetic counseling, but the revised model requires genetic counseling both before and after testing. The revised model requires counseling and adopts value transparency and non-directive counseling. In this model, genetic counselors should use a decision tree, which is a tool to look at all the information that goes into a decision to undergo pleiotropic genetic testing.[230] In this case, Morgan needs to analyze his risk of CAD, his increased exercise level from triathlon training, and his possible susceptibility to Alzheimer's disease.

Voluntariness is the third aspect of the current and revised models. First, in the current model, there are no specific measures to address or avoid multiple sources of external pressures which increase the possibility of coercion upon the individual. However, the revised model addresses external pressures on the patient and the fam-

---

[226] Tom Beauchamp and James Childress, *Principles of Biomedical Ethics,* 127.

[227] Robert Wachbroit, "The Question Not Asked: The Challenge of Pleiotropic Genetic Tests," 138.

[228] Zachary Cooper, Robert Nelson, and Lainie Ross, "Informed Consent for Genetic Research Involving Pleiotropic Genes: An Empirical Study of ApoE Research," 6–9.

[229] Robert Wachbroit, "The Question Not Asked: The Challenge of Pleiotropic Genetic Tests," 138.

[230] Thomas Goetz, *The Decision Tree,* xii–xiii, 47–48, 197.

ily (such as pressures by the family for the patient to be tested and pressure upon the family regarding testing outcomes) to alleviate or resolve external coercion upon the patient. In this case, before participating in PGT, the doctors and counselors should inquire into the reasons Morgan wants to get tested in order to eliminate the idea of possible sources of coercion.[231] Second, the current model does not take into consideration all family-related implications which can lead to coercion of family members. In this case, there are multiple family-related implications because of the risk of Alzheimer's disease. As a result, the revised model includes family-related concerns before testing and identifies ways to help the patient struggle with family-related PGT information. In this case, Morgan needs to discuss the implications of APOE testing with his family since it could produce results for Alzheimer's disease.[232] The doctors and counselors should encourage discussion of family implications.

Patient safety is the last component of the revised model. This aspect is a new component which is not found in the current model. First, the revised model encourages internal and external accountability by promoting communication among medical departments and institutional policies. In this case, the accountability of pleiotropic genetic testing is important to Morgan's decision in order to encourage safety. Second, the revised model requires transparency with physician discussions and consent requirements. In this case, Morgan's doctor should be transparent with his discussions and the consent forms. Third, the revised model encourages trust in the organizations and physicians by having open discussions with patient participation in the revised consent process. Because Morgan's doctor already encouraged open discussions, trust can be promoted in this case study even further by having additional discussions with the counselor as well. Fourth, in the revised model, patient safety is fostered by having systems of accountability and transparency to establish preventive measures as systems that promote the safety of patients considering PGT. Morgan's doctor can encourage patient safety when he describes to Morgan the systems of accountability and transparency within the revised model of consent in order to encourage an appropriate decision for pleiotropic testing.[233]

In this case study, Morgan needs to take into consideration all of the aspects of the revised model of consent, which includes comprehension, disclosure, voluntariness, and patient safety. After analyzing each area, Morgan should be able to make an appropriate, ethical decision about PGT for the APOE gene. By applying the revised model of consent to his decision, he can decide whether or not he needs to have the testing performed before he continues training for the triathlon.

---

[231] Linda Farber Post, Jeffrey Blustein, and Nancy Neveloff Dubler, *Handbook for Health Care Ethics Committees*, 42–43.

[232] Martin Richards, "How Distinctive is Genetic Information?" 681.

[233] George Lundberg, *Severed Trust: Why American Medicine Hasn't Been Fixed*, 176; Colleen McBride, Deborah Bowen, Lawrence Brody, et al., "Future Health Applications of Genomics: Priorities for Communication, Behavioral, and Social Sciences Research," 563.

C. Conclusion

The revised model involves the foundational aspects of consent.[234] In each section, the components of the revised model of consent (comprehension, disclosure, voluntariness, and patient safety) were applied to a specific topic. The first topic was DTC genetic testing. This section analyzed what happens when research and medical care merge. Miller and Wertheimer say that unless specifically stated, consent for medical care does not carry over into consent for research.[235] While this statement seems obvious, with some tests like DTC genetic testing, the results can illustrate a level of interdependence between medical care and research. Thus, any time genetic tests for patient care has an association with genetic research, the individuals should be aware of that fact and be able to consent accordingly. The second topic was pleiotropic genetic testing. This section addresses how multiple findings for a genetic test can affect informed consent. Because of the nature of pleiotropic genes, Ellen Wright Clayton explains that incidental findings which include the ideas of pleiotropy should certainly be addressed in informed consent.[236] If the individual understands that pleiotropic genetic testing will yield results about multiple diseases and if this information is disclosed before participating in the test, a person should be able to make an informed choice.

With all the new technologies and genetic tests being created, sometimes the new tests can create some serious concerns. In order to be able to continue the advances of medicine, it is important to balance the protection of patients and research participants with the innovation of the medical and research fields. Informed consent plays an important role in the ethical decision making of patients and research participants. As a result, the revised model of informed consent can help to eliminate some of the harms that might arise from the progression of medicine and research.[237]

References

23andMe. "About Us." Accessed May 5, 2010. https://www.23andme.com/.

23andMe. "Personal Genome Service: How it Works." Accessed May 4, 2010. https://www.23andme.com/howitworks/.

Aktan-Collan, Katja, Jukka-Pekka Mecklin, Albert de la Chapelle, et al. "Evaluation of a Counselling Protocol for Predictive Genetic Testing for Hereditary Non-Polyposis Colorectal Cancer." *Journal of Medical Genetics* 37:2 (February 2000): 108–113.

---

[234] Barbara Bowles Biesecker, "Privacy in Genetic Counseling," 110.

[235] Franklin Miller and Alan Wertheimer, *The Ethics of Consent*, 377–379; Albert Jonsen, *The Birth of Bioethics*, 143.

[236] Ellen Wright Clayton, "Incidental Findings in Genetics Research Using Archived DNA," 290.

[237] Tony McGleenan, "Genetic Testing for Cancer Predisposition- An Ongoing Debate- Genetic Screening Forum," 122–123.

American College of Medical Genetics/American Society of Human Genetics Working Group on ApoE and Alzheimer disease. "Statement on Use of Apolipoprotein E Testing for Alzheimer Disease." *The Journal of the American Medical Association* 274:20 (1995): 1627–1629.

American Heart Association. "Coronary Artery Disease- Coronary Heart Disease." Accessed July 21, 2013. http://www.heart.org/HEARTORG/Conditions/More/MyHeartandStrokeNews/Coronary-Artery-Disease--The-ABCs-of-CAD_UCM_436416_Article.jsp.

American Medical Association. "Direct-to-Consumer Genetic Testing." Accessed May 3, 2010. http://www.ama-assn.org/ama1/pub/upload/mm/464/dtc-genetic-test.pdf.

Andrews, Lori B. "Gen-Etiquette: Genetic Information, Family Relationships, and Adoption." In *Genetic Secrets: Protecting Privacy and Confidentiality in the Genetic Era*, edited by Mark Rothstein, 255–280. New Haven, CT: Yale University Press, 1997.

Arnold, Robert M. and Charles W. Lidz. "Informed Consent: Clinical Aspects of Consent in Health Care." In *Taking Sides: Clashing Views on Bioethical Issues*, edited by Carol Levine, 4–14. Boston: McGraw Hill Higher Education, 2010.

Ball, David, Audrey Tyler, and Peter Harper. "Predictive Testing of Adults and Children." In *Genetic Counselling*, edited by Angus Clarke, 63–94. New York: Routledge, 1994.

Beal, Kathy. "Statement on Direct-to-Consumer Genetic Testing: Genetics Professionals Should Be Part of Genetic Testing Process Says American College of Medical Genetics." *American College of Medical Genetics* (September 24, 2007): 1–2.

Beauchamp, Tom L. "Informed Consent: Its History, Meaning, and Present Challenges." *Cambridge Quarterly of Healthcare Ethics* 20 (2011): 515–523.

Beauchamp, Tom and James Childress. *Principles of Biomedical Ethics*. New York: Oxford University Press, 2001.

Berdik, Chris. "Genetic Tests Give Consumers Hints About Disease Risk; Critics Have Misgivings." *Washington Post*. (January 26, 2010): Special, 1–2.

Biesecker, Barbara Bowles. "Privacy in Genetic Counseling." In *Genetic Secrets: Protecting Privacy and Confidentiality in the Genetic Era*, edited by Mark Rothstein, 108–125. New Haven, CT: Yale University Press, 1997.

Bredenoord, Annelien L., Hester Y. Kroes, Edwin Cuppen, et al. "Disclosure of Individual Genetic Data to Research Participants: The Debate Reconsidered." *Trends in Genetics* 27:2 (February 2011): 41–47.

Buccafurni, Diana. "Reconsidering the Facilitation of Autonomous Decision Making in Genetic Counseling." PhD diss., University of Utah, August, 2008.

Burgess, Michael. "Beyond Consent: Ethical and Social Issues in Genetic Testing." In *Contemporary Issues in Bioethics*, edited by Tom Beauchamp and LeRoy Walters, 507–512. Belmont, CA: Wadsworth Publishing Company, 1999.

Carter, Ashley and Andrew Nguyen. "Antagonistic Pleiotropy as a Widespread Mechanism for the Maintenance of Polymorphic Disease Alleles." *BMC Medical Genetics* 12:160 (2011): 1–13.

Cassidy, Michael, J. Scott Roberts, Thomas Bird, et al. "Comparing Test-Specific Distress of Susceptibility versus Deterministic Genetic Testing for Alzheimer's Disease." *Alzheimer's & Dementia* 4 (2008): 406–413.

Cervantes, Sebastián, Lluís Samarancha, José Manuel Vidal-Taboadaa, et al. "Genetic Variation in *APOE* Cluster Region and Alzheimer's Disease Risk." *Neurobiology of Aging* 32 (2011): 2107.e7–2107.e17.

Chamberlain, Matt, Paul Baird, Mohamed Dirani, et al. "Unraveling a Complex Genetic Disease: Age-related Macular Degeneration." *Survey of Ophthalmology* 51:6 (November-December 2006): 576–586.

Clarke, Angus. "Genetic Counseling." In *The Concise Encyclopedia of the Ethics of New Technologies*, edited by Ruth Chadwick, 131–146. San Diego, CA: Academic Press, 2001.

Clayton, Ellen Wright. "Incidental Findings in Genetics Research Using Archived DNA." *Journal of Law, Medicine & Ethics* (Summer 2008): 286–291.

Cobb, Leonard and W. Douglas Weaver. "Exercise: A Risk for Sudden Death in Patients with Coronary Heart Disease." *Journal of the American College of Cardiology* 7:1 (January 1986): 215–219.

Collins, Francis. *The Language of Life*. New York: Harper Collins Publishers, 2010.

Cooper, Zachary, Robert Nelson, and Lainie Ross. "Informed Consent for Genetic Research Involving Pleiotropic Genes: An Empirical Study of ApoE Research." *IRB: Ethics and Human Research* 28:5 (September/October 2006): 1–11.

Dawson, Ellen A., Greg P. Whyte, Mark A. Black, et al. "Changes in Vascular and Cardiac Function after Prolonged Strenuous Exercise in Humans." *Journal of Applied Physiology* 105 (November 2008): 1562–1568.

Evans, Jeff. "DTC Genetic Tests Seen as Problematic." *Internal Medicine News* 42:17 (October 1, 2009): Genetic Tests 4.

Farkas, Daniel, and Carol Holland. "Direct-to-Consumer Genetic Testing: Two Sides of the Coin." *Journal of Molecular Diagnostics* 11:4 (2009): 263–265.

Fulda, KG and Lykens K. "Ethical Issues in Predictive Genetic Testing: A Public Health Perspective." *Journal of Medical Ethics* 32:3 (March 2003): 143–147.

Gaff, Clara, Elly Lynch, and Lesley Spencer. "Predictive Testing of Eighteen Year Olds: Counseling Challenges." *Journal of Genetic Counseling* 15:4 (August 2006): 245–251.

Gillette, Hope. "Strenuous Exercise Puts Heart Health at Risk, Study Says." Last modified June 11, 2012. http://www.voxxi.com/strenuous-exercise-heart-health-risks/.

Goetz, Thomas. *The Decision Tree*. New York: Rodale Inc., 2010.

Goodwin, Kristine. "Information Overload? National Conference of State Legislatures." *State Legislatures Magazine*, September 2008. Accessed December 10, 2011. http://www.ncsl.org/issues-research/health/state-legislatures-magazine-information-overload.aspx.

Govindaraju, Diddahally, L. Adrienne Cupples, William B. Kannel, et al. "Genetics of the Framingham Heart Study Population." *Advances in Genetics* 62 (2008): 33–65.

Guillaume, Frederic and Sarah Otto. "Gene Functional Trade-Offs and the Evolution of Pleiotropy." *Genetics* 192 (December 2012): 1389–1409.

Harris, Marion, Ingrid Winship, Merle Spriggs. "Controversies and Ethical Issues in Cancer-Genetics Clinics." *Lancet Oncology* 6 (2005): 301–310.

Hayes, Catherine. "Genetic Testing for Huntington's Disease—A Family Issue." *The New England Journal of Medicine* 327:20 (November 12, 1992): 1449–1451.

Henderson, Mark. "Cashing in on Your Genes." *The Times* (January 7, 2010): 2.

Hsiung, Ging-Yuek Robin and A. Dessa Sadovnick. "Genetics and Dementia: Risk Factors, Diagnosis, and Management." *Alzheimer's & Dementia* 3 (2007): 418–427.

Hubbard, Ruth and R.C. Lewontin "Genetic Testing for Disease Predisposition, Pitfalls of Genetic Testing," In *Intervention and Reflection*, edited by Ronald Munson, 352–354. Belmont, CA: Wadsworth Publishing, 2007.

Jonsen, Albert. *The Birth of Bioethics*. New York: Oxford University Press, 1998.

Kahn, Jeffrey. "Informed Consent in the Context of Communities." *The Journal of Nutrition* 135:4 (April 2005): 918–920.

Kaye, Jane. "The Regulation of Direct-to-Consumer Genetic Tests." *Human Molecular Genetics* 17:2 (2008): R180–183.

Kilner, John, Rebecca Pentz, Frank Young, eds. *Genetic Ethics*. Grand Rapids, MI: William B Eerdmans Publishing Company, 1997.

Kraft, Peter, Ph.D., David Hunter. "Genetic Risk Prediction – Are We There Yet?" *The New England Journal of Medicine*. 360:17 (April 23, 2009): 1701–1703.

Lei, Hsien-Hsien, Dr. "Dr. Robert Marion on Direct-to-Consumer Genetic Testing." *Books About DNA, DNA Testing, Personalities with DNA*, August 26, 2009. Accessed September 2, 2011. www.eyeondna.com/2009/08/26/dr-robert-marion-on-direct-to-consumer-genetic-testing/.

Lo, Bernard. *Resolving Ethical Dilemmas*. Philadelphia, PA: Lippincott Williams and Wilkins, 2005.

Lundberg, George. *Severed Trust: Why American Medicine Hasn't Been Fixed*. New York: Basic Books, 2000.

Macklin, Ruth. "The Inner Workings of an Ethics Committee: Latest Battle over Jehovah's Witnesses." In *Bioethics: An Introduction to the History, Methods, and Practice*, edited by Nancy

Jecker, Albert Jonsen, and Robert Pearlman, 232–235. Sudbury, MA: Jones and Bartlett Publishers, 2007.

Marietta, Cynthia and Amy McGuire. "Direct-to-Consumer Genetic Testing: Is It the Practice of Medicine?" *Journal of Law, Medicine & Ethics* 37:2 (Summer 2009): 369–374.

Markel, Dorene S. and Beverly M. Yashar. "The Interface Between the Practice of Medical Genetics and Human Genetic Research: What Every Genetic Counselor Needs to Know," *Journal of Genetic Counseling*, 13:5 (October 2004): 351–368.

Marteau, Theresa, Scott Roberts, Susan LaRusse, et al. "Predictive Genetic Testing for Alzheimer's Disease: Impact upon Risk Perception." *Risk Analysis* 25:2 (2005): 397–404.

Martin, Douglas and Heather Greenwood. "Public Perceptions of Ethical Issues Regarding Adult Predictive Genetic Testing." *Health Care Analysis* 18:2 (2010): 103–112.

Matloff, Ellen, Arthur Caplan. "Direct to Confusion: Lessons Learned from Marketing BRCA Testing." *The American Journal of Bioethics* 8:6 (2008): 5–8.

Mayeux, R., M. Saunders, S. Shea, et al. "Utility of the Apolipoprotein E Genotype in the Diagnosis of Alzheimer's Disease." *New England Journal of Medicine* 338:8 (1998): 506–511.

McBride, Colleen, Deborah Bowen, Lawrence Brody, et al. "Future Health Applications of Genomics: Priorities for Communication, Behavioral, and Social Sciences Research." *American Journal of Preventive Medicine* 38:5 (2010): 556–565.

McGleenan, Tony. "Genetic Testing for Cancer Predisposition- An Ongoing Debate- Genetic Screening Forum." *The Lancet Oncology* 1 (October 2000): 118–124.

Messner, Donna. "Informed Choice in Direct-to-Consumer Genetic Testing for Alzheimer and Other Diseases: Lessons from Two Cases." *New Genetics in Sociology* 30:1 (2011): 59–72.

Miller, Franklin and Alan Wertheimer. *The Ethics of Consent.* New York: Oxford University Press, 2010.

Mitchell, Philip, Bettina Meiser, Alex Wilde, et al. "Predictive and Diagnostic Genetic Testing in Psychiatry." *Psychiatric Clinics of North America* 33:1 (March 2010): 225–243.

Nassar, Bassam, Kenneth Rockwood, Susan Kirkland, et al. "Improved Prediction of Early-onset Coronary Artery Disease using APOE ε4, BChE-K, PPARγ2 Pro12 and ENOS T-786C in a Polygenic Model." *Clinical Biochemistry* 39 (2006): 109–114.

Navigenics. "How our Services Work." Accessed May 4, 2010. http://www.navigenics.com/visitor/what_we_offer/how_it_works/.

Nelson, William A., Julia Neily, Peter Mills, et al. "Collaboration of Ethics and Patient Safety Programs: Opportunities to Promote Quality Care." *HEC Forum*, 20:1 (2008): 15–27.

Noakes, Timothy. "Sudden Death and Exercise." *Sportscience* 2:4 (November 1998). Accessed January 10, 2013. http://www.sportsci.org/jour/9804/tdn.html.

Orentlicher, David. "Genetic Privacy in the Patient-Physician Relationship." In *Genetic Secrets: Protecting Privacy and Confidentiality in the Genetic Era*, edited by Mark Rothstein, 77–91. New Haven, CT: Yale University Press, 1997.

Pollack, Andrew. "Consumers Slow to Embrace the Age of Genomics." *New York Times* (March 20, 2010): B1.

Post, Linda Farber, Jeffrey Blustein, and Nancy Neveloff Dubler. *Handbook for Health Care Ethics Committees.* Baltimore: The John Hopkins University Press, 2007.

Prainsack, B., and J. Reardon. "Misdirected precaution." *Nature* 456:7218 (November 6, 2008): 34–35.

Pray, Leslie. "DTC Genetic Testing: 23andMe, DNA Direct and Genelex." *Nature Education* 1:1 (2008): 1–4.

Richards, Martin. "How Distinctive is Genetic Information?" *Studies in History and Philosophy of Biological & Biomedical Sciences* 32:4 (2001): 663–687.

Roberts, J. Scott and Wendy Uhlmann. "Genetic Susceptibility Testing for Neurodegenerative Diseases: Ethical and Practice Issues." *Progress in Neurobiology* 110 (2013): 89–101. Accessed March 10, 2013. http://dx.doi.org/10.1016/j.pneurobio.2013.02.005.

Runciman, Bill, Alan Merry, and Merrilyn Walton. *Safety and Ethics in Healthcare.* Burlington, VT: Ashgate Publishing Company, 2007.

Schipper, Hyman. "Presymptomatic Apolipoprotein E Genotyping for Alzheimer's Disease Risk Assessment and Prevention." *Alzheimer's & Dementia* 7 (2011): e118-e123.

Sharpe, Neil F. and Ronald Carter. *Genetic Testing: Care, Consent, and Liability*. Hoboken, New Jersey: John Wiley & Sons, Inc., 2006.

Shedden, Mary. "Genetic Screenings are no Replacement for Medical Advice." *The Tampa Tribune* (April 1, 2010): 1.

Shipe, Michael. "Exercising with Coronary Heart Disease." *American College of Sports Medicine*. Last modified January 19, 2012. http://www.acsm.org/access-public-information/articles/2012/01/19/exercising-with-coronary-heart-disease.

Shore, David. *The Trust Prescription for Healthcare: Building Your Reputation with Consumers*. Chicago: Health Administration Press, 2005.

Singer, Emily. "Off-the-Shelf Genetic Testing on Display." *Technology Review*, June 9, 2009. Accessed October 2, 2011. http://www.technologyreview.com/news/413745/off-the-shelf-genetic-testing-on-display/2/.

Sivakumaran, Shanya, Felix Agakov, Evropi Theodoratou, et al., "Abundant Pleiotropy in Human Complex Diseases and Traits," *The American Journal of Human Genetics* 89 (November 11, 2011): 607–618.

St. George-Hyslop, Peter and Agnes Petit. "Molecular Biology and Genetics of Alzheimer's Disease." *C. R. Biologies* 328 (2004): 119–130.

Stearns, Frank. "One Hundred Years of Pleiotropy: A Retrospective." *Genetics* 186 (November 2010): 767–773.

Tauber, Alfred. *Patient Autonomy and the Ethics of Responsibility*. Cambridge, MA: The MIT Press, 2005.

Trepanier, Angela, Mary Ahrens, Wendy McKinnon, et al. "Genetic Cancer Risk Assessment and Counseling: Recommendations of the National Society of Genetic Counselors." *Journal of Genetic Counseling* 13:2 (April 2004): 83–114.

U.S. National Library of Medicine. "What is Direct-to-Consumer Genetic Testing?" Accessed May 3, 2010. http://ghr.nlm.nih.gov/handbook/testing/directtoconsumer.

Vaughn, Lewis. *Bioethics: Principles, Issues, and Cases*. New York: Oxford University Press, 2009.

Wachbroit, Robert. "The Question Not Asked: The Challenge of Pleiotropic Genetic Tests." *Kennedy Institute of Ethics Journal* 8:2 (June 1998): 131–144.

Wear, Stephen. *Informed Consent: Patient Autonomy and Clinician Beneficence within Health Care*. Washington, DC: Georgetown University Press, 1998.

Wells, Rebecca Erwin and Ted J. Kaptchuk. "To Tell the Truth, the Whole Truth, May Do Patients Harm: The Problem of the Nocebo Effect for Informed Consent." *American Journal of Bioethics* 12:3 (March 2012): 22–29.

Wexler, Alice. "On Not Taking the Test." Huntington's Disease Society of America. Accessed October 2, 2011. http://www.hdsa.org/images/content/1/1/11710.pdf.

Chapter 6
Conclusion

This book develops a revised model of informed consent for PGT. The need for this model arises from distinguishing characteristics of PGT, which make it distinctive from other forms of health-related testing. These characteristics are: the difficulty in understanding genetic risks and probabilities; the problem of treatment options for diagnosed genetic traits; and the concern with family-related genetic information.

Since none of the literature has merged the current components of consent (understanding, disclosure, and voluntariness) and the distinguishing characteristics of PGT together in order to form a revised model, this book addresses an important facet for modification. Given the setting of the literature, the book's thesis is distinctive, because it establishes a revised model by aligning the three distinguishing characteristics of PGT with the three widely recognized components in the current model.

The first chapter introduces the topic and outline. The second chapter explains PGT to identify these characteristics that shape the revised model of consent. The third chapter explores the history of consent to identify the widely recognized components of consent (understanding, disclosure, and voluntariness) that represent the current model. The fourth chapter explains the revised model by aligning the three distinguishing characteristics of PGT with the three widely recognized components in the current model. In the fifth chapter, the revised model is applied to DTC and pleiotropic genetic testing. In the sixth chapter, the conclusion looks at implementation of the revised model and a comparison of the current and revised models of consent.

A. Implementation of the Revised Model of Informed Consent

The revised model of informed consent for PGT tries to emphasize and clarify the expectations, goals, and challenges of implementation to encourage better medical treatment for individuals. This section of implementation involves a discussion of

© Springer International Publishing Switzerland 2015
J. Minor, *Informed Consent in Predictive Genetic Testing,*
DOI 10.1007/978-3-319-17416-7_6

the responses to failed attempts at reform, system changes, reimbursement changes, and measuring the effectiveness of implementation.

1. Response to Failed Attempts at Reform

The first part will look at some responses to failed attempts at reforming consent and the research that has been done to improve consent. Sometimes attempts to improve informed consent can fail, because the consent either did not meet standards or those standards are unrealistic. Responses to failure can include looking for lower, more practical standards; confirming current standards and keep going with existing clinical and research practices; and/or rethinking and transforming informed consent.[1] Like the authors of the book *Rethinking Informed Consent in Bioethics*, this book chooses to rethink and transform informed consent in the area of PGT. Instead of continuing on with the current model, this book adopts a revised model of informed consent for PGT that addresses the inconsistencies among the current model and the ethical ideals for informed consent.

Catharine Lucey and Wiley Souba suggest that in order to resolve complex problems, new measures need to be implemented. The authors promote identifying new information to help solve difficulties. However, while the novel knowledge and changes to the current way of thinking can be helpful, implementing new measures could also result in unpredictable and/or inconsistent results.[2] Because implementing completely new changes could encourage additional and unnecessary problems, this book promotes a revised model. As a result, this work merges both current practices and new practices for consent in order to make up the revised model of informed consent for PGT. This foundation is important to the implementation of the revised model.

2. System Changes

Implementation of the revised model of informed consent for PGT involves a new way of thinking. This new way of thinking involves system changes. Catherine Lucey and Wiley Souba suggest that often changes to solve complex problems include establishing new "rules and regulations or demanding more resources."[3] However, the authors suggest that those typical implementations might not change the fundamental difficulties and challenges that occur. While the authors are emphasizing the problems of professionalism in this article, the underlying principles of solving complex problems are still the same.

---

[1] Neil C. Manson and Onora O'Neill, *Rethinking Informed Consent in Bioethics*, 185–186, 198.

[2] Catherine Lucey and Wiley Souba, "The Problem with the Problem of Professionalism," 1019.

[3] Catherine Lucey and Wiley Souba, "The Problem with the Problem of Professionalism," 1019.

Since the previous chapters have shown that there are still inadequacies of the current model, the current model does not seem to adequately address the essential problems of consent. Thus, in order for the revised model to be implemented adequately, the revised model encourages system changes. System changes can address some of the fundamental challenges to informed consent. By implementing system changes, those changes can also help the individual's attitudes and behaviors to change as well over time. Implementing the revised model requires changes to the system of consent.

The revised model encourages a proactive approach to consent instead of a reactive approach. Kathryn M. Taylor and Merrijoy J. Kelner in the *Canadian Medical Association Journal* conclude that if professionals want to implement "proactive" instead of "reactive" measures towards PGT, then medical organizations and staff have to "define clearly the expectations and prerogatives of all physicians. If not, physicians will be obligated to respond to rules and regulations imposed from outside the profession, to which they are unlikely to adhere."[4] Thus, consistent and appropriate system changes need to be implemented before the revised model can be effective. If there is not adequate thought given to the system changes, there can be problems with the implementation and adherence of the revised model of consent.

3. Reimbursement Changes

In 1982, the President's Commission concluded that people were interested in knowing their options and discussing their choice and values.[5] That idea has generally stayed constant to encourage disclosure and choices for treatments. Accordingly, Katz and Veatch encourage patient participation in choosing treatment options. As a result, increased communication through genetic counselors can assist in selecting a suitable treatment option for PGT even if the course of action is just continual surveillance.[6]

Another aspect to address before implementing the revised model is the reimbursement policies for counseling. In the current mode, the reimbursement policies typically emphasize diagnosis and treatment over prevention.[7] The current system pays for treatments and testing, but not necessarily patient discussions and counseling measures.[8] Arnold and Lidz suggest that the current model has the potential to discourage doctors and counselors from spending enough time discussing their

---

[4] Kathryn M. Taylor and Merrijoy J. Kelner, "The Emerging Role of the Physician in Genetic Counselling and Testing for Heritable Breast, Ovarian and Colon Cancer," 1158.

[5] Hana Osman, "History and Development of the Doctrine of Informed Consent," 45–46.

[6] Jay Katz, "Physicians and Patients: A History of Silence," 138; Robert Veatch, "Abandoning Informed Consent," 12.

[7] Stephen Wear, *Informed Consent,* 62; James Evans, "Health Care in the Age of Genetic Medicine," 1.

[8] Thomas Goetz, *The Decision Tree,* 122; Stephen Wear, *Informed Consent,* 62.

options with patients.[9] Hence, disclosure in order to select an appropriate treatment option can be compromised.

However, the revised model has more of an emphasis on prevention in order to reduce some of the challenging organizational aspects of the current model. Goetz suggests that prevention can help to facilitate appropriate institutional and reimbursement policies for counseling and education.[10] As a result, insurance companies can reimburse for proper counseling instead of just diagnosis and procedures.[11] Right now in the United States, doctors are not reimbursed well for talking to patients; they are reimbursed more for invasive tests.[12] Since the revised model is a process, this model will allow more time in order to promote patient reflection about the possible options.[13] It takes time to help patients understand their illness, clarify the therapeutic goals, elucidate any false perceptions, decide on treatment plan, and answer questions.[14] As a result, this model encourages counselors to set up multiple meetings with patients to discuss any questions or concerns. In the United Kingdom, the genetic counseling process involves a flexible amount of time with the patients to promote better decision-making about treatment and family disclosure options.[15] Because the revised model encourages more time and multiple counseling sessions, in order to adequately implement the revised model, there should be more genetic counselors.[16] However, there cannot be more genetic counselors unless the reimbursement policies of counseling change. If counselors are being encouraged to spend more time and take on more individuals, in order to implement the revised model appropriately, health care systems and insurance organizations need to ensure that counselors are reimbursed adequately. If not, the implementation of the revised model can suffer.

---

[9] Robert M. Arnold and Charles W. Lidz, "Informed Consent: Clinical Aspects of Consent in Health Care," 6–8; Eugene C. Rich, Wylie Burke, Caryl J. Heaton, et al., "Reconsidering the Family History in Primary Care," 277.

[10] Thomas Goetz, *The Decision Tree,* xiv–xvi; Stephen Wear, *Informed Consent,* 62.

[11] Eugene C. Rich, Wylie Burke, Caryl J. Heaton, et al., "Reconsidering the Family History in Primary Care," 277.

[12] Robert M. Arnold and Charles W. Lidz, "Informed Consent: Clinical Aspects of Consent in Health Care," 6–8; Thomas Goetz, *The Decision Tree,* xiv–xvi.

[13] Katja Aktan-Collan, Jukka-Pekka Mecklin, Albert de la Chapelle, et al., "Evaluation of a Counselling Protocol for Predictive Genetic Testing for Hereditary Non-Polyposis Colorectal Cancer," 111; Michael Arribas-Ayllon, Srikant Sarangi, and Angus Clarke, *Genetic Testing: Accounts of Autonomy, Responsibility and Blame,* 124; Thomas Goetz, *The Decision Tree,* xvii, 47, 67–68, 142, 197, 215; Neil C. Manson and Onora O'Neill, *Rethinking Informed Consent in Bioethics,* 85; Michael Hayden, "Predictive Testing for Huntington's Disease: A Universal Model?" 141.

[14] Robert M. Arnold and Charles W. Lidz, "Informed Consent: Clinical Aspects of Consent in Health Care," 6–8; Angela Trepanier, Mary Ahrens, Wendy McKinnon, et al., "Genetic Cancer Risk Assessment and Counseling: Recommendations of the National Society of Genetic Counselors," 93.

[15] Michael Arribas-Ayllon, Srikant Sarangi, and Angus Clarke, *Genetic Testing: Accounts of Autonomy, Responsibility and Blame,* 124.

[16] J. Scott Roberts and Wendy Uhlmann, "Genetic Susceptibility Testing for Neurodegenerative Diseases: Ethical and Practice Issues," 93.

4. Measuring the Effectiveness of Implementation

The last section looks at how the effectiveness of implementation is measured and analyzed. Being able to look at the effectiveness of informed consent is a crucial aspect. An article in the American Psychological Association Ethics Rounds suggests that there is a relationship between ethics and clinical care. Dr. Stephen Behnke of the American Psychological Association says "good ethics can promote good clinical care."[17] The revised model of informed consent for PGT can improve medical treatments, patient outcomes, and ethical decision making about proposed treatments and testing.[18] The improvement of medical care and decision making is one of the most important ways to measure the success of the revised model. Because the revised model adds the patient safety component to informed consent, the revised model encourages the promotion of safety in clinical and research care.

Also another way to measure the success of the revised model is the addition of communication. Because increased communication is promoted in every component, the revised model can be analyzed by the level of communication. Since the revised model promotes better communication about decision making, the value of communication should be the measure by which the model is analyzed instead of by many of the current legalistic rules.[19] Clarke suggests that patient satisfaction is a bad way to measure success of counseling, because often patients are receiving bad news.[20] While the satisfaction of the patient might not be high right after receiving certain information, if there is increased communication after receiving those results, many patients still feel the informed consent was successful. Looking at patient outcomes and the success of communication can be an appropriate method of analyzing the success of the revised model of informed consent.

In order to encourage a more effective revised model, Lucey and Souba suggest "continuous learning and adaptation."[21] The revised model encourages individuals to apply each component of consent to their decision-making process.[22] While changes of systems and attitudes can be difficult, the revised model strives to promote a more ethical approach to decision making for informed consent of PGT. The revised process model should be a continual "process where patient insight is developed and re-assessed" instead of the bureaucratic interferences.[23]

---

[17] Dr. Stephen Behnke, "Informed Consent and APA's New Ethics Code: Enhancing Client Autonomy, Improving Client Care," 80–81.

[18] Robert M. Arnold and Charles W. Lidz, "Informed Consent: Clinical Aspects of Consent in Health Care," 5.

[19] Neil C. Manson and Onora O'Neill, *Rethinking Informed Consent in Bioethics*, 198.

[20] Angus Clarke, "Genetic Counseling," 140–141.

[21] Catherine Lucey and Wiley Souba, "The Problem with the Problem of Professionalism," 1019.

[22] Bill Runciman, Alan Merry, and Merrilyn Walton, *Safety and Ethics in Healthcare*, 159.

[23] Robert M. Arnold and Charles W. Lidz, "Informed Consent: Clinical Aspects of Consent in Health Care," 4–5; Stephen Wear, *Informed Consent*, 95.

B. Comparison Comparison of the Current and Revised Models

In order to recognize the contribution of the revised model of informed consent, both models are summarized. This section will look at both the current and revised model's approach to each component including comprehension, disclosure, voluntariness, and patient safety. By pointing out the differences among the models, this section will be able to identify the role of the revised model and the importance of adopting the revised model of consent for PGT. The differences among the models demonstrate the disparities between reality and the ethical ideal.[24]

1. Comprehension

Comprehension of risk assessment includes autonomy, understanding genetic risks, and the doctor-patient relationship. Arnold and Lidz suggest that autonomy and beneficence are crucial aspects of both informed consent and "good medicine."[25] The current model uses a standardized approach to consent that typically focuses on the autonomous patient signing a consent form without much discussion. Since this model emphasizes the consent form, there is insufficient time and communication for understanding the meaning of PGT risk. The current doctor-patient relationship focuses upon the patient freely signing the consent form without sufficient education of the patient about the meaning of PGT. On the other hand, the revised model adopts a personalized approach to consent that emphasizes extensive discussion with the patient as an autonomous agent. The revised model focuses on a process that provides time for communication to foster an understanding of the complex meaning of PGT risk. The revised model emphasizes the doctor-patient relationship as an interactive process to ensure sufficient education of the patient about the meaning of PGT. Howard Brody suggests that today's culture can help to promote the doctor-patient relationship. He says that "When the physician builds a relationship with the patient in which the power can be shared over time, the ground is prepared for ensuring that the patient gets the most benefit out of medical care and also exercises autonomy to optimal degree."[26]

2. Disclosure

Disclosure to select an appropriate treatment option involves disclosure and genetic counseling. The current model focuses on medical information in a standardized approach of consent. The current model recommends non-directive counseling, and

---

[24] Catherine Lucey and Wiley Souba, "The Problem with the Problem of Professionalism," 1018.
[25] Robert M. Arnold and Charles W. Lidz, "Informed Consent: Clinical Aspects of Consent in Health Care," 8.
[26] Howard Brody, "The Physician-Patient Relationship," 96.

does not require counseling. Whereas, the revised model addresses not only medical information but all other relevant information for the patient to consider for consent, including the fact that some PGT diseases might not have any available treatment. The revised model requires counseling and adopts value transparency and non-directive counseling. Genetic counseling along with patient assessment and feedback mechanisms can encourage appropriate decision-making.[27]

3. Voluntariness

While autonomy is promoted for comprehension, too much emphasis on individual autonomy can lead to a harmful impact on a patient's level of voluntariness.[28] One lesson that can be learned from the Nazi experiments is the fact that no single principle should be focused on exclusively and those principles should always be applied to actual settings and not too theoretical in nature. Sometimes ethical principles can become too abstract and devoid of meaning for individual patients. Glover warns against this type of thinking, because this can sometimes cause problems for thinking that leads to a possible disconnect between the theoretical and practical ethics principles for consent.[29]

Voluntariness of consent discusses coercion and family-related implications. In the current model, there are no specific measures to address or avoid multiple sources of external pressures (such as pressures from relatives, the medical staff and community, and/or societal influences) which increase the possibility of coercion upon the individual. The current model does not take into consideration all family related implications which can lead to coercion of family members. Conversely, the revised model addresses external pressures on the patient and the family (such as pressures by the family for the patient to be tested and pressure upon the family regarding testing outcomes) to alleviate or resolve external coercion upon the patient. Because genetic information impacts the family, the revised model includes family-related concerns before testing and identifies ways to help the patient struggle with family-related PGT information.

4. Patient Safety

Patient safety consists of accountability, transparency, trust, and patient safety. This is a new component that is not in the current model. Stephen Wear says that even with all the regulating bodies and peer review committees for research that were developed in the past, some of the improvements "were not accomplished without the growth of a residual distrust within the society that physicians might use patients as guinea pigs."[30] This last component of consent addresses those issues.

---

[27] Thomas Goetz, *The Decision Tree,* xvii, 141–142, 197, 215; Stephen Wear, *Informed Consent,* 12, 95.

[28] Allen Buchanan, "From Chance to Choice: Genetics and Justice," 490.

[29] Jonathan Glover, "Eugenics: Some Lessons from the Nazi Experience," 471.

[30] Stephen Wear, *Informed Consent,* 31.

The revised model of consent requires nationally established systems of accountability for PGT that implement the revised components of consent in a transparent manner to foster trust in the emerging system of genetic-related services. The revised model encourages internal and external accountability by promoting communication among medical departments and institutional policies. The revised model requires transparency with physician discussions and consent requirements. The revised model encourages trust in the organizations and physicians by having open discussions with patient participation in the revised consent process. In the revised model, patient safety is fostered by having systems of accountability and transparency to establish preventive measures as systems that promote the safety of patients considering PGT.

While everyone agrees that informed consent is important, Sugarman, Jeremy, Douglas C. McCrory, Donald Powell, et al. question the reality and adequacy of informed consent. The authors state that there is "uncertainty" about the effectiveness of implementation, the impact of the current "theoretical understanding" on the value and reasonableness of consent, and the measures that might promote meaningful consent.[31] However, the revised model of consent addresses each one of those aspects in the previous chapters. The revised model of informed consent discusses the inadequacies of the current model and identifies ways to resolve the underlying problems in order to encourage ethical decision making in the informed consent process for PGT.

C. Contribution and Future Research

This book promotes a revised model of informed consent that specifically addresses the issues that arise from PGT. Since PGT is a little different than other types of genetic testing, having a revised approach to informed consent can help individuals come to a better decision about testing. Since PGT often produces a greater level of information, the revised model strives to help individuals address and handle appropriately the amount of information that results. Often the current model does not handle the amount of information well, and often times as a result, the individual is confused and makes inappropriate decisions about PGT. However by adopting the revised model, individuals can have a greater level of understanding PGT in general, and thus the individual will be able to make ethical decisions without coercion and misunderstandings. Also by having the new component of patient safety in the revised model, the individual considering PGT for research or medical purposes should be able to have a greater degree of trust in the medical system and health professionals. Because the current model does not specifically emphasize patient safety, the contribution of the revised model to safety can greatly impact the future of informed consent.

---

[31] Jeremy Sugarman, Douglas C. McCrory, Donald Powell, et al., "Empirical Research on Informed Consent: An Annotated Bibliography," S1.

The revised model for PGT emphasizes understanding the test, being able to make an appropriate decision based on adequate information, eliminating possible sources of coercion including family-related coercion, and promoting patient safety through new systems. The goal of the revised model of consent is to encourage an ethical decision making-process that specifically addresses the distinctive issues of PGT.

While this book provides the basic components of the revised model of consent (comprehension, disclosure, voluntariness, and patient safety), the revised model can be strengthened further by encouraging additional research. First, further research can be done analyzing the specific methods of encouraging each component. While this work gives specific methods of implementation for each component, additional research can propose more methods for encouraging comprehension, disclosure, voluntariness, and patient safety. Second, more research should be done to look into the revised process of genetic counseling for PGT. Since the revised model of consent handles genetic counseling differently, additional research should be done. Research can study how to implement the revised approach to counseling, how to handle the reimbursement of genetic counseling, and how to get more genetic counselors into the field of PGT. Third, more research is needed in order to fully implement a proactive and organizational approach to patient safety in informed consent. While many professionals might recognize the benefits of taking proactive measures, the health system has not completely conformed to this approach yet. Thus, additional research can look into how to encourage the application of a systematic, proactive approach to medicine and PGT. Since the revised model of consent for PGT cannot be fully implemented until there are system changes, this area should encourage significant research for the future.

Fourth, after implementation of the revised model of PGT, research should be conducted analyzing the specific successes and/or failures of the model. Then, if there are any risks or failures identified, research can be done to address those failures and seek new ways to handle the problems. Fifth, after implementation, research should be done comparing and contrasting the effectiveness of both the current and revised model of consent in specific situations such as DTC genetic testing and pleiotropic genetic testing. These are only a couple of areas identified to encourage additional research. However after analyzing and addressing each area, the revised model of consent can be strengthened even further to produce an effective process of informed consent for PGT.

References

Aktan-Collan, Katja, Jukka-Pekka Mecklin, Albert de la Chapelle, et al. "Evaluation of a Counselling Protocol for Predictive Genetic Testing for Hereditary Non-Polyposis Colorectal Cancer." *Journal of Medical Genetics* 37:2 (February 2000): 108–113.
Arnold, Robert M. and Charles W. Lidz. "Informed Consent: Clinical Aspects of Consent in Health Care." In *Taking Sides: Clashing Views on Bioethical Issues*, edited by Carol Levine, 4–14. Boston: McGraw Hill Higher Education, 2010.

Arribas-Ayllon, Michael, Srikant Sarangi, and Angus Clarke. *Genetic Testing: Accounts of Autonomy, Responsibility and Blame.* Abingdon, Oxon Oxford: Routledge Taylor and Francis Group, 2011.

Behnke, Stephen, Dr. "Informed Consent and APA's New Ethics Code: Enhancing Client Autonomy, Improving Client Care." *Ethics Rounds. American Psychological Association* 35:6 (June 2004): 80–81.

Brody, Howard. "The Physician-Patient Relationship." In *Medical Ethics*, edited by Robert Veatch, 75–101. Sudbury, MA: Jones and Bartlett Publishers, 1997.

Buchanan, Allen. "From Chance to Choice: Genetics and Justice." In *Contemporary Issues in Bioethics*, edited by Tom Beauchamp and LeRoy Walters, 485–495. Belmont, CA: Wadsworth Publishing Company, 1999.

Clarke, Angus. "Genetic Counseling." In *The Concise Encyclopedia of the Ethics of New Technologies*, edited by Ruth Chadwick, 131–146. San Diego, CA: Academic Press, 2001.

Evans, James. "Health Care in the Age of Genetic Medicine." *Genetics in Medicine* 10:1 (January 2008): 1–3.

Glover, Jonathan. "Eugenics: Some Lessons from the Nazi Experience." In *Contemporary Issues in Bioethics*, edited by Tom Beauchamp and LeRoy Walters, 467–472. Belmont, CA: Wadsworth Publishing Company, 1999.

Goetz, Thomas. *The Decision Tree.* New York: Rodale Inc., 2010.

Hayden, Michael. "Predictive Testing for Huntington's Disease: A Universal Model?" *The Lancet Neurology* 2 (March 2003): 141–142.

Katz, Jay. "Physicians and Patients: A History of Silence." In *Contemporary Issues in Bioethics*, edited by Tom Beauchamp and LeRoy Walters, 135–138. Belmont, CA: Wadsworth Publishing Company, 1999.

Lucey, Catherine and Wiley Souba. "The Problem with the Problem of Professionalism." *Academic Medicine* 85:6 (June 2010): 1018–1024.

Manson, Neil C. and Onora O'Neill. *Rethinking Informed Consent in Bioethics.* New York: Cambridge University Press, 2007.

Osman, Hana. "History and Development of the Doctrine of Informed Consent." *The International Electronic Journal of Health Education* 4 (2001): 41–47.

Rich, Eugene C., Wylie Burke, Caryl J. Heaton, et al. "Reconsidering the Family History in Primary Care." *Journal of General Internal Medicine* 19 (March 2004): 273–280.

Roberts, J. Scott and Wendy Uhlmann. "Genetic Susceptibility Testing for Neurodegenerative Diseases: Ethical and Practice Issues." *Progress in Neurobiology* 110 (2013): 89–101. Accessed March 10, 2013. http://dx.doi.org/10.1016/j.pneurobio.2013.02.005.

Runciman, Bill, Alan Merry, and Merrilyn Walton. *Safety and Ethics in Healthcare.* Burlington, VT: Ashgate Publishing Company, 2007.

Sugarman, Jeremy, Douglas C. McCrory, Donald Powell, et al. "Empirical Research on Informed Consent: An Annotated Bibliography." *A Hastings Center Report* (January- February 1999): S1–S42 Special Supplement.

Taylor, Kathryn M. and Merrijoy J. Kelner. "The Emerging Role of the Physician in Genetic Counselling and Testing for Heritable Breast, Ovarian and Colon Cancer." *Canadian Medical Association Journal* 154:8 (April 15, 1996): 1155–1158.

Trepanier, Angela, Mary Ahrens, Wendy McKinnon, et al. "Genetic Cancer Risk Assessment and Counseling: Recommendations of the National Society of Genetic Counselors." *Journal of Genetic Counseling* 13:2 (April 2004): 83–114.

Veatch, Robert. "Abandoning Informed Consent." *The Hastings Center Report* 25:2 (1995): 5–12.

Wear, Stephen. *Informed Consent: Patient Autonomy and Clinician Beneficence within Health Care.* Washington, DC: Georgetown University Press, 1998.

Index

Printed in the United States
By Bookmasters